Feline Ophthalmology

The Manual

For this English edition:

Feline Ophthalmology - The Manual

Copyright © 2015 Grupo Asís Biomedia, S.L.
Plaza Antonio Beltrán Martínez nº 1, planta 8 - letra I
(Centro empresarial El Trovador)
50002 Zaragoza - Spain

First printing: May 2015

Illustrator:
Jacob Gragera Artal

ISBN: 978-84-16315-11-6
D.L.: Z 637-2015

Design, layout and printing:
Servet editorial - Grupo Asís Biomedia, S.L.
www.grupoasis.com
info@grupoasis.com

Warning:

Veterinary science is constantly evolving, as are pharmacology and the other sciences. Inevitably, it is therefore the responsibility of the veterinary clinician to determine and verify the dosage, the method of administration, the duration of treatment and any possible contraindications to the treatments given to each individual patient, based on his or her professional experience. Neither the publisher nor the author can be held liable for any damage or harm caused to people, animals or properties resulting from the correct or incorrect application of the information contained in this book.

Feline
Ophthalmology
The Manual

NATASHA MITCHELL
JAMES OLIVER

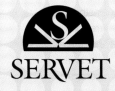
SERVET

Acknowledgments

This work would not have been possible without the contributions of so many friends and colleagues – many more than can be individually named here. Clinicians across the globe have generously shared their precious images so that they might be included in this semi-atlas and be made available to a global audience. These dedicated clinicians and keen photographers are acknowledged throughout the book. We would, however, like to give special mention to a few people who have donated their expert advice and, more importantly, their valuable time to greatly enhance this manual. We extend our heartfelt thanks to Dr Carl Bradbrook and Mr James Gasson for their insightful reviews on the chapter on anaesthesia and surgery and to Dr Fabio Stabile who provided his expertise without hesitation in his review of the neuro-ophthalmology chapter. Finally, the authors would like to acknowledge the overwhelming and significant contribution to the images contained in this book made by the Animal Health Trust. Without the contribution of those clinicians, past and present, to the Animal Health Trust archive of clinical images, this book would probably never have seen the light of day.

Authors

Dr James Oliver

BVSc CertVOphthal DipECVO MRCVS

James graduated from the University of Bristol in 2002 and, after five years in general practice, undertook a residency in veterinary ophthalmology at Davies Veterinary Specialists, Hertfordshire, UK. Now a European and RCVS Recognised Specialist in Veterinary Ophthalmology, James serves on the scientific committee of the British Association of Veterinary Ophthalmologists and is Co-chair of the Education & Residency Committee of the European College of Veterinary Ophthalmologists. James has published widely in the peer-reviewed literature and performs editorial and review work for several veterinary journals. He currently works as Senior Ophthalmologist at the Animal Health Trust, where he divides his time between clinical practice, teaching and genetics research.

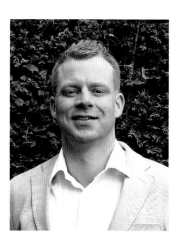

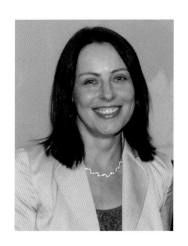

Dr Natasha Mitchell

MVB DVOphthal MRCVS

Natasha graduated from the University College Dublin in 1998. She worked for several years in general practice in the UK and Australia and obtained the RCVS Certificate in Veterinary Ophthalmology. She then undertook an alternative residency at the Eye Vet Clinic in Herefordshire and obtained the RCVS Diploma in Veterinary Ophthalmology. Natasha is a Veterinary Council of Ireland Recognised Specialist in Veterinary Ophthalmology. She is joint secretary of the British Association of Veterinary Ophthalmologists. She runs her own referral ophthalmology service, Eye Vet, in Limerick, Ireland, with a varied small animal and equine caseload.

Foreword

It is both a pleasure and an honor to be asked to write the foreword for this new and exciting textbook of Feline Ophthalmology. I would first like to congratulate the authors, Drs Natasha Mitchell and James Oliver on a most complete and well-illustrated textbook on the subject of feline ophthalmology.

As veterinarians and veterinary ophthalmologists over the years we have come to realize that the subject of veterinary ophthalmology is a diverse and varied one. In the early years, textbooks on the subject of veterinary ophthalmology focused primarily on diseases and treatment of the canine eye, with brief chapters on other species such as feline and equine. With experience, we have come to understand that these species deserve equal and specific attention of their own. Cats are not simply small dogs and their ophthalmic diseases and treatment are often unique to the species. Congenital, inherited, infectious and inflammatory diseases of the feline eye and ophthalmic manifestations of feline systemic disease must be understood as they pertain specifically to the feline eye and cannot simply be extrapolated from the canine any more than canine ophthalmology can be extrapolated from human ophthalmology.

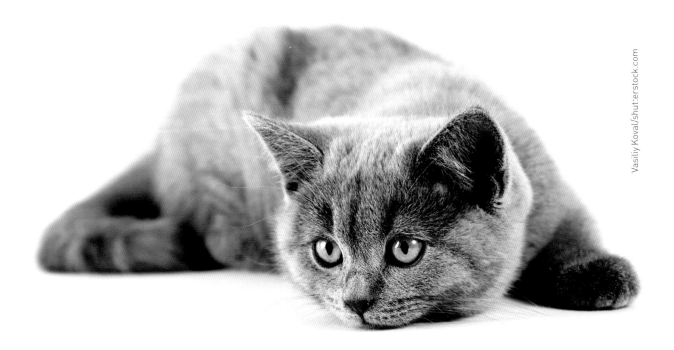

Vasiliy Koval/shutterstock.com

In this new textbook, the authors have done an excellent job, using text, illustrations and marvelous clinical images to equip the practicing veterinarian with the tools to examine, interpret, diagnose and treat common diseases of the feline eye. The first three chapters cover the techniques required for a complete ophthalmic examination of the feline eye, the techniques and principles as they pertain to ophthalmic anesthesia and surgery and, finally, medications used for treatment of ophthalmic disease. This is followed by nine chapters that are divided by specific anatomic locations such as orbit, cornea, lens, with each of the chapters beginning with anatomy and function, and followed by disease and treatment. The text is written in a logical, reader friendly and clinically applicable fashion. At each step, the text is extensively illustrated with diagrams and clinical photographs that match the text as the reader progresses. Finally, current and extensive references are provided to the reader should they wish to review a subject in greater depth.

In conclusion, I would highly recommend this textbook of Feline Ophthalmology as a clinical and reference textbook that should be in the library of all feline, small animal and mixed animal practices. The authors are to be commended for the extensive work they have done to assist veterinarians and students in the understanding of the unique and fascinating feline eye.

David A. Wilkie
DVM, MS, Diplomate ACVO
Professor, The Ohio State University

X

Preface

From the outset, we aimed for *Feline Ophthalmology – The Manual* to be an up-to-date semi-atlas style text encompassing all areas of clinical feline ophthalmology. The manual is intended to provide a detailed outline of feline ophthalmology for veterinary students, practitioners with an interest in feline ophthalmology and those undertaking more specialist training in veterinary ophthalmology.

The manual takes a logical approach to the discipline beginning with the fundamental platform of the ophthalmic examination, which must be mastered to enable disease recognition, before taking a largely tissue-based approach to ophthalmic disease with reference to clinically relevant anatomy and physiology. We also decided to include chapters on ocular therapeutics, anaesthesia and surgery, as these are all essential ancillary topics with which the ophthalmologist must be familiar and use on a day-to-day basis, but are so often neglected in clinical ophthalmology texts. For those techniques commonly encountered in feline practice, step-by-step photographs and/or illustrations have been provided for the reader to follow whilst providing guidance of when specialist advice or referral should be sought.

Advanced diagnostic imaging has become increasingly available with more and more practitioners having access to CT and MRI scanners since the publication of previous similar texts and atlases. To reflect this, many of the clinical photographs in the chapters on the orbit and neuro-ophthalmology are accompanied by case-specific annotated CT or MRI images.

At the end of each chapter, a list of references is provided. However, this is by no means exhaustive and the budding veterinary ophthalmologist is advised to consult further texts to expand his knowledge and understanding of this diverse and fascinating field.

Finally, this book is dedicated to all those with an interest in feline ophthalmology for whom we hope it proves to be a useful resource or, at the very least, an enjoyable read!

James Oliver
Natasha Mitchell

Table of contents

Ocular examination

Introduction

It is often possible to make a diagnosis through clinical ocular examination, as many of the structures of the eye can be directly or indirectly visualised and many diagnostic tests are simple to perform. Familiarity with the clinical appearance of the normal eye is required to differentiate abnormalities from natural variation. This chapter provides an ordered systematic approach to the ocular examination and outlines the basic principles of commonly performed diagnostic tests.

Background

It is important to have a room that can be darkened and is in a quiet area to minimise stress. Cats should be handled gently and calmly, and those that are not compliant generally relax when wrapped in a towel for restraint (Fig. 1). Sedation should be avoided unless absolutely necessary, as it may cause downward rotation of the globe, protrusion of the nictitans, change the pupil size or alter the results of diagnostic testing such as the Schirmer tear test (STT) and tonometry. Signalment is important, as certain conditions are more common in specific breeds or in particular age ranges. A good history should include background information about previous and current morbidities, current medications, vaccinations, parasite control, in-contact animals and travel. Regarding the eye problem, information about onset and duration of clinical signs, laterality, concurrent systemic signs and details of any previous therapy and response are all important. A systemic clinical examination should be performed in addition to the ocular examination.

➜ Examine both eyes to avoid missing abnormalities of the seemingly unaffected eye, and because a normal contralateral eye acts as a useful comparative control.

Equipment

Requirements for a basic ocular examination include:
- A light source: focal illumination is best provided with a transilluminator (e.g. Finhoff). Other light sources include a pen-torch, direct ophthalmoscope and otoscope.
- Magnification: ideally a slit-lamp biomicroscope, but alternatives are the direct ophthalmoscope, otoscope and loupes.
- Disposables: Schirmer tear test (STT) strips, fluorescein and Rose Bengal test strips or single dose vials, sterile swabs with transport medium, 0.9 % saline for ocular irrigation, topical anaesthetic (e.g. 0.5 % proxymetacaine/proparacaine) and a mydriatic (0.5-1 % tropicamide).

Examination tip

Topical anaesthesia facilitates ocular surface procedures and examination when there is ocular surface pain. Maximum effect is achieved within 60 seconds of application and lasts 5 minutes.

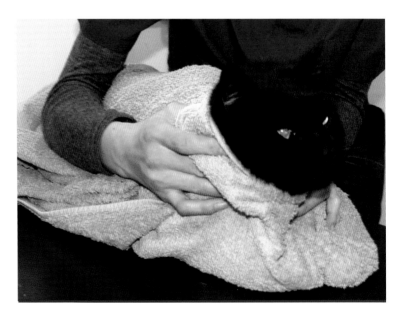

Figure 1. Towel-wrapping is an effective means of feline restraint.

Ocular examination

It is best to adhere to a step-by-step approach, examining all parts of the eye in order. By following such a routine, it is less likely that abnormalities will be missed. While the protocol is kept relatively consistent, not every diagnostic test is required for each patient, and the choice of appropriate tests is made during the examination. The recommended order of a thorough eye examination is as follows.

Examination in ambient lighting

Distant examination is referred to as the 'hands-off' approach. Usually this involves observing the cat initially in the carrier, and then on the examination table with no, or only minimal, restraint. The appearance and symmetry of the head and eyes, especially the periocular areas, are noted. The eyelids are observed for position (relationship to the globe), blepharospasm and the presence of any ocular discharge. The globe is observed for size, position (presence of strabismus) and movement (presence of nystagmus or restricted movement). The size and shape of the pupils are noted.

If ulceration and foreign bodies are absent, the globes may be gently retropulsed via the closed upper eyelids, to check for any resistance that would indicate a retrobulbar space-occupying lesion (Fig. 2).

Schirmer tear test

The Schirmer tear test (STT) is a quantitative measurement of the aqueous component of the tear film. Standardised filter paper strips are available that are calibrated with a millimeter scale and impregnated with a blue dye for easy visualisation of the result. The STT I measures both the basal and reflex secretion of aqueous tears. The STT II is performed after application of topical anaesthetic. It measures only basal and residual tears, and thus it is lower than STT I. The STT I is much more widely used, and most reported normal values refer to this test. The notched end of the strip is hooked over the lateral aspect of the lower eyelid, contacting the palpebral conjunctiva and the cornea (Fig. 3). The distance traveled by the tears on the test strip in sixty seconds is recorded. Cats

have variable results and a value of < 10 mm wetting per minute is considered significant if accompanied by ocular surface disease, such as ocular discharge, conjunctival hyperaemia, corneal vessels or ulceration and a lack-lustre appearance of the ocular surface. Comparison of the results of the two eyes may be useful. A published value in normal adult cats is 14.3 ± 4.7 mm/minute (Cullen et al., 2005).

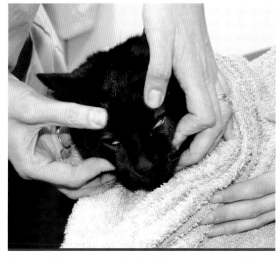

Figure 2. Globe retropulsion. Gentle digital pressure is applied through the upper eyelids onto the globe, resulting in nictitans protrusion. Any resistance is noted.

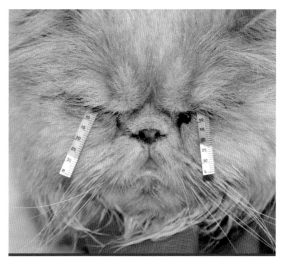

Figure 3. Correct placement of a STT strip at the lateral to middle third of the lower eyelid.

Laboratory sample collection

Microbiological sampling

Cotton-tipped sterile swabs are carefully applied to the desired sampling site (for example the conjunctival fornix or corneal surface) before placement in the appropriate container and transport medium (Fig. 4). Samples to be submitted for culture should be collected before application of topical anaesthetic, which can affect viability of microorganisms. Samples for virus isolation should also be taken prior to the application of diagnostic dyes as these can inhibit viral replication. PCR testing is not affected by the use of topical anaesthetic or ophthalmic dyes.

Cytological sampling

Corneal and conjunctival scraping is carried out after application of topical anaesthetic, using a cytobrush (Fig. 5), the blunt end of a scalpel blade or a Kimura spatula. Pressure applied should be just firm enough to yield some surface cells, usually from the lower conjunctival fornix or the edge of a corneal ulcer. The harvested cells are spread onto a clean microscope slide, air-dried and then cytology can be performed, usually after applying stains such as Gram stain or Diff-Quik®. Immediate in-house examination of specimens allows for rapid diagnosis and initial treatment selection.

Neuro-ophthalmic examination

The neuro-ophthalmic examination is an essential component of the overall ocular examination. The pathways and techniques involved in the neuro-ophthalmic examination are discussed in detail in Chapter 12 and are just summarised here.

Vision testing

Cats can be uncooperative patients and so multiple tests may be required to ascertain vision status.

The menace response

The menace response is learned and may not be present in normal cats younger than 12 weeks of age. Movement of the hand towards the eye is expected to evoke a reaction including eyelid closure, nictitans protrusion due to globe retraction or head avoidance

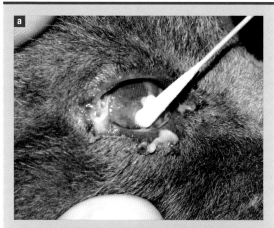
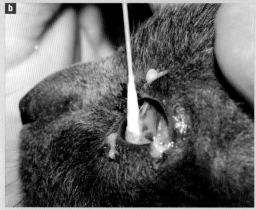

Figure 4. Microbiological sampling. a) A saline-soaked cotton-tipped swab is being gently rolled across the corneal surface to harvest the ocular discharge. b) A saline-soaked cotton-tipped swab in being firmly rubbed in the ventral conjunctival fornix.

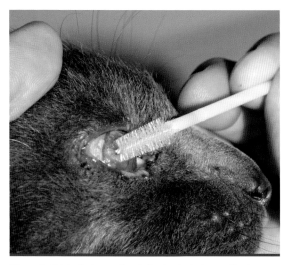

Figure 5. Cytological sampling. Following topical anaesthesia, a cytobrush is gently rolled across the corneal surface to harvest cellular material before rolling onto a glass microscope slide.

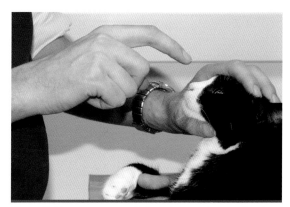

Figure 6. Menace response. A finger is moved across the visual field towards the eye, taking care not to create an air current or to touch any vibrissae.

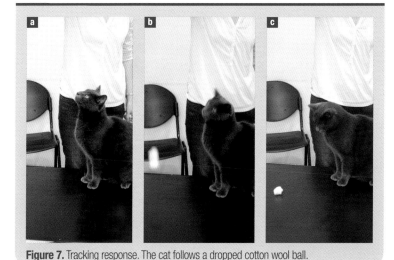

Figure 7. Tracking response. The cat follows a dropped cotton wool ball.

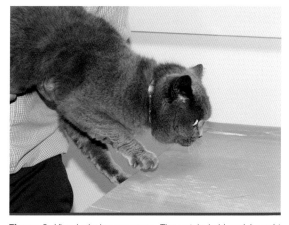

Figure 8. Visual placing response. The cat is held and brought towards a table edge. A visual cat should reach for the table surface before coming into contact with it.

movement (Fig. 6). A positive response infers vision is present. A negative response infers blindness, facial nerve paralysis or cerebellar lesions.

The tracking response

A kinetic stimulus without sound or smell is selected, such as a dropped cotton wool ball or moving laser pointer (Fig. 7). Cats with vision should detect the motion and follow it with their eyes, although can appear disinterested and not partake.

The visual placing response

Covering one eye at a time, a cat may be carried towards the edge of a table. Cats with vision should extend their forelimbs towards the table (Fig. 8).

Maze tests and obstacle courses

Maze testing is not usually an objective test of vision in cats due to their typically stoic behaviour.

Light reflexes

The pupillary light reflex

The reflex has a subcortical pathway, involving the optic nerve as the afferent arm and parasympathetic fibres within the oculomotor nerve as the efferent arm. The fibres cross at the optic chiasm and in the pretectum before influencing both oculomotor nuclei, and the pathway is illustrated in Chapter 12. A bright light shone into one eye should cause both pupils to constrict (the direct and consensual responses). A negative PLR can be due to retinal, optic nerve or oculomotor nerve lesions, as well as pharmacological mydriasis, glaucoma, synechiae, extreme stress or iris atrophy (not common in cats). The swinging flashlight test is a modification of the PLR test and is discussed in Chapter 12.

→ Normal PLRs do not always infer vision, and absence of PLRs does not always imply blindness.

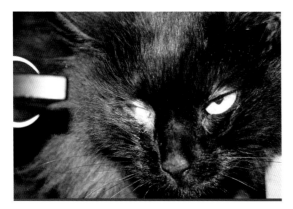

Figure 9. Dazzle reflex. The right eye is being illuminated with a bright light source. There is bilateral partial eyelid closure, more pronounced on the illuminated side.

The dazzle reflex

Shining a bright focused light into a normal eye is expected to evoke partial or complete eyelid closure with globe retraction (Fig. 9). The reflex shares some of the same pathways as the menace response and the PLR, but it is subcortical. Therefore a negative response indicates either facial nerve paralysis or subcortical blindness.

The palpebral reflex

The medial and lateral canthi are lightly touched, which normally elicits a complete blink and globe retraction. It is important to establish a normal blink response before judging the results of the menace response and dazzle reflex, to ensure that the animal is capable of responding in the expected way. A normal result confirms an intact sensory pathway (trigeminal nerves) and motor pathway (facial and abducent nerves). An abnormal result (lack of a blink) indicates poor sensation or, more commonly, facial nerve paralysis.

The vestibulo-ocular reflex and physiological nystagmus

In normal patients, moving the head from side to side and then up and down induces a physiological nystagmus. These normal saccadic ocular movements preserve image stability on the retina. The vestibulo-ocular reflex is considered normal when the fast phase of jerk nystagmus occurs in the same direction as head movement, with a slower phase in the opposite direction. It assesses the function of the extraocular muscles and their respective nerves.

Distant direct ophthalmoscopy

This technique is quick and simple to perform. The room is darkened and the direct ophthalmoscope lens is set to 0 D. The ophthalmoscope is placed very close to the observer's eye (Fig. 10). The tapetal reflection, through the pupil, is obtained at an arm's length from the patient. The size, shape and symmetry of the pupils, along with the direction of gaze, are observed and compared between the two eyes. Any opacity of the ocular media will be highlighted as a black obstruction viewed against the reflection from the tapetum (Fig. 11). Distant direct ophthalmoscopy may reveal the following abnormalities:

- Anisocoria (difference between the size of the pupils)
- Dyscoria (abnormal pupil shape)
- Absence of tapetal reflection either due to the presence of large opacities or lack of tapetum
- Focal opacities on or within the eye
- Aphakic crescent if the lens is subluxated or luxated
- Strabismus (abnormal direction of gaze)
- Nuclear sclerosis

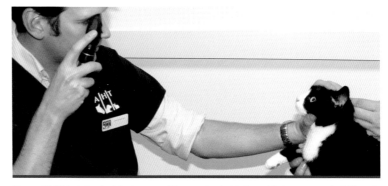

Figure 10. Distant direct ophthalmoscopy. The examiner holds the ophthalmoscope, set at 0 D, up to his eye. The tapetal reflection from behind the pupils is observed from an arm's distance.

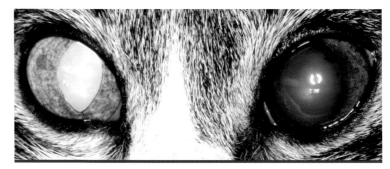

Figure 11. An example of a view obtained on distant direct ophthalmology. The right eye is normal, and a bright tapetal reflection is seen from behind the pupil. The left eye has a mature cataract and uveitis. No tapetal reflection can be seen because a cataract obscures the light. Anisocoria is appreciated as the left pupil is abnormally dilated due to secondary glaucoma.

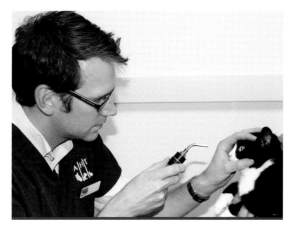

Figure 12. General examination of the eye with a Finhoff transilluminator.

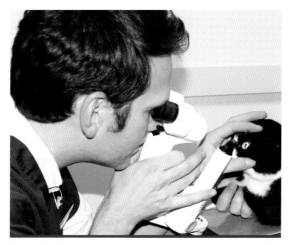

Figure 13. Use of a portable slit-lamp biomicroscope for magnified examination of the anterior segment and localisation of lesion depth.

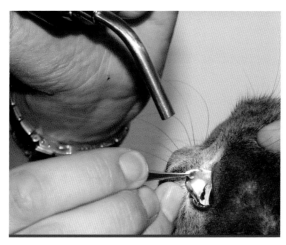

Figure 14. Examination behind the nictitans using a thumb forceps after application of topical anaesthetic.

Close examination in dim light or darkness

Close inspection of the eye and adnexa is then carried out, using a focal light source (Fig. 12). The direct ophthalmoscope can be used, making use of the different lens settings to focus at different depths within the eye. For the emmetropic observer, the eyelids and cornea will be in focus at approximately +20 D, the lens at +10 D and the vitreous +4 D. However, the slit-lamp biomicroscope provides a superior view although the high cost of the instrument renders it unattainable for many general practices. It combines a biomicroscope with a bright light source and allows for a much more detailed examination of the anterior segment, lens and anterior vitreous (Fig. 13). Depending on the model used, magnification up to 16× is possible with hand-held instruments. It contains a beam of light which can be altered from narrow to wide, and is used to provide an optical section view which is highly focused and magnified, allowing the depth of lesions in transparent tissues to be determined.

It is best to proceed from external to internal. The position of the eyelids and presence of any defects or abnormal hairs are observed. The palpebral as well as the bulbar conjunctiva should be assessed for colour, integrity, chemosis or surface irregularities. The presence and location of lacrimal puncta are observed. The nictitans is observed for position, thickness, and any irregularities of the margin or surfaces. If a more detailed inspection of the posterior aspect is required, it may be grasped with atraumatic forceps and carefully retracted from the globe (Fig. 14). The episclera, sclera and limbus are examined next. The normal cornea should be transparent. Loss of transparency may be due to vascularisation, cellular infiltration, pigmentation, fibrosis, keratic precipitates, or lipid or mineral deposition. The contour and surface are observed for regularity. The anterior chamber should be optically clear, and free from blood (hyphaema), turbidity (implying aqueous flare or lipaemic aqueous), cellular material (e.g. hypopyon or keratic precipitates), fibrin or structures such as foreign bodies or the lens. The iris is observed for altered colour and texture, and for the presence of any swellings or irregularities. The pupil should be round when dilated and a regular vertically-orientated slit shape when constricted. If the pupil size is suspected to be abnormal, this is further verified using observation in light and dark, PLR and swinging flashlight tests followed by distant direct ophthalmoscopy. The axial lens is observed behind the pupil but detailed examination requires mydriasis.

In order to examine the lens, vitreous and fundus thoroughly, the pupil should be pharmacologically dilated, using a short acting mydriatic such as 0.5-1 % tropicamide topically. It takes 20 minutes to achieve sufficient dilation. Atropine is not a suitable mydriatic for diagnostics as pupil dilation is slower, the effect lasts much longer than is required and it may cause copious salivation due to its bitter taste, reaching the mouth through the nasolacrimal duct.

Fundus examination

It is important to become familiar with the appearance of the normal anatomical variants of the feline fundus (see Chapter 11). Normal variation results from differences in colour and extent of the tapetum, pigmentation of the nontapetal fundus and retinal vascular pattern. The fundus is examined using direct and/or indirect ophthalmoscopy, and darkness is required. With direct ophthalmoscopy, the image obtained is upright, small and highly magnified. The disadvantage is that only a very small area of the fundus can be examined at a time. The image obtained using indirect ophthalmoscopy is inverted and reversed, but it is a larger image due to a wider field of view and less magnification. The latter technique takes a little longer to learn, but is very rewarding as the view obtained is easier to interpret and lesions are less likely to be missed.

Examination tip

Fundus examination techniques are complementary. Indirect ophthalmoscopy may be used to obtain an overview followed by direct ophthalmoscopy to examine any abnormalities at higher magnification.

Direct ophthalmoscopy

The lens dial is set to 0 D, although spectacle-wearers may use the lens dial to compensate for their degree of refractive error. The light level is adjusted using the rheostat, using the minimal amount of illumination required to perform the examination. The ophthalmoscope is placed very close to the observer's eye. The tapetal reflection is obtained from a short distance away to align the image, and then the observer and instrument move forward until the instrument is close to the cat's cornea (Fig. 15). The optic nerve head is identified and examined, and then the rest of the tapetal and nontapetal fundus is examined in quadrants, taking note of the retinal vasculature and any abnormal lesions. The green (red-free) light enhances contrast, and therefore is useful to distinguish retinal pigment from haemorrhage.

Indirect ophthalmoscopy

Monocular indirect ophthalmoscopy requires just a focal light source and a handheld condensing lens. Higher dioptre lenses provide less magnification but a wider field of view. The 20D lens and 30D lens are often used, and the Pan Retinal® 2.2 lens is very useful as it combines magnification of the 20D lens with the wider field of view of the 30D lens. The light is directed into the eye from an arm's distance away, until the tapetal reflection is obtained (Fig. 16). The condensing lens is placed approximately 5 cm in front of the cat's eye. The image is inverted and reversed, therefore practice is required to be able to navigate around the fundus. Binocular indirect ophthalmoscopy is carried out using a head-mounted indirect ophthalmoscope (Fig. 17). The stereoscopic view obtained is superior, and the second hand is free to help stabilise the cat's head.

Another form of monocular indirect ophthalmoscope is provided with the PanOptic® ophthalmoscope which provides a wider field of view than the direct ophthalmoscope, and the image is upright and not reversed. The advantages are that it is easy to use and to orientate the images obtained and it is possible to get a reasonable view of the fundus through an undilated pupil (Fig. 18). Examples of the views obtained using the three different techniques are shown in Figure 19.

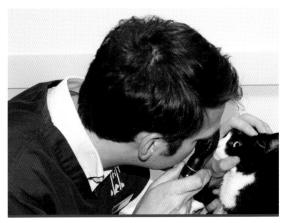

Figure 15. Fundus examination using direct ophthalmoscopy. The instrument is close to the observer's eye and the observer is close to the cat's cornea.

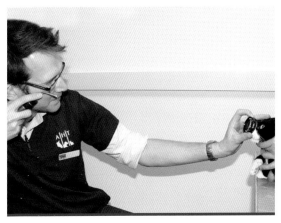

Figure 16. Fundus examination using monocular indirect ophthalmoscopy. A light source (in this case a Finhoff transilluminator) is held close to the observer's eye. A hand-held condensing lens is held approximately 5 cm in front of the cat's cornea.

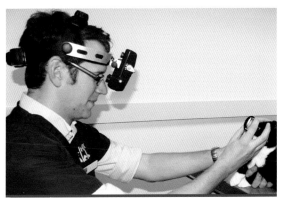

Figure 17. Fundus examination using binocular indirect ophthalmoscopy with a wireless head-mounted indirect ophthalmoscope. The observer holds the cat's head with one hand and the condensing lens approximately 5 cm in front of the cat's cornea with the other hand.

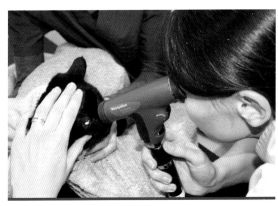

Figure 18. Fundus examination using a PanOptic® ophthalmoscope through an undilated pupil.

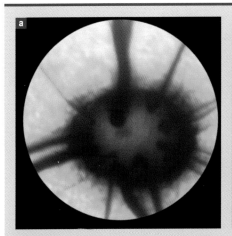
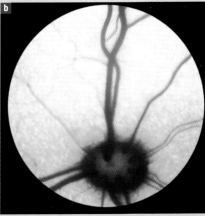
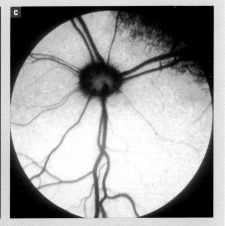

Figure 19. Typical views of the feline fundus. a) With a direct ophthalmoscope. b) With a monocular indirect (PanOptic®) ophthalmoscope. c) With a 30 D indirect condensing lens.

Examination tip

Indirect ophthalmoscopy can be performed very inexpensively using just a pen torch and an acrylic condensing lens.

Ophthalmic dyes

Fluorescein

Fluorescein is a water-soluble ophthalmic dye available as a solution and as impregnated paper strips. The dye is highly lipophobic and hydrophilic, and therefore does not penetrate an intact corneal epithelium due to the phospholipid cell membranes. The dye has several uses in clinical ophthalmology:

Detection of corneal epithelial defects (ulceration)

One drop is applied before irrigation of the ocular surface. If there is a full-thickness corneal epithelial defect, the dye is absorbed into the exposed hydrophilic stroma where it can be observed as 'uptake' (Fig. 20). Descemet's membrane does not uptake fluorescein; therefore a clear area at the base of a deep defect in the cornea most likely indicates a descemetocoele. A blue light such as a cobalt blue filter, present in many direct ophthalmoscopes, greatly enhances visualisation of the dye.

Tear film break-up time

Tear film break-up time (TFBUT) is a noninvasive qualitative tear film test used to obtain a measurement of the time taken for evaporation of the tear film from an exposed corneal surface, and is measured in seconds. It correlates with the stability of the preocular tear film. One drop of fluorescein is applied to the cornea and then the eyelids are closed. On opening, the corneal surface is immediately observed using a cobalt blue light source, and the time taken until dark spots start to appear within the dye is measured. The TFBUT indirectly measures tear film mucin and/or lipid quantity and quality. A normal mean published value is 21 ± 12 seconds in adult cats (Grahn et al., 2005). TFBUT was found to be significantly lower in cats with conjunctivitis at 8.5 ± 4.7 seconds (Lim and Cullen, 2005).

The Seidel test

The Seidel test is used to assess corneal integrity. Fluorescein is applied liberally and distributed by a forced blink motion so that the entire corneal surface is covered with a thin film of green dye. A corneal wound will retain fluorescein but any aqueous that leaks out of the corneal wound will dilute the film of green dye on the ocular surface, appearing as a gradually expanding dark rivulet (Fig. 21). Very gentle pressure can be applied to the globe via the upper eyelid if the test is initially negative to assess if the wound is stable, or if it will open and leak if the IOP increases.

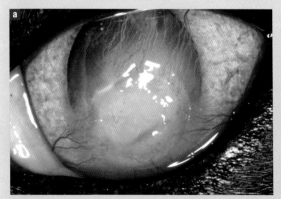
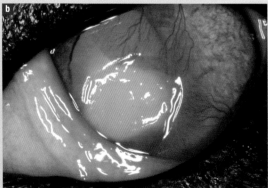

Figure 20. Corneal ulcer, before and after fluorescein staining. a) Corneal vascularisation extends into a central irregular area with oedema. b) Fluorescein staining highlights the area of the cornea with the epithelial defect (corneal ulcer).

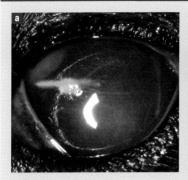
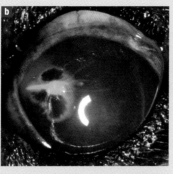

Figure 21. Seidel test. a) A linear corneal perforation injury stains positive with fluorescein dye. b) Positive Seidel test depicting aqueous leaking from the corneal wound and diluting the green fluorescein dye with a black rivulet, both above and below the wound. Courtesy of Rob Lowe.

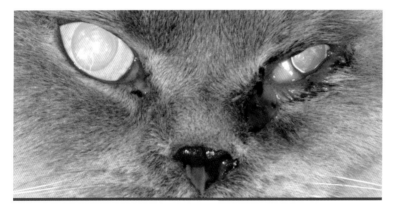

Figure 22. Fluorescein passage test. Fluorescein dye has been applied to both eyes. On the right side, fluorescein has drained to the naris within five minutes, indicating nasolacrimal duct patency. On the left side, fluorescein dye has not drained to the naris and is spilling over the medial canthus. There is a smaller palpebral aperture and nictitans protrusion on this side, along with symblepharon over the lacrimal puncta, all due to previous feline herpesvirus-1 infection.

Fluorescein drainage test (Jones' test)

The passage of fluorescein from the conjunctival sac to the ipsilateral naris confirms anatomical and physiological patency of the nasolacrimal drainage system. It is expected to occur within five minutes (Fig. 22). A negative Jones' test is therefore not conclusive of a nasolacrimal obstruction although it is suggestive if unilateral in the presence of compatible clinical signs. Conformational differences in the nasolacrimal duct also exist. In brachycephalic cats, it follows a steep V-shaped course around the canine tooth (Schlueter et al., 2009), which will alter drainage (see Chapter 5, Fig. 66).

Rose Bengal

Rose Bengal (dichlorotetraiodo fluorescein) is used as a diagnostic aid for tear film disorders and defects in the superficial corneal epithelium. It is available both as an impregnated paper strip and as a solution (Fig. 23). It stains dead and degenerating cells and mucous. It also has a dose-dependent ability to stain normal cells, which is usually prevented by tear film components. Therefore uptake of stain may indicate tear film abnormalities (such as a mucin deficiency) more accurately than lack of cell viability. It is examined with a normal white light, and magnification enhances the ability to detect uptake. It can be more useful than fluorescein for highlighting small dendritic ulcers that are sometimes seen with feline herpetic keratitis. This is because these ulcers may not be full-thickness epithelial defects and therefore fluorescein would not gain access to the stroma. Other indications include keratoconjunctivitis sicca and qualitative tear film defects, which occur much less commonly in cats than in dogs.

→ Clinical analysis of the tear film requires performance of multiple tests, including the Schirmer tear test-1, tear film breakup time and fluorescein and Rose Bengal staining.

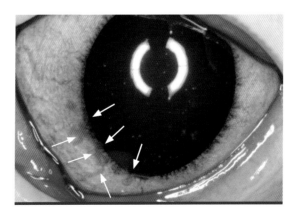

Figure 23. Rose Bengal dye has been applied to the eye of a stray kitten that presented with sneezing, conjunctival hyperaemia and chemosis. There is uptake of the dye in a branching dendritic pattern (arrows) due to FHV-1 infection.

Aesthesiometry

Corneal touch threshold (CTT) is the minimum corneal stimulation required to elicit a blink response and is a measurement of corneal sensitivity. Pressure is applied to the cornea by means of a nylon monofilament in the aesthesiometer (see Chapter 12, Fig. 8). The monofilament length can be adjusted, and as it is made shorter, it becomes stiffer. A pressure significant enough to stimulate sufficient corneal sensory nerve endings causes a blink response. Higher CTT, with shorter monofilament length, correlates with lower corneal sensitivity. Normal values for the sensitivity of the central cornea in cats have been established; the mean CTT value in 26 normal cats was 42.82 ± 2.94 mm of filament length centrally (Kafarnik et al., 2004). Reduced corneal sensitivity is associated with increased susceptibility to corneal ulcers, keratitis and possibly corneal sequestra.

Tonometry

Tonometry is the estimation of IOP which in normal cats if generally 10-25 mmHg (see Chapter 9). The most commonly used tonometers are the applanation Tono-Pen®, the rebound TonoVet® and the indentation Schiotz (Fig. 24). Topical anaesthesia is required for the Schiotz and Tono-Pen® tonometers. Gentle patient handling is essential to avoid excitement and jugular compression which could induce a temporary increase in the IOP and lead to a false diagnosis of glaucoma. IOP can be influenced by many factors including age, sex, reproductive status, time of day, drugs and type of tonometer used (see Chapter 9). It is used for the diagnosis of glaucoma (raised IOP, usually > 25mmHg), uveitis (lowered IOP, usually < 10mmHg) and for monitoring response to treatment.

Gonioscopy

Gonioscopy is the visual assessment of the iridocorneal (drainage) angle at the junction between the iris and cornea. It is possible to view the angle directly in the cat using a light source and magnification, but the view is greatly enhanced with the use of a goniolens and a slit-lamp biomicroscope (Fig. 25). Topical anaesthetic should be applied to the cornea prior to placement of a goniolens which is filled with a liquid medium, for example saline or methylcellulose solution. Gonioscopy is used in the investigation of glaucoma and other disease processes which may involve the iridocorneal angle.

→ Normal feline intraocular pressure is 10-25 mmHg, but a difference of more than 5 mmHg between the eyes is also potentially significant and warrants further investigation.

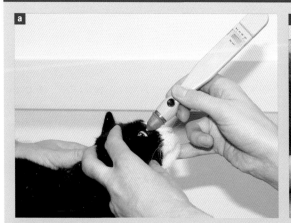
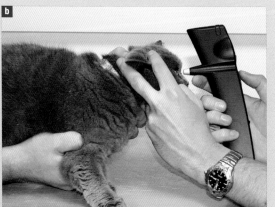

Figure 24. Tonometry. a) Applanation tonometry using the Tono-Pen®. Topical anaesthesia is required. b) Rebound tonometry using the TonoVet®. Topical anaesthesia is not required.

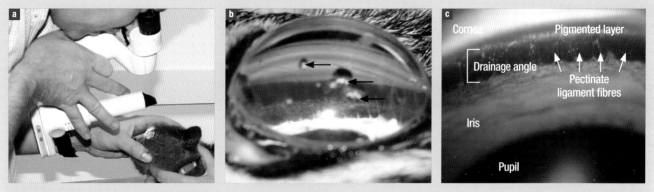

Figure 25. Gonioscopy. a) A Koeppe goniolens is on the ocular surface. The drainage angle is being viewed using a portable slit-lamp biomicroscope. b) The typical feline iridocorneal drainage angle as seen through a Koeppe goniolens during gonioscopy. Some air bubbles are present (arrows) within the methylcellulose solution. c) Anatomy of the iridocorneal drainage angle.

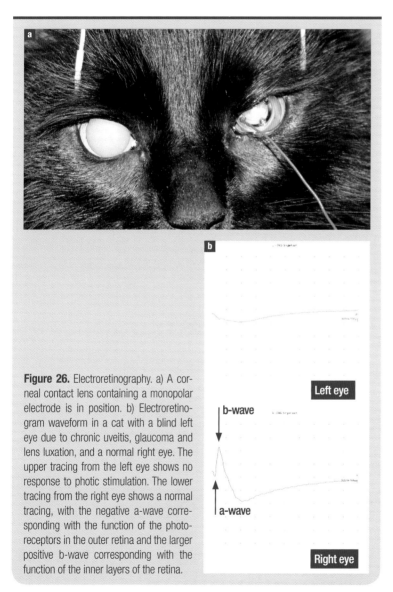

Figure 26. Electroretinography. a) A corneal contact lens containing a monopolar electrode is in position. b) Electroretinogram waveform in a cat with a blind left eye due to chronic uveitis, glaucoma and lens luxation, and a normal right eye. The upper tracing from the left eye shows no response to photic stimulation. The lower tracing from the right eye shows a normal tracing, with the negative a-wave corresponding with the function of the photoreceptors in the outer retina and the larger positive b-wave corresponding with the function of the inner layers of the retina.

Electroretinography

Electroretinography (ERG) is used to measure the electrical activity generated by the retina in response to light stimuli (Fig. 26). Standardised protocols and conditions are used to minimise variability and therefore increase reliability of results. It is usually performed under sedation or general anaesthesia. Clinically it may be used prior to cataract surgery when funduscopy is not possible; to determine the retinal response to flashes of light, and therefore assess retinal function. It is also indicated for sudden onset blindness where the retina looks normal, to confirm whether the blindness is central or at the level of the retina.

Diagnostic imaging

Radiology

Radiology is most useful for investigation of bony diseases of the orbit and maxillary dental arcade and for the presence of metallic foreign bodies. Contrast studies are used to investigate lacrimal duct conditions (dacryocystorhinography). Radiography of the chest and abdomen may be required to complement investigation of uveitis or ocular neoplasia.

Ultrasonography

Ultrasonography is a noninvasive procedure allowing useful imaging of the eye and retrobulbar region, and can usually be carried out with gentle manual restraint without sedation. After applying topical anaesthetic and coupling gel, the probe may be directly applied to the cornea (Fig. 27). A B-mode scanner with a 10 MHz sector probe provides good detail with high near-field axial resolution. Ocular ultrasonography is indicated when opacity of the ocular media prevents intraocular examination. It is also used in the investigation of orbital disease, measuring globe size and determining the patency of persistent embryonic vessels.

Computerised tomography and magnetic resonance imaging

Computerised tomography (CT) and magnetic resonance imaging (MRI) are advanced cross-sectional imaging techniques which offer superior image quality to conventional radiography and ultrasonography. CT is of particular use in investigation of pathology of the bony orbit. MRI is the technique of choice for investigation of soft tissue conditions of the orbit, periorbit and brain. Contrast studies are routinely used for both CT and MRI after IV infusion of contrast agents.

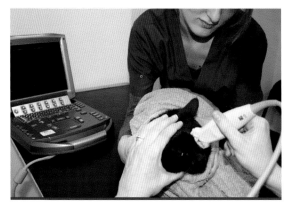

Figure 27. Ocular ultrasonography in an unsedated cat. After applying topical anaesthetic to the ocular surface, a sector ultrasound probe with coupling gel is applied directly to the cornea.

In summary

→ The majority of the eye is readily examinable often allowing for rapid diagnosis in the consulting room.

→ Use a systematic approach.

→ Examine both the affected and unaffected eye.

→ Dilate the pupil with 0.5-1 % tropicamide for examination of the lens, vitreous and fundus 20 minutes later.

→ When the diagnosis is not clear seek advice from a veterinary ophthalmologist.

References

ARNETT BD, BRIGHTMAN AH 2ND, MUSSELMAN EE (1984). Effect of atropine sulfate on tear production in the cat when used with ketamine hydrochloride and acetylpromazine maleate. *Journal of the American Veterinary Medical Association*; 185:214-215.

CULLEN CL, LIM C, SYKES J (2005). Tear film breakup times in young healthy cats before and after anesthesia. *Veterinary Ophthalmology*; 8:159-165.

GRAHN BH, SISLER S, STOREY E (2005). Qualitative tear film and conjunctival goblet cell assessment of cats with corneal sequestra. *Veterinary Ophthalmology*; 8:167-170.

KAFARNIK C, ALLGOEWER I, REESE S (2004). Innervation of the feline and canine cornea in correlation to corneal sensitivity (abstract); *DOK/ECVO/ESVO Meeting, Munich.*

LIM CC, CULLEN CL (2005). Schirmer tear test values and tear film break-up times in cats with conjunctivitis. *Veterinary Ophthalmology*; 8:305-310.

SCHLUETER C, BUDRAS KD, LUDEWIG E et al. (2009). Brachycephalic feline noses: CT and anatomical study of the relationship between head conformation and the nasolacrimal drainage system. *Journal of Feline Medicine and Surgery*; 11:891-900.

2

Anaesthesia and surgery

Introduction

Certain minor ocular surgical procedures can be successfully carried out under topical anaesthesia or with sedation. However, general anaesthesia is inevitably required to treat some conditions, particularly in cats, for ethical or practical reasons. Anaesthesia of the ophthalmic patient presents some unique aspects including considerations of intraocular pressure (IOP), the oculo-cardiac reflex and ocular pain. Monitoring of these patients under anaesthesia presents many challenges because of the position and the lack of access to the head and forelimbs for venous access. Specific surgical instruments are required for eye surgery, with particular design considerations and maintenance requirements.

Anaesthesia and analgesia

Preanaesthetic assessment

A thorough preanaesthetic assessment should be undertaken in advance of all elective procedures. The assessment should include a careful evaluation of the cat's history, including previous and current drug administration, and details of any prior anaesthetics.

A complete physical examination should be performed which, together with the signalment and history, will dictate whether further diagnostic tests are indicated – the results of which may influence the formulation of the anaesthetic plan. When blood testing is necessary in a cat with a fragile eye, the contralateral jugular vein should be used to minimise the effects of ipsilateral venous compression on IOP.

Geriatric patients requiring ophthalmic procedures may have extensive comorbidities which require investigation and appropriate management to enable safe anaesthesia. Systemic conditions requiring stabilisation prior to general anaesthesia are summarised in Table 1.

Cats with ocular trauma (e.g. from road traffic accidents and dog attacks) must be assessed for potentially life-threatening systemic organ damage which would take priority over ophthalmic injury. Factors that will influence anaesthetic management decision-making are summarised in Table 2.

Analgesia and analgesics

Pain must be treated for both humane and practical reasons. Good analgesia is associated with reduction of fear and aggression and reduces self-trauma. Preexisting pain should be treated prior to induction of anaesthesia and preemptive analgesia is more effective before surgical stimulation of nociceptors, although providing effective analgesia throughout the perioperative period is considered most important. A multimodal approach to analgesia, involving the use of drugs from more than one analgesic class, is more effective than if a single drug is used and allows reduction in total dose, and therefore side effects, of each individual drug.

Table 1. Systemic conditions requiring attention prior to general anaesthesia.

Systemic conditions	• Severe hypovolaemia • Severe dehydration • Hypoproteinaemia (albumin < 15 g/L) • Anaemia (PCV < 20 %) • Pneumothorax • Oliguria/anuria • Congestive heart failure • Cardiac arrhythmias • Acid-base disturbance (pH < 7.2) • Electrolyte disturbances

Table 2. Factors that influence anaesthetic management decision-making.

Patient factors	• Brachycephalia • Age • IOP • Fragile eye • Comorbidity • Previous anaesthetic history • Current and previous medications • Preoperative pain
Procedure to be undertaken	• Centrally positioned eye required • Painful procedure

Opioids

Opioids may be administered by a variety of routes. Systemic morphine should be avoided because cats have limited ability to convert it to its active metabolite and because it may cause emesis, which is likely to increase IOP. In addition, a recent study has shown no clear analgesic efficacy of morphine, when used topically to treat corneal pain (Thomson et al., 2013). Buprenorphine appears to be quite effective in cats and may be administered via the oral transmucosal route at standard intravenous and intramuscular doses. Methadone appears to be an effective analgesic in cats, but may occasionally cause dysphoria making patient management difficult. Oral tramadol, although it may seem appealing as it can be administered at home, is not tolerated well in cats due to poor palatability.

Nonsteroidal antiinflammatory drugs

Nonsteroidal antiinflammatory drugs (NSAIDs) exert their action by inhibition of the cyclooxygenase enzymes COX-1 and COX-2 which are involved in prostaglandin synthesis. Prostaglandins act as mediators of inflammation peripherally and as neurotransmitters centrally. Thus, NSAIDs have both antiinflammatory and analgesic properties. Meloxicam, carprofen and robenacoxib are licenced in cats in many countries and meloxicam is particularly attractive owing to its license for chronic use. The most common side effect of NSAIDs is gastrointestinal irritation, although nephroxicity is also a concern. Care should be taken to ensure normovolaemia and normotension prior to NSAID administration. It may be prudent to avoid administering NSAIDs prior to anaesthesia and wait until blood pressure is measured as normal, or until the end of anaesthesia.

Local anaesthetics

Topically applied local anaesthetics are useful facilitators of various diagnostic and surgical procedures. They should not be used as a treatment for ocular surface pain, however, owing to their negative effects on tear production and corneal health. Proxymetacaine (proparacaine), available as a 0.5 % solution, is the most commonly used topical local anaesthetic and, in cats, onset of action occurs after one minute and lasts for 25 minutes (Binder and Herring, 2006).

Retrobulbar injection of local anaesthetic agents provides both analgesia and globe akinesia, and may be used prior to enucleation. A concentration of 2 % lidocaine (rapid onset, short acting; up to 1 mg/kg) is often combined with 0.5 % bupivacaine (slower onset, longer acting; up to 1 mg/kg), and a maximum total volume of 1 ml is administered to the retrobulbar space. A special needle designed for use in humans can be used (Fig. 1). The best technique is unknown

→ Topical anaesthesia is only suitable for short-term use and should not be used as a treatment, as continued use can lead to significant conjunctival and corneal disease.

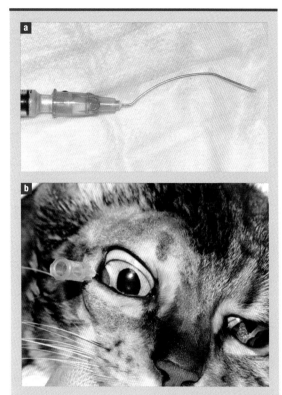

Figure 1. a) A curved 25 G retrobulbar needle designed for human use. The straight portion measures 11.0 mm and the curved portion measures 24.0 mm. b) Ventrolateral positioning of the needle prior to retrobulbar block.

for cats, although recent studies have suggested that a peribulbar injection technique may be more reliable than a retrobulbar approach (Shilo-Benjamini et al., 2013 and 2014).

Complications may be higher than in dogs owing to the relatively lower volume of the retrobulbar space, and include globe perforation and inadvertent intravascular or intrathecal injection. The latter has been associated with brainstem anaesthesia (Oliver and Bradbrook, 2012).

Alpha-2 adrenoreceptor agonists

Alpha-2 adrenoreceptor agonists are extremely useful sedatives with analgesic properties. They can be particularly useful in the premedication of fractious cats but can have serious cardiovascular side effects. Medetomidine (10 µg/kg) and dexmedetomidine (3-5 µg/kg) given intramuscularly are effective as adjunctive drugs when used at low doses.

Ketamine

Ketamine is a potent analgesic. Potential side effects include elevation in IOP, mydriasis and a central eye position. These latter two side effects may be useful for certain ophthalmic procedures.

Anaesthesia for ophthalmic surgery

Premedication

Premedication is used to achieve sedation prior to induction of anaesthesia in combination with analgesia. Appropriate premedication will assist with patient restraint for intravenous cannulation. It is particularly important to have a calm patient, especially with brachycephalic individuals and those with fragile globes. A complete list of possible drugs used as premedicants is beyond the scope of this text. Typically, however, premedication will include an opioid such as buprenorphine or methadone combined with acepromazine or a low dose of an alpha-2 agonist such as medetomidine.

Induction, intubation and maintenance of anaesthesia

In cats, induction is best achieved by intravenous administration of an induction agent to effect. Although intravenous catheters are often placed in a cephalic vein, for ophthalmic procedures in which access to the front of the animal may be limited, a saphenous vein may be preferred.

How to avoid drying of the ocular surfaces during general anaesthesia

→ The operated eye should be regularly irrigated (e.g. with balanced saline solution) or lubricated.

→ Lubrication should be applied to the contralateral eye also to reduce the risk of corneal ulceration.

→ Ensure that the eyelids are not left open underneath a bright surgical light for a prolonged period, which would dry the ocular surfaces and potentially damage the light-sensitive retina.

Commonly used intravenous agents include propofol and alfaxalone. These are administered until jaw tone is sufficiently relaxed to enable tracheal intubation. The induction agent should ideally abolish the laryngeal reflex prior to intubation, and the risk of laryngospasm (which causes undesirable increase in IOP) is further reduced by the topical application of lidocaine to the larynx.

Red rubber endotracheal tubes are not recommended in cats as the high pressure-low volume cuffs are likely to lead to tracheal damage. Many ophthalmic procedures require neck ventroflexion for positioning which can cause tube kinking. Armoured endotracheal tubes may help reduce this risk as can 90° connectors, but the latter will increase dead space.

Maintenance of general anaesthesia is usually achieved with the use of a volatile agent, such as isoflurane. The amount of agent delivered to the patient should be the minimum required to maintain an adequate plane of anaesthesia for the procedure being undertaken, and is adjusted in response to continued monitoring of the patient.

There is usually complete lack of access to the head during ophthalmic procedures, which may delay detection of inappropriate anaesthetic plane or patient disconnection from the breathing system. The correct use of blood pressure monitoring, capnography and pulse oximetry together is therefore of extreme importance and will allow detection of the vast majority of anaesthesia-related complications. An oesophageal stethoscope is also useful.

Recovery is often the most critical phase of a general anaesthetic and close monitoring is vital. The cat should be transferred to a well-trained and dedicated nurse for monitoring until it can be safely left unattended for short periods. An incubator is often used in which maintenance of normothermia will accelerate a smooth and rapid recovery, and oxygen may be supplied if necessary.

Neuromuscular blockade

For ophthalmic surgeons that routinely perform corneal and intraocular surgery, the use of nondepolarising neuromuscular blocking agents to paralyse the extraocular muscles, can be extremely useful.

For ophthalmic procedures, the aims of neuromuscular blockade are threefold. Firstly, they achieve a central eye position without the need for stay sutures or deeper planes of anaesthesia. Secondly, they reduce pressure on the globe and hence IOP (of particular importance in fragile eyes and during intraocular surgery). Thirdly, they eliminate small muscular movements which could interfere with surgery.

Commonly used nondepolarising neuromuscular blocking agents include atracurium, vecuronium and rocuronium, which are administered intravenously. These agents will paralyse all skeletal muscles and so mechanical positive pressure ventilation will be required until the effects of the drug are fully worn off and the patient is able to breathe unassisted.

The degree of neuromuscular blockade is assessed using a peripheral nerve stimulator, e.g. by stimulation of the peroneal nerve and evaluation of the cranial tibial muscle (Fig. 2). The use of neuromuscular blocking agents is regarded as specialist anaesthesia and should only be performed by well-trained and experienced individuals.

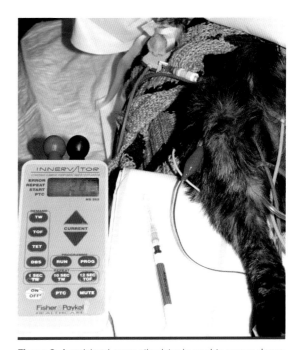

Figure 2. A peripheral nerve stimulator is used to assess degree of neuromuscular blockade achieved by intravenous administration of atracurium. In this case, the peroneal nerve, which supplies the cranial tibial muscle, is being assessed.

Surgical preparation for ophthalmic procedures

Hair removal

In veterinary surgery, clippers are generally used to remove hair from the surgical site. The periocular skin, however, is thin and prone to lacerations. Poor clipping technique is associated with inflammation and irritation which can lead to self-trauma, and also with increased resident bacterial populations with a corresponding increased risk of surgical site infection.

A good compromise is to clip only over the site of the proposed incision and its immediate surrounding area, followed by careful aseptic preparation which extends beyond the clip site followed by the use of adhesive occlusive drapes. Thus, clipping is only used for the eyelids and periocular area. For nictitans, ocular surface and intraocular procedures, only particularly long cilia adjacent to the eyelid margins need to be removed, and scissors are best employed for this purpose using a lubricating gel to protect the ocular surface and entrap loose hairs before irrigating the ocular surface.

Ocular disinfection

Aerobic bacteria can be isolated from approximately 40 % of normal feline eyes which may act as opportunistic infectious agents. In order to reduce bacterial load prior to surgery, an antiseptic agent is needed. Dilute aqueous solutions (not alcohol solution or surgical scrub, which damage the corneal epithelium) of povidone-iodine are widely used for ophthalmic surgical preparation.

The 10 % aqueous solution is diluted 1:50 (0.2 % solution) for preparation of the ocular surface, and to 1:20-1:10 (0.5-1 % solution) for the eyelids and periocular skin. In cases of ocular perforation, povidone-iodine should be avoided because severe endothelial toxicity has been demonstrated and sterile 0.9 % NaCl solution is preferred.

Chlorhexidine gluconate is also safe at a concentration of 0.05 %, and is as effective an antiseptic as 0.2 % povidone-iodine, but higher concentrations are irritant. It is unstable in saline, and should be diluted with sterile water. Chlorhexidine diacetate is toxic to the corneal epithelium and should never be used.

→ Avoid using disinfectants on the ocular surface that contain alcohol or surgical scrub.

→ If the cornea is perforated, the use of gel or disinfectants is contraindicated. Instead, the eye should be gently flushed with sterile saline or balanced salt solution.

Draping

Good draping technique is of utmost importance in ophthalmic surgery, in which there is usually a very narrow aseptically prepared surgical field. Hair, although microbiologically relatively unimportant, is objectionable in any surgical site.

Drape types include cloth, woven fabric, synthetic and plastic. Cloth drapes allow for absorption of irrigation fluids but provide a risk of contamination of the surgical site. Paper drapes provide good barriers to moisture and are now more popular for general surgical use in most referral hospitals (Fig. 3). Adhesive plastic drapes are particularly useful in ophthalmic procedures as they can precisely isolate the surgical site and prevent surrounding hairs from entering it and can be combined with a fluid collection pouch. When used for corneal and intraocular surgery, the adhesive plastic drape is used to isolate the eyelids from the ocular surface with the precise use of a speculum (Fig. 4).

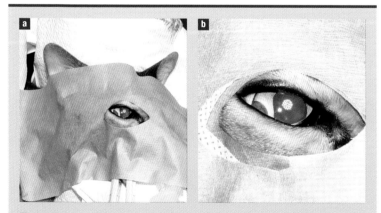

Figure 3. a) and b) A series of adhesive paper drapes is used to isolate the surgical site prior to enucleation.

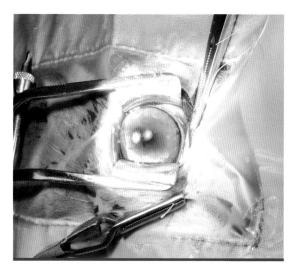

Figure 4. When used for corneal and intraocular surgery, the adhesive plastic drape is used to isolate the eyelids from the ocular surface with the precise use of a speculum.

The operating room

Magnification

The most appropriate source of magnification for an individual surgeon will vary according to the type of surgical procedure performed and also, to some extent, to the caseload. For adnexal (eyelid, conjunctival, nictitans and orbital) procedures, head-mounted loupes are usually sufficient. Loupes are available in a range of magnifications. An important consideration when selecting loupes is the trade-off between magnification and focal length. As magnification increases, focal length decreases which limits the surgeon's working distance and field of view of the surgical site. For the majority of adnexal procedures a magnification of 2.5-3.5× is sufficient for most surgeons and allows a working distance of 400-460 mm. When purchasing a pair of loupes, another important consideration is surgeon comfort, as some procedures will last in excess of one hour. Some loupes have an in-built source of illumination which, although very useful, will add to the overall weight of the loupes and therefore may increase the potential for discomfort over time (Fig. 5).

For surgeons with advanced interest in corneal and intraocular surgery, an operating microscope will be an essential part of the operating room furniture. Corneal and intraocular surgeries require the use of microsurgical instruments and sutures as fine as 10/0 rendering the magnification afforded by loupes inadequate. Operating microscopes may be table, floor or ceiling mounted (Fig. 6). The main body of the microscope consists of focus, zoom and illumination systems and a beam splitter which allows for observation by an assistant. A connected footplate allows for surgeon-directed adjustment of focus, zoom and illumination levels, along with limited movement of the surgeon's view about the X and Y axes. Level of magnification varies but 10-20× is most common and useful and the most common working distance afforded is 200-250 mm.

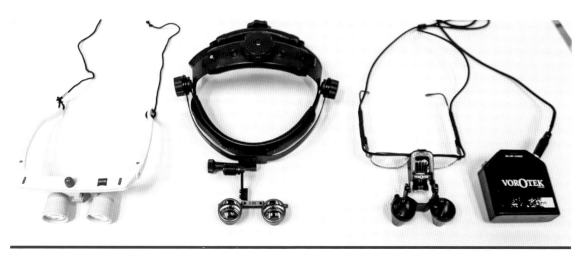

Figure 5. Three different types of surgical loupes. Loupes vary in the level of magnification afforded and the presence/absence of an in-built light source.

Operating microscopes have in-built illumination systems. Additional illumination, for example in the form of ceiling mounted operating lamps, are useful in all operating rooms for either illumination of the surgical site, for example when surgical loupes are used, or illumination of the surgical trolley, when the surgeon prefers the main theatre lights to be dimmed/off.

Seating of the surgeon

For eyelid and adnexal procedures, the use of a chair depends on the individual surgeon's preference. For corneal and intraocular surgery, however, the surgeon should be seated as very precise hand and finger movements are required. The chair or stool should be height-adjustable by surgeon-operated hydraulics, and adjustable back and arm rests are very useful for operating chairs.

Above all of these considerations, the chair should be comfortable to help avoid surgeon fatigue, which can play a part in surgical misadventure.

Head positioning of the patient

Adnexal procedures are usually performed with the patient in either sternal or lateral recumbency. In this situation, where loupes are typically used, head position may be supported by sandbags, towels or cushions. An alternative is a vacuum-aided bead-filled cushion. This is particularly useful in maintaining very precise positioning for corneal and intraocular surgery which is performed in dorsal recumbency under an operating microscope (Fig. 6).

Surgical instrumentation

Instruments

Typically, instruments are divided into those required for enucleation, those required for adnexal surgery and those required for corneal and intraocular surgery. Tables 3-5 present some suggested instrumentation to be included in the various surgical kits but are not exhaustive. Instruments that may be less familiar to the reader are depicted. Disposables commonly used in ophthalmic surgery are listed in Table 6.

Suture material and needles

Choice of suture material depends on tissue type, presence of infection and inflammation, strength of closure required and need for suture removal. For most ophthalmic procedures, relatively small suture material is used and, to avoid tissue drag, needles are swaged-on to the suture. Absorbable suture material is widely used in veterinary ophthalmic surgery, even in the skin, as suture removal would often otherwise require sedation. Commonly used suture materials along with their properties and uses are presented in Table 7.

The three main types of needle tip design used in ophthalmic surgical procedures are reverse cutting, taper point and spatulated. Conventional cutting needles are not suitable for the eyelids. Their design and typical uses are represented in Table 8. Spatulated needles are specifically designed for use in lamellar tissues such as the cornea and sclera.

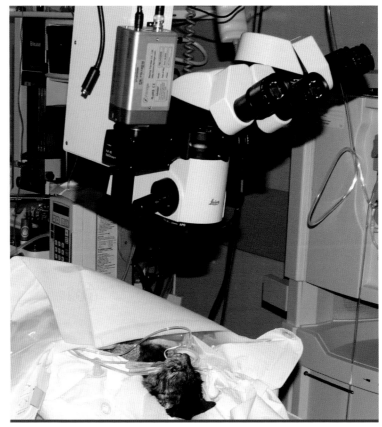

Figure 6. Ceiling mounted microscope used to facilitate cataract surgery. The cat's head is positioned using a vacuum-aided cushion.

Table 3. Instrumentation for enucleation.

Instrument	Function
Fine toothed forceps e.g. Brown-Adson (Fig. 7)	Skin and conjunctival fixation
Curved Steven's tenotomy scissors	Conjunctival, eyelid and orbital tissue dissection
Curved and straight haemostats	Blood vessel haemostasis
Bard-Parker scalpel handle	Skin cutting (with blade, initial incision)
Straight Metzenbaum scissors	Skin cutting (to achieve full thickness incision)
Needle holders e.g. Castroviejo (nonlocking), Derf (Fig. 8)	Needle fixation
Eyelid speculum e.g. Castroviejo, Barraquer (Fig. 11)	Globe exposure for transconjunctival incision, and extraocular muscle and optic nerve transection

Table 4. Instrumentation for eyelid and adnexal surgery.

Instrument	Function
Allis tissue forceps	Eyelid fixation (especially lateral canthus)
Fine toothed forceps e.g. Bishop-Harmon, Castroviejo, Hoskin (Fig. 7)	Skin fixation
Bard-Parker and Beaver scalpel handles (Fig. 10)	Eyelid margin and skin cutting (with blade, initial incision)
Steven's tenotomy scissors (Fig. 9)	Skin cutting (to achieve full thickness incision)
Straight Metzenbaum scissors	Skin cutting (to achieve full thickness incision)
Straight haemostats	Blood vessel haemostasis
Needle holders e.g. Castroviejo (nonlocking), Derf (Fig. 8)	Needle fixation
Eyelid speculum (Fig. 11)	Globe exposure for, in particular, surgery of the nictitans
Chalazion forceps (Fig. 12)	Eyelid stabilisation and haemostasis
Jeweller's forceps	Cilia removal following follicle destruction of distichia
Bennet's forceps	Atraumatic manipulation of eyelids and nictitans
Callipers e.g. Jameson, Castroviejo	Accurate measurement of planned tissue resection
Jaeger lid plate (Fig. 13)	Eyelid stabilisation to assist accurate sharp incision
Chalazion curette	Curettage of chalazia
Nettleship's dilator	Enlargement of nasolacrimal puncta

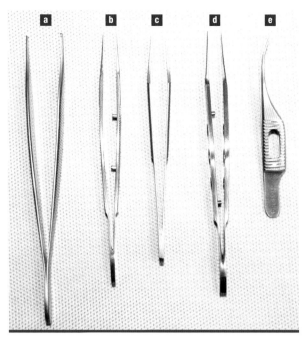

Figure 7. Forceps used in ophthalmic surgery. a) Brown-Adson. b) Castroviejo. c) Hoskins. d) Bishop-Harmon. e) Colibri.

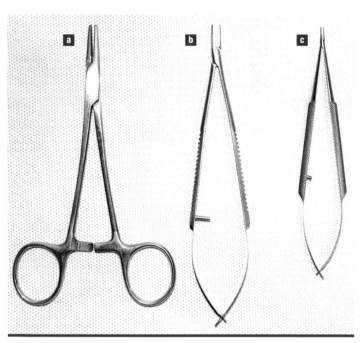

Figure 8. Needle holders used in ophthalmic surgery. a) Derf. b) Castroviejo. c) Micro-surgical Castroviejo.

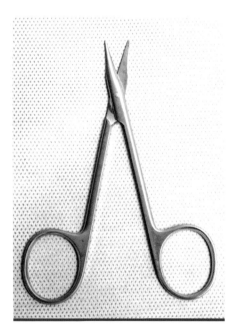

Figure 9. Steven's tenotomy scissors.

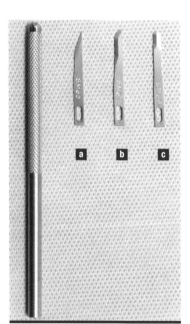

Figure 10. A Beaver scalpel handle with assorted blades. a) No. 65 is used to make full-thickness corneal, limbal and scleral incisions. b) and c) Nos 67 and 69 are used to make partial thickness incisions in cornea, limbus and sclera.

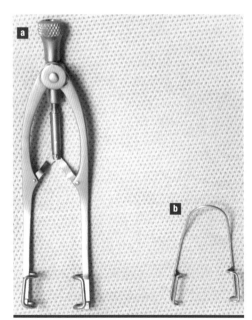

Figure 11. Eyelid specula. a) Castroviejo speculum. b) Wire Barraquer speculum.

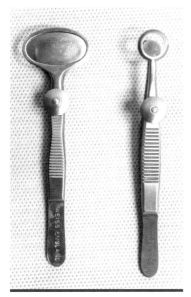

Figure 12. Chalazion clamps are available in a variety of sizes. The smaller, round, 12 mm diameter clamp on the right is most suitable for use in the cat.

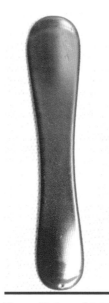

Figure 13. Jaeger lid plate. Placed in the conjunctival fornix to stabilise the eyelid to facilitate its incision.

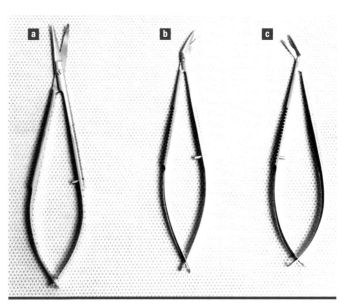

Figure 14. a) Westcott's tenotomy scissors. b) Left corneal scissors. c) Right corneal scissors.

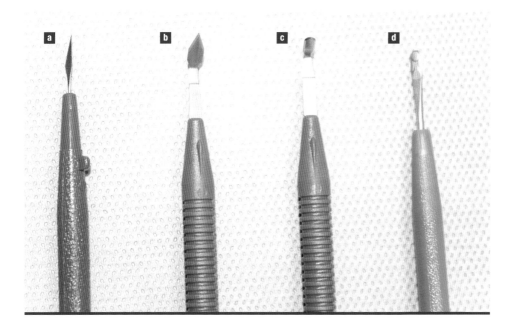

Figure 15. Corneal knives. a) 15° knife, most commonly used to make a full thickness side-port incision to facilitate intraocular surgery. b) 3.2 mm knife used to make full-thickness corneal incision. Most commonly for introduction of the phacoemulsification hand-piece into the anterior chamber. c) Crescent knife for corneal lamellar dissection. d) 300 μm restricted depth knife for keratectomy.

Table 5. Instrumentation for corneal and intraocular surgery.

Instrument	Function
Fine toothed forceps e.g. Bishop-Harmon, Hoskins (Fig. 7)	Skin and conjunctival fixation
Colibri forceps (Fig. 7)	Conjunctival and corneal fixation
Beaver scalpel handle (Fig. 10)	Anchoring blade for corneal sharp incision
Steven's tenotomy scissors (Fig. 9)	Lateral canthotomy
Westcott's tenotomy scissors (Fig. 14)	Conjunctival and corneal incision
Left and right corneal scissors (Fig. 14)	Corneal incision
Iris scissors	Iris incision
Needle holders e.g. Castroviejo (nonlocking) (Fig. 8)	Needle fixation
Eyelid speculum e.g. Barraquer, Castroviejo (Fig. 11)	Globe exposure
Additional instruments for phacoemulsification surgery	
Phacoemulsification hand-piece	Lens cutting and fragment removal
Irrigation/aspiration hand-piece	Removal of lens cortex and viscoelastic
Vannus scissors	Extending initial lens capsule incision
Utrata forceps	Capsulorhexis
Lens manipulator	Mobilisation of lens during phacoemulsification and aspiration
Intraocular lens introducer	Introduction of intraocular lens

Table 6. Disposables for ophthalmic surgery.

Item	Function
No. 15 Bard-Parker scalpel blade	Skin incision
Beaver blades (Nos. 64, 65, 67) (Fig. 10)	Eyelid skin, conjunctival, corneal and scleral incision
Cellulose-tipped spears	Swabbing fluid and debriding epithelium
Restricted depth corneal knife e.g. 300 μm (Fig. 15)	Fixed depth corneal incision
2.8-3.2 mm corneal stab knife (Fig. 15)	Fixed length entry into anterior chamber
Crescent corneal knife (Fig. 15)	Corneal lamellar dissection
Cannulae (23 G and 25 G)	Ocular surface and intracameral irrigation and drug administration
Syringes	Ocular surface and intracameral irrigation and drug administration
Insulin syringes	Subconjunctival injections, capsulotomy
Suture material and needles (see next page)	

Table 7. Types of suture material suitable for ocular and adnexal surgery.

Suture	Properties	Size	Use
Nylon	Nonabsorbable, monofilament, strong	3/0 to 5/0	Skin, lateral canthal stabilisation, stay sutures, temporary tarsorrhaphy
		8/0 to 10/0	Cornea (uncommonly in cats)
Silk	Nonabsorbable, multifilament, strong, induces strong tissue reaction	4/0 to 6/0	Skin
		7/0	Stay sutures
Polyglactin 910	Absorbable, multifilament or monofilament (smaller sizes)	4/0 to 6/0	Skin, subcutaneous tissues
		8/0 to 10/0	Conjunctiva, cornea
Polyglycolic acid (PGA)	Absorbable, multifilament, weaker than polyglactin 910 but slower absorption rate	5/0 to 7/0	Subcutaneous tissues, subconjunctival tissues, sclera
Polydioxanone (PDS)	Absorbable, slower absorption rate than polyglactin 910	5/0 to 7/0	Subcutaneous tissues, subconjunctival tissues, sclera

Table 8. Types of needle tip design suitable for ocular and adnexal surgery.

Needle type	Tip cross-section	Properties	Use
Reverse cutting		Triangle in cross-section Sharp tip and sides Traumatic to tissue	Skin including eyelids
Taper point		Sharp tip but smooth sides Minimal tissue trauma	Conjunctiva
Spatulated		Flat in cross-section	Cornea Sclera

References

Barton-Lamb AL, Martin-Flores M, Scrivani PV et al. (2013). Evaluation of maxillary arterial blood flow in anesthetized cats with the mouth closed and open. *The Veterinary Journal*; 196:325-331.

Binder DR, Herring IP (2006). Duration of corneal anesthesia following topical administration of topical proparacaine hydrochloride solution in clinically normal cats. *American Journal of Veterinary Research*; 67:1780-1782.

Oliver JA, Bradbrook C (2012). Suspected brainstem anaesthesia following retrobulbar block in a cat. *Veterinary Ophthalmology*; 16:225-228.

Pypendop BH, Siao KT, Ilkiw JE (2009). Effects of tramadol hydrochloride on the thermal threshold in cats. *American Journal of Veterinary Research*; 70:1465-1470.

Shilo-Benjamini Y, Pascoe PJ, Maggs DJ et al. (2013). Retrobulbar and peribulbar regional techniques in cats: a preliminary study in cadavers. *Veterinary Anaesthesia and Analgesia*; 40:623-631.

Shilo-Benjamini Y, Pascoe PJ, Maggs DJ et al. (2014). Comparison of peribulbar and retrobulbular regional anaesthesia with bupivacaine in cats. *American Journal of Veterinary Research*; 75:1029-1039.

Stiles J, Weil AB, Packer RA and Lantz GC (2012). Postanaesthetic cortical blindness in cats: twenty cases. The Veterinary Journal; 193:367-373.

Thomson S, Oliver JA, Gould DJ et al. (2010). Preliminary investigations into the analgesic efficacy of topical ocular morphine in dogs and cats. *Veterinary Anaesthesia and Analgesia*; 40:632-640.

3

Ocular therapeutics

Drug delivery to the eye and adnexa

Drugs can be delivered to the eye and its adnexa by a variety of routes. The route of administration chosen will need to take into account several factors including the intended site of drug action, potential barriers to drug distribution, possible adverse side effects, required frequency of drug administration and, of particular importance in the cat, patient cooperation.

The topical route is preferred for treatment of ocular surface disease, and is also usually employed, together with the systemic route, for treatment of anterior segment pathology and certain adnexal diseases. To penetrate the intact cornea, the drug must possess both lipophilic and hydrophilic properties. Penetration can be enhanced by increasing drug concentration, increasing drug contact time with the ocular surface and through combination of the drug with esters and certain preservatives. Topical ophthalmic preparations include solutions, suspensions, gels and ointments. In general, the more viscous the preparation, the longer the drug contact time with the ocular surface, potentially reducing the frequency of administration required. Topically applied drugs do not usually achieve therapeutic concentrations in the posterior segment of the eye and so the systemic route is employed for diseases in this location and also for diseases of the orbit and ocular adnexa.

Less commonly used routes of administration include subconjunctival, intracameral and intravitreal.

Subconjunctival drug administration is useful for uncooperative cats in which application of topical medications is not possible and where enhanced penetration of the anterior segment is required, but this requires sedation. Typically, 0.2-0.5 ml of solution or suspension is injected under the dorsal bulbar conjunctiva via a 25-27 G needle, following the application of topical anaesthetic (Fig. 1).

The intracameral route is most commonly used during intraocular surgery but is also used to treat fibrin accumulation in the anterior chamber in cases of anterior uveitis. Under heavy sedation and topical anaesthesia, an injection of 25 µg of tissue plasminogen activator (tPA) is injected intracamerally across the corneoscleral limbus (Fig. 2).

Intravitreal gentamicin has been suggested as a treatment for end-stage glaucoma but has unpredictable results and has been associated with intraocular sarcoma formation and, thus, is best avoided.

Ocular medications

Antibacterials

Topical antibiotics are indicated for ocular surface infections and as prophylaxis in cases of ulcerative keratitis and following corneal and intraocular surgery. Systemic antibiotics are indicated for infections of the eyelids, orbit and posterior segment. Table 1 summarises the most commonly used antibacterials in feline ophthalmology.

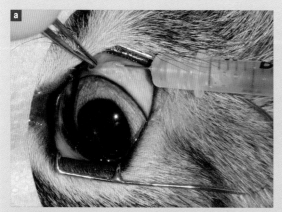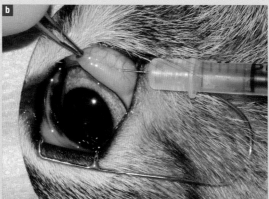

Figure 1. Subconjunctival injection carried out under sedation, following aseptic preparation of the ocular surface and application of topical anaesthetic. a) The dorsal bulbar conjunctiva is grasped and tented with fine forceps. A 27 G needle is then inserted under the conjunctiva. b) 0.2-0.5 ml of the desired formulation is steadily injected to form a bleb.

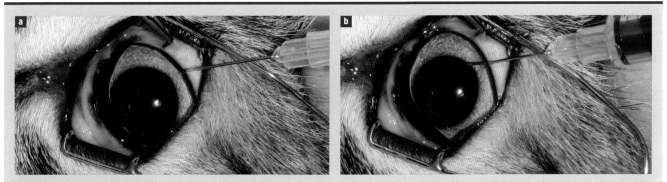

Figure 2. Intracameral injection carried out under heavy sedation, following aseptic preparation of the ocular surface and application of topical anaesthetic. a) Fine forceps are used to stabilise the eye by grasping the conjunctiva and underlying Tenon's capsule adjacent to the corneoscleral limbus. b) A 27 G needle is then passed obliquely across the corneoscleral limbus into the anterior chamber taking care to avoid contact with the iris, lens and corneal endothelium. 0.1-0.2 ml of the desired drug is then slowly administered.

Table 1. Commonly used antibacterials in feline ophthalmology.

Antibiotic class	Spectrum of activity	Commonly used drug examples	Indications	Comments
Beta-lactamase penicillins and cephalosporins	Bactericidal Broad spectrum	Amoxycillin/ clavulanate Cephalexin Cefazolin	Infections of eyelids, orbit and globe Perioperative prophylaxis	Used systemically
Aminoglycosides	Bactericidal Gram-negative	Gentamicin Tobramycin Neomycin	Melting corneal ulcers	Used topically
Fluoroquinolones	Bactericidal Broad spectrum Good Gram-negative activity Good corneal penetration when used topically	Enrofloxacin Ciprofloxacin Ofloxacin	Infections of eyelids, orbit and globe (enrofloxacin) Melting corneal ulcers (ciprofloxacin and ofloxacin)	Enrofloxacin has been associated with retinal degeneration when used systemically at high doses Not to be used prophylactically
Tetracyclines	Bacteriostatic Broad spectrum	Doxycycline Tetracycline Chlortetracycline	Chlamydial, mycoplasmal and rickettsial disease Melting corneal ulcers	Doxycycline has good intraocular penetration Topical tetracyclines have good activity against matrix metalloproteinases (MMPs)
Macrolides and lincosamides	Bacteriostatic Gram-positive Parasiticide activity	Clindamycin Azithromycin	Toxoplasmosis (clindamycin) *Chlamydophila* spp. (azithromycin)	
Polypeptide antibiotics	Bactericidal Poor corneal penetration	Bacitracin Polymyxin B	Gram-positive ocular surface infections (bacitracin) Gram-negative ocular surface infections (polymyxin B)	Often used topically in combination for mixed ocular surface infections
Chloramphenicol	Bacteriostatic Broad spectrum Good corneal penetration	Chloramphenicol	Ocular surface infections Perioperative prophylaxis	Used topically Excellent first-line choice for uncomplicated corneal ulcers and prophylaxis
Fusidic acid	Bactericidal Gram-positive	Fusidic acid	Ocular surface infections Perioperative prophylaxis	Used topically Excellent first-line choice for uncomplicated corneal ulcers Can be used once or twice daily

> → Topical antibiotics are always indicated in cases of corneal ulceration.
>
> → Appropriate first-line antibiotic choices for uncomplicated corneal ulcers include chloramphenicol and fusidic acid.
>
> → Choice of antibiotic is ideally initially made following cytology, pending result of bacterial culture and susceptibility testing.

The penicillins have bactericidal effects. Ampicillin and amoxicillin have relatively broad spectrum activity but are readily inhibited by bacterial beta-lactamases. Combination of a penicillin with a lactamase inhibitor such as clavulanic acid or sulbactam protects against this. Amoxicillin/clavulanic acid is perhaps the most commonly used systemic preparation for ophthalmic infections but does not penetrate the noninflamed eye well. Amoxicillin/clavulanic acid may be useful in cats with *Chlamydophila felis* infections where doxycycline is contraindicated (Sturgess et al., 2001).

Cephalosporins are also bactericidal and have a very similar mode of action to penicillins. In cats, the most commonly used examples are cefazolin and cephalexin which are mainly effective against Gram-positive bacteria.

Aminoglycosides are bactericidal and are active against both Gram-positive and Gram-negative bacteria. Topical gentamicin and tobramycin are good choices for the treatment of ulcers associated with infections with susceptible Gram-negative bacteria such as *Pseudomonas aeruginosa*. Neomycin is active against Gram-negative bacteria and staphylococci but this drug has been associated with contact hypersensitivity when used topically. Amikacin is often effective against *Pseudomonas* spp. that are resistant to tobramycin and gentamicin.

Fluoroquinolones exert a bactericidal effect on Gram-negative and some Gram-positive bacteria. Enrofloxacin and marbofloxacin are available as injectable and oral formulations and are licensed for use in cats in most countries. Enrofloxacin has been associated with acute retinal degeneration in cats when used above the manufacturer's current dosing recommendations (Fig. 62) (Ford et al., 2007). Ofloxacin and ciprofloxacin are available as topical ophthalmic solutions and are frequently used in cats, although ofloxacin tends to be better tolerated and has enhanced corneal penetration.

Tetracyclines are bacteriostatic agents with activity against Gram-positive and Gram-negative bacteria, mycoplasmas, rickettsiae and *Chlamydophila* spp. Oral doxycycline has been recommended as the treatment of choice for feline chlamydial and mycoplasmal conjunctivitis (10 mg/kg q24h for 21 days). Possible side effects include enamel discoloration in growing kittens and reflux oesophagitis with resultant stricture formation. Topical tetracyclines are available in some countries and are beneficial in the treatment of feline chlamydial conjunctivitis and in melting corneal ulcers owing to their ability to inhibit matrix metalloproteinases (MMPs).

Macrolides and lincosamides are bacteriostatic. Erythromycin, azithromycin and clarithromycin are all macrolides with activity against Gram-positive bacteria, mycoplasmas, rickettsiae, bartonellas and *Chlamydophila* spp. Oral azithromycin is effective in the treatment of *Chlamydophila felis* infections (50 mg/kg q24h for 21 days) but is less effective than doxycycline. Clindamycin, a lincosamide, is particularly useful as a treatment for toxoplasmosis. It is administered orally at 12.5 mg/kg q12h for 21-28 days.

Bacitracin and polymyxin B are polypeptide antibiotics with bactericidal activity. Bacitracin is mainly effective against Gram-positive bacteria whilst polymyxin B has mainly Gram-negative activity. Bacitracin and polymyxin B are available as a combined topical preparation to provide broad spectrum activity for mixed ocular surface infections. One study has reported anaphylactic events in cats receiving topical ophthalmic preparations which all included polymyxin B although no causal association was proved (Hume-Smith et al., 2011).

> → In cats, enrofloxacin has been associated with acute retinal degeneration when used above manufacturer's dosing recommendations.

Chloramphenicol has bacteriostatic activity against both Gram-positive and Gram-negative bacteria. It is available as a 0.5 % ophthalmic solution and 1 % ointment and is an excellent choice in the topical treatment of bacterial conjunctivitis and as prophylaxis for corneal ulceration. Owing to its lipophilic nature, it penetrates the cornea well and achieves therapeutic concentrations in the aqueous, and thus is often used prophylactically following intraocular surgery.

Fusidic acid is bactericidal and its main activity is against Gram-positive bacteria, in particular staphylococci. It is available as a 1 % gel and is indicated for the treatment of ocular surface infections, has good corneal penetration and is effective even when given only once daily and so may be an attractive choice for the uncooperative feline patient. In some countries, where topical chloramphenicol and fusidic acid are unavailable, combination antibiotic preparations (e.g. neomycin/polymixin B/bacitracin) are often used as a first-line treatment. However, such polypharmacy is best avoided if at all possible.

Antiviral agents

Treatment of feline herpesvirus-1 (FHV-1) infections has been reviewed by Gould (2011). Topical antivirals usually need to be applied frequently as they are virustatic rather than virucidal. Those investigated and used in feline ophthalmology are summarised in Table 2.

Trifluorothymidine (trifluridine, TFT) and cidofovir have excellent *in vitro* activity against FHV-1 and are arguably the best choices for topical therapy. Cidofovir has the benefit of a long half-life enabling it to reduce viral shedding significantly when applied only twice daily (Fontenelle et al., 2008). No commercially available products exist for these antivirals in most countries, however, and so ophthalmic preparations have to be compounded. Ganciclovir (0.15 %) and aciclovir (3 %) are both commercially available and ganciclovir has good activity against FHV-1. Aciclovir has poor *in vitro* activity against FHV-1 but may have some clinical benefit when applied five times daily (Williams et al., 2005). Famciclovir is available in an oral tablet formulation and may be of use when topical therapy is not possible or when systemic herpetic disease is present. The active metabolite of famciclovir, penciclovir, has good *in vitro* activity against FHV-1 (Groth et al., 2014). Oral famciclovir has been shown to reduce the severity of clinical signs in cats experimentally infected with FHV-1 when given at a dose of 90 mg/kg q8h (Thomasy et al., 2011).

Although some clinicians advocate the use of oral L-lysine as a treatment for FHV-1 infections, there is, however, very little evidence of the benefits of this treatment and, in fact, the largest studies have shown either no benefit or an increase in severity of clinical signs and viral shedding in cats supplemented with L-lysine (Maggs et al., 2007; Rees and Lubinski, 2008; Drazenovich et al., 2009).

Table 2. Commonly used antivirals in feline ophthalmology.

Drug	Formulation	Route, dose and frequency of administration	FHV-1 *in vitro* activity	Clinical utility	Relative cost	Commercial availability
Aciclovir	3 % ointment	Topically 1 drop q4-6h	Poor	Moderate	Low	Available
Ganciclovir	0.15 % gel	Topically 1 drop q4-6h	Good	Good	Low	Available
Trifluorothymidine	1 % solution	Topically 1 drop q4-6h	Excellent	Excellent	High	Unavailable
Cidofovir	0.5 % solution	Topically 1 drop q8-12h	Excellent	Excellent	Very high	Unavailable
Famciclovir	125 mg and 250 mg tablets	Orally 15-90 mg/kg q8-24h	Excellent	Good	Very high	Available

The use of interferons (IFNs) has also been suggested for FHV-1 infections. However, whereas feline IFN-ω and human IFN-α have good *in vitro* activity against FHV-1, pretreatment with topical feline IFN-ω had no beneficial effect on the course of experimental FHV-1 infection in cats and no controlled clinical trials have been performed (Siebeck et al., 2006; Haid et al., 2007).

Antifungal agents

Fungal disease of the ocular surface is extremely rare in the cat. Cryptococcosis is the most common systemic and intraocular fungal infection, and is caused by the *Cryptococcus neoformans-Cryptococcus gattii* species complex (Pennisi et al., 2013). Cats are also susceptible to histoplasmosis, blastomycosis and coccidioidomycosis.

Amphotericin B, ketoconazole, fluconazole and itraconazole have all been used to treat systemic fungal diseases in cats. Fluconazole has enhanced intraocular penetration and may be useful for the treatment of intraocular cryptococcosis. Amphotericin B is available as an injectable formulation and is sometimes used in conjunction with other antifungals in the treatment of intraocular mycotic infections. It should be noted that antifungal agents are generally fungistatic rather than fungicidal, thus requiring protracted therapy and being reliant on a functional host immune system to clear the infection.

Parasiticides

Selamectin has been used off-licence to treat feline scabies caused by *Notoedres cati* (Itoh et al., 2004) and amitraz or 2 % lime sulphur dips can be used to treat generalised demodecosis taking care to avoid contact with the ocular surfaces. Current dermatological texts should be consulted for more detailed treatment protocols for these diseases.

Pentavalent antimonials, such as sodium stibogluconate and/or allopurinol are used systemically to treat ocular and systemic leishmaniasis.

Encephalitozoon cuniculi has been reported as a cause of focal anterior cortical cataract and uveitis in cats and effective treatment can be achieved using oral fenbendazole in combination with other medications and phacoemulsification surgery (Benz et al., 2011).

Successful treatment of thelaziasis with a topical dermatological preparation containing 10 % imidacloprid and 2.5 % moxidectin has been reported (Bianciardi and Otranto, 2005). An alternative treatment of thelaziasis is oral milbemycin oxime at 2 mg/kg (Motta et al., 2012), see Chapter 6.

Antiinflammatory and immunomodulatory drugs

The nonsteroidal antiinflammatory drugs (NSAIDs) meloxicam, carprofen and robenacoxib are licensed for systemic use in cats in several countries. There are no licensed topical NSAIDs for use in cats although ketorolac, flurbiprofen and diclofenac are widely used in the treatment and prevention of intraocular inflammation, especially when corticosteroids are contraindicated. In cats, 0.1 % diclofenac was as effective as 1 % prednisolone and more effective than 0.03 % flurbiprofen and 0.1 % dexamethasone, in controlling experimentally induced intraocular inflammation (Rankin et al., 2011). Diclofenac and flurbiprofen, however, were found to increase intraocular pressure significantly and should be used with caution in cats with ocular hypertension. In addition, because NSAIDs may inhibit platelet function, they should be used with caution in cats with coagulopathies or when intraocular haemorrhage is present.

In the eye, corticosteroids reduce cell and protein exudation, inhibit chemotaxis and neovascularisation, and stabilise lysosomal membranes and the blood-aqueous barrier. Corticosteroids should be used with caution in the presence of infection, and topical corticosteroids are contraindicated in the presence of corneal ulceration. Several topical ophthalmic corticosteroids are available, which differ in their potency and corneal penetration. Prednisolone acetate has excellent corneal penetration and is widely used in the treatment of anterior uveitis. Dexamethasone phosphate penetrates the cornea less effectively, and is more suitable for the treatment of immune-mediated diseases of the ocular surface such as eosinophilic keratoconjunctivitis and stromal keratitis. Topical corticosteroids may be associated with systemic signs including polydipsia and polyuria, and diabetic cats may be difficult to stabilise during their use. Chronic use of topical corticosteroids has also been associated with subcapsular cataract formation in cats (Zhan et al., 1992).

Ciclosporin and tacrolimus are calcineurin inhibitors. They bind to intracytosolic immunophilins in T-helper lymphocytes and block the production of lymphokines necessary for T-lymphocyte activation. Topical ciclosporin is useful in the treatment of stromal keratitis and eosinophilic keratoconjunctivitis (Spiess et al., 2009). Oral megoestrol acetate has been used as a treatment for feline eosinophilic keratoconjunctivitis which is refractory to first-line topical treatments but is not without the risk of potentially serious systemic side effects.

Antiglaucoma drugs

Carbonic anhydrase inhibitors (CAIs) reduce the production of aqueous humour and are frequently used in the management of feline glaucoma. They are administered topically owing to potential serious adverse side effects when given systemically. Dorzolamide and brinzolamide are both available as topical ophthalmic preparations and are usually applied every 8-12 hours. In normal cats and those with primary congenital glaucoma, dorzolamide significantly reduces intraocular pressure (IOP) (Sigle et al., 2011). Brinzolamide has no effect on IOP in normal cats (Gray et al., 2003).

Topical beta-blockers are also used fairly commonly in the management of glaucoma in cats. Beta-blockers may reduce IOP via several mechanisms, although their main effect is from the blockade of beta-adrenergic receptors in the nonpigmented ciliary epithelium. Commercially available topical beta-blockers include timolol, betaxalol, carteolol, levobunolol and metripranolol. Timolol is the most widely used and is available as 0.25 % and 0.5 % solutions and is usually applied every 8-12 hours. Timolol is also available in combination with dorzolamide and brinzolamide. Timolol has not been evaluated in glaucomatous cats, but in normotensive cats it reduces IOP by around 20 % (Wilkie and Latimer, 1991). Ocular side effects include local irritation, conjunctival hyperaemia and miosis. Adverse systemic side effects include bradycardia and hypotension, and thus it has been suggested that the lower 0.25 % solution may be more appropriate in cats.

Prostaglandin analogues are very effective in reducing IOP in dogs but are not very effective in cats owing to the differences in relative distribution and type of prostanoid receptors between the eyes of these species.

Mydriatics and cycloplegics

Pharmacological pupil dilation is effected by either stimulating the sympathetic nervous supply to the iridal dilator muscle or by interrupting the parasympathetic supply to the iridal sphincter muscle. Sympathomimetic (adrenergic) agents include adrenaline and phenylephrine. They are poorly effective mydriatics in the cat when used topically and have potentially serious adverse effects on the cardiovascular system (Franci et al., 2011). Adrenaline is, however, useful when administered intracamerally during intraocular surgery for both mydriasis and haemostasis. It can either be directly injected at a dilution of 1:10,000 or added to the irrigating fluids at a 1:1,000,000 dilution.

→ Atropine is a potent mydriatic and cycloplegic, but poorly tolerated in cats due to its bitter taste which may induce hypersalivation.

Agents that work in a parasympatholytic fashion (anticholinergics) also cause cycloplegia, making them useful in the treatment of anterior uveitis. Tropicamide, available as a 0.5 % or 1 % solution, is both used diagnostically owing to its rapid onset (20-40 minutes) and relatively short duration of action (8-9 hours), and also therapeutically. Although it produces less cycloplegia and stabilisation of the blood-aqueous barrier than atropine, it is much better tolerated in cats. Side effects include increase in IOP in both the treated and untreated eye, and transient reduction in Schirmer tear test (STT) readings (Stadtbaumer et al., 2002 and 2006; Margadant et al., 2003; Gomes, 2011).

Atropine is a potent mydriatic and cycloplegic but is not well tolerated in cats owing to its bitter taste. A less concentrated 1 % ointment preparation may be better tolerated in this species, or the drug can be applied at the conclusion of any diagnostic or surgical procedures performed under sedation or general anaesthesia.

Tear substitutes

Keratoconjunctivitis sicca is rare in the cat but tear substitutes are still frequently needed. Aqueous tear substitutes, such as hydroxypropylmethylcellulose, require too frequent application (every 1-2 hours) to be useful for treatment in cats. Polyacrylic acid (Carbomer 980), a mucinomimetic, is one of the most effective artificial tear preparations in cats replacing both the aqueous and mucin layers of the tear film. It is usually applied 4-6 times daily.

Sodium hyaluronate, an example of a viscoelastic, is involved in wound healing and increases corneal epithelial migration. It has prolonged ocular retention time owing to its high viscosity and is becoming an increasingly popular choice as a tear substitute in cats as it requires less frequent application than aqueous substitutes and mucinomimetics.

Lanolin, petrolatum and mineral oil mimic the lipid layer of the tear film and reduce evaporation of the tear film. Excellent corneal retention means that they only require application 3-4 times daily. However, they can be difficult to apply and cause blurring of vision.

Anticollagenases

Anticollagenases are used to inhibit the enzymes (matrix metalloproteinases or MMPs, and serine proteases) involved in melting corneal ulceration. Examples of frequently used anticollagenases in cats include serum, tetracyclines and EDTA.

Autologous serum is the anticollagenase of choice owing to its ready availability and broad spectrum activity. Serum is preferred over plasma as it contains higher concentrations of epithelial growth factor, platelet-derived growth factor and vitamin A which are all thought to be important in corneal wound healing. Initially, autologous serum is applied every 1-2 hours until the process of melting has arrested. Thereafter, frequency of application can be reduced.

Tetracycline antibiotics have anticollagenase effects independent of their antimicrobial activity. Topical therapy, although commercially available products may not be available in all countries, is preferred to ensure adequate drug concentration at the intended site of action.

Preparation of autologous serum eye drops

→ A blood sample (5-10 ml) is collected from the jugular vein of the patient in an aseptic manner and added to plain or serum-gel blood collection tubes. If the affected eye is fragile, the contralateral jugular vein should be used to avoid the increase in ipsilateral IOP, which occurs with jugular vein compression.

→ The blood is allowed to coagulate at room temperature for 30 minutes.

→ It is then centrifuged and the supernatant (serum) is harvested and transferred to a sterile dropper bottle.

→ It is then stored in a refrigerator at 4 °C. Owing to the lack of preservatives, it should be discarded after 96 hours owing to the risk of contamination by microorganisms.

Note: Donor serum can be collected if the patient is too fractious or if the eye is in serious danger of rupturing. Owing to the risk of transmitting infectious agents such as FIV and FeLV, homologous donors should be screened for infection with these agents. Alternatively, the use of a healthy heterologous donor such as the dog or horse could be considered.

EDTA owes its anti-MMP activity to its ability to chelate zinc and calcium ions required as cofactors for the enzymes. A 0.2 % solution is applied to the eye initially every 1-2 hours.

Fibrinolytics

Fibrin within the eye can cause formation of anterior and posterior synechiae which, in turn, can lead to glaucoma. Tissue plasminogen activator (tPA), a serine protease, is commonly used to dissolve fibrin as an intracameral injection and exerts its effect within 15-30 minutes. Doses should not exceed 25 µg owing to the risk of intraocular toxicity (Hrach et al., 2000). It should not be used within 48 hours of an intraocular bleed owing to its potential to precipitate further haemorrhage.

References

BENZ P, MAASS G, CSOKAI J et al. (2011). Detection of *Encephalitozoon cuniculi* in the feline cataractous lens. *Veterinary Ophthalmology*; 14(Suppl 1):37-47.

BIANCIARDI P, OTRANTO D (2005). Treatment of dog thelaziosis caused by *Thelazia callipaeda* (Spirurida, Thelaziidae) using a topical formulation of imidacloprid 10 % and moxidectin 2.5 %. *Veterinary Parasitology*; 129:89-93.

BINDER DR, HERRING IP (2006). Duration of corneal anaesthesia following topical administration of 0.5 % proparacaine hydrochloride solution in clinically normal cats. *American Journal of Veterinary Research*; 67:1780-1782.

DRAZENOVICH TL, FACETTI AJ, WESTERMEYER HD et al. (2009). Effects of dietary lysine supplementation on upper respiratory and ocular disease and detection of infectious organisms in cats within an animal shelter. *American Journal of Veterinary Research*; 70:1391-1400.

FONTENELLE JP, POWELL CC, VEIR JK et al. (2008). Effect of topical ophthalmic application of cidofovir on experimentally induced primary ocular feline herpesvirus-1 infection in cats. *American Journal of Veterinary Research*; 69:289-293.

FORD MM, DUBIELZIG RR, GIULIANO EA et al. (2007). Ocular and systemic manifestations after oral administration of a high dose of enrofloxacin in cats. *American Journal of Veterinary Research*; 68:190-202.

FOWLER JD, SCHUH JCL (1992). Preoperative chemical preparation of the eye: a comparison of chlorhexidine diacetate, chlorhexidine gluconate, and povidone iodine. *Journal of the American Animal Hospital Association*; 28:451-457.

FRANCI P, LEECE EA, MCCONNELL JF (2011). Arrhythmias and transient changes in cardiac function after topical administration of one drop of phenylephrine 10 % in an adult cat undergoing conjunctival graft. *Veterinary Anaesthesia and Analgesia*; 38:208-212.

GOMES FE, BENTLEY E, LIN TL et al. (2011). Effects of unilateral topical administration of 0.5 % tropicamide on anterior segment morphology and intraocular pressure in normal cats and cats with primary congenital glaucoma. *Veterinary Ophthalmology*; 14(Suppl 1):75-83.

GOULD DJ (2011). Feline herpesvirus 1. Ocular manifestations, diagnosis and treatment options. *Journal of Feline Medicine and Surgery*; 13:333-346.

GRAY HE, WILLIS AM, MORGAN RV (2003). Effects of topical administration of 1 % brinzolamide on normal cat eyes. *Veterinary Ophthalmology*; 6:285-290.

GROTH AD, CONTRERAS MT, KADO-FONG HK et al. (2014). *In vitro* cytotoxicity and antiviral efficacy against feline herpesvirus type 1 of famciclovir and its metabolites. *Veterinary Ophthalmology*; 17:268-274.

HAID C, KAPS S, GÖNCZI E et al. (2007). Pretreatment with feline interferon omega and the course of subsequent infection with feline herpesvirus in cats. *Veterinary Ophthalmology*; 10:278-284.

HRACH CJ, JOHNSON MW, HASSAN AS et al. (2000). Retinal toxicity of commercial intravitreal tissue plasminogen activator solution in cat eyes. *Archives of Ophthalmology*; 118:659-663.

HUME-SMITH KM, GROTH AD, RISHNIW M et al. (2011). Anaphylactic events observed within 4h of ocular application of an antibiotic-containing ophthalmic preparation: 61 cats (1993-2010). *Journal of Feline Medicine and Surgery*; 13:744-751.

ITOH N, MURAOKA N, AOKI M et al. (2004). Treatment of *Notoedres cati* infestation in cats with selamectin. *Veterinary Record*; 154:409.

MAGGS DJ, SYKES JE, CLARKE HE et al. (2007). Effects of dietary lysine supplementation in cats with enzootic upper respiratory disease. *Journal of Feline Medicine and Surgery*; 9:97-108.

MARGADANT DL, KIRKBY K, ANDREW SE et al. (2003). Effect of topical tropicamide on tear production as measured by Schirmer's tear test in normal dogs and cats. *Veterinary Ophthalmology*; 6:315-320.

MOTTA B, SCHNYDER M, BASANO F et al. (2012). Therapeutic efficacy of milbemycin oxime / praziquantel oral formulation (Milbemax) against *Thelazia callipaeda* in naturally infested dogs and cats. *Parasit Vectors*; 5:85.

NASISSE MP, GUY JS, DAVIDSON MG et al. (1989). *In vitro* susceptibility of feline herpesvirus-1 to vidarabine, idoxuridine, trifluridine, acyclovir, or bromovinyldeoxyuridine. *American Journal of Veterinary Research*; 50:158-160.

PENNISI MG, HARTMANN K, LLORET A et al. (2013). Cryptococcosis in cats: ABCD guidelines on prevention and management. *Journal of Feline Medicine and Surgery*; 15:611-618.

RANKIN AJ, KHRONE SG, STILES J (2011). Evaluation of four drugs for inhibition of paracentesis-induced blood-aqueous humor barrier breakdown in cats. *American Journal of Veterinary Research*; 72:826-832.

REES TM, LUBINSKI JL (2008). Oral supplementation with L-lysine did not prevent upper respiratory infection in a shelter population of cats. *Journal of Feline Medicine and Surgery*; 10:510-513.

SIEBECK N, HURLEY DJ, GARCIA M et al. (2006). Effects of human recombinant alpha-2b interferon and feline recombinant omega interferon on *in vitro* replication of feline herpesvirus-1. *American Journal of Veterinary Research*; 67:1406-1411.

SIGLE KJ, CAMAÑO-GARCIA G, CARRIQUIRY AL et al. (2011). The effect of dorzolamide 2 % on circadian intraocular pressure in cats with primary congenital glaucoma. *Veterinary Ophthalmology*; 14(Suppl 1):48-53.

STADTBAUMER K, FROMMLET F, NELL B (2006). Effect of mydriatics on intraocular pressure and pupil size in the normal feline eye. *Veterinary Ophthalmology*; 9:233-237.

STADTBAUMER K, KOSTLIN RG, ZAHN KJ (2002). Effects of topical 0.5 % tropicamide on intraocular pressure in normal cats. *Veterinary Ophthalmology*; 5:107-112.

STURGESS CP, GRUFFYDD-JONES TJ, HARBOUR DA et al. (2001). Controlled study of the efficacy of clavulanic acid-potentiated amoxicillin in the treatment of *Chlamydia psittaci* in cats. *Veterinary Record*; 149:73-76.

THOMASY SM, LIM CC, REILLY CM et al. (2011). Evaluation of orally administered famciclovir in cats experimentally infected with feline herpesvirus type-1. *American Journal of Veterinary Research*; 72:85-95.

WILKIE DA, LATIMER CA (1991). Effects of topical administration of timolol maleate on intraocular pressure and pupil size in cats. *American Journal of Veterinary Research*; 52:436-440.

WILLIAMS DL, ROBINSON JC, LAY E et al. (2005). Efficacy of topical aciclovir for the treatment of feline herpetic keratitis: results of a prospective clinical trial and data from *in vitro* investigations. *Veterinary Record*; 157:254-257.

ZHAN G-L, MIRANDA OC, BITO LZ (1992). Steroid glaucoma: corticosteroid-induced ocular hypertension in cats. *Experimental Eye Research*; 54:211-218.

4

The orbit and globe

Anatomy and function

The feline orbit is approximately 24.0 mm wide and 26.0 mm high and offers protection to the globe which measures approximately 21.3 mm anterio-posteriorly and 20.6 mm equatorially. The orbit encases all but the anterior globe and is delineated by bone and soft tissue. The bony orbit is classified as 'open' as it is incomplete dorsolaterally and ventrally, with these orbital boundaries being composed of soft tissues. Dorsolaterally, the short orbital ligament connects the frontal process of the zygomatic bone to the zygomatic process of the frontal bone. Masticatory muscles provide further boundaries to the orbit with the temporal muscle located dorsally, the masseter muscle lying medial and ventral to the zygomatic arch and the pterygoid muscle forming the orbital floor. The orbital septum is a fascial barrier that is continuous with and extends anteriorly from the periorbital fascial sheath. It forms the anterior border of the orbit separating the orbital contents from the eyelids.

The bony orbital fossa is composed of seven bones: the lacrimal, zygomatic, frontal, sphenoid, palatine, ethmoidal and maxillary bones (Fig. 1). Foramina

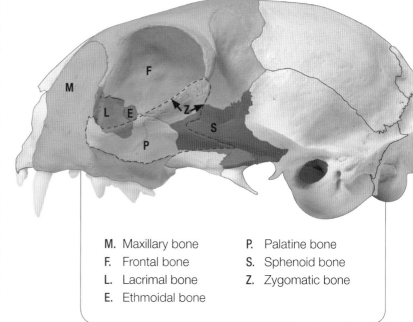

M. Maxillary bone
F. Frontal bone
L. Lacrimal bone
E. Ethmoidal bone

P. Palatine bone
S. Sphenoid bone
Z. Zygomatic bone

Figure 1. The bones of the feline orbit.

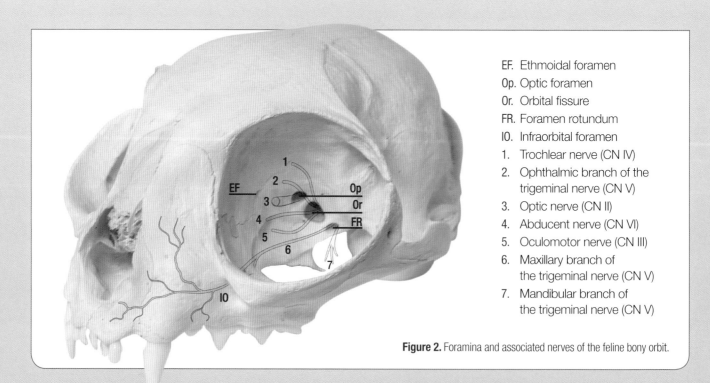

EF. Ethmoidal foramen
Op. Optic foramen
Or. Orbital fissure
FR. Foramen rotundum
IO. Infraorbital foramen
1. Trochlear nerve (CN IV)
2. Ophthalmic branch of the trigeminal nerve (CN V)
3. Optic nerve (CN II)
4. Abducent nerve (CN VI)
5. Oculomotor nerve (CN III)
6. Maxillary branch of the trigeminal nerve (CN V)
7. Mandibular branch of the trigeminal nerve (CN V)

Figure 2. Foramina and associated nerves of the feline bony orbit.

and fissures offer bony conduits for blood vessels and nerves between the orbit and the cranial cavity and alar canal (Fig. 2). Of particular clinical significance is the thin septum of frontal bone which separates the orbit from the nasal cavity and frontal sinus. This septum is sometimes breached during neoplastic and severe inflammatory disease processes.

The orbit is divided into intraconal and extraconal regions by the periorbital fascial sheath which envelops the four rectus muscles which arise from the orbital apex and insert on the globe posterior to the corneoscleral limbus. The respective contents of these regions are illustrated in Figure 4.

Diagnosis of orbital disease

Introduction

The steps in diagnosis of orbital disease can be summarised as follows:

- Obtaining a thorough clinical history
- General physical examination
- Orbital and ophthalmic examination
- Diagnostic imaging
- Collection and laboratory examination of samples

Relevant elements of the patient's history include onset of clinical signs (acute vs chronic) and reluctance to eat (which may be indicated by pain when opening the jaw). An initial diagnosis of orbital disease can usually be made through clinical examination, by paying attention to the classical signs (see below). Definitive diagnosis is achieved by diagnostic imaging and laboratory examination of any collected samples.

Examination and clinical signs

Patient examination begins with a 'hands-off' approach with careful observation of the position of the globe and any gross abnormalities of the adnexa, signs of pain or ocular discharge. The feline orbit is relatively limited in its potential space compared with that of the canine, and so any space occupying lesion results in gross clinical signs of orbital disease early on in the disease process. Feline orbital disease is usually unilateral in presentation and so any asymmetry between the two sides should be noted. Gentle palpation of the periocular region, including the orbital rim and ligament, may yield signs of pain, crepitus or emphysema. Simultaneous bilateral retropulsion of the globes (via the upper eyelids) usually

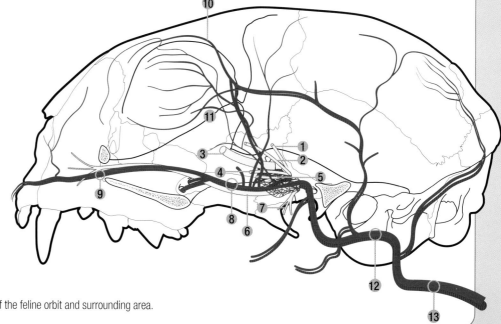

1. Trochlear nerve (CN IV)
2. Ophthalmic branch of the trigeminal nerve (CN V)
3. Optic nerve (CN II)
4. Abducent nerve (CN VI)
5. Oculomotor nerve (CN III)
6. Maxillary branch of the trigeminal nerve (CN V)
7. Mandibular branch of the trigeminal nerve (CN V)
8. Maxillary vessels
9. Infraorbital vessels
10. Palpebral vessels
11. Ethmoidal vessels
12. External carotid vessels
13. Common carotid vessels

Figure 3. Blood vessels and nerves of the feline orbit and surrounding area.

DO. Dorsal oblique
DR. Dorsal rectus
LR. Lateral rectus
RB. Retractor bulbi
VR. Ventral rectus
VO. Ventral oblique
ON. Optic nerve
LG. Lacrimal gland
ZG. Zygomatic gland
OS. Orbital septum
PO. Periorbital fascia
OF. Orbital fat

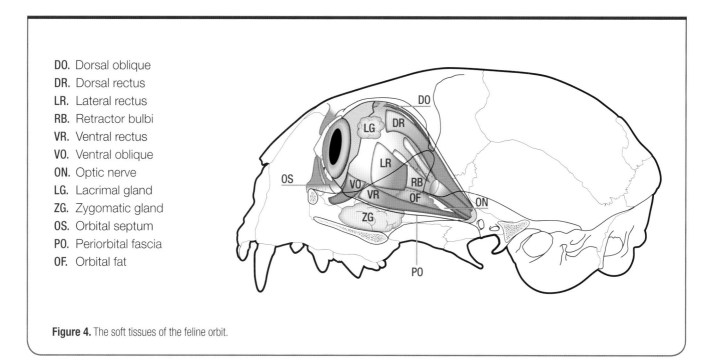

Figure 4. The soft tissues of the feline orbit.

reveals restriction of movement on the affected side. Exophthalmos, globe deviation (strabismus) and protrusion of the nictitans are hallmark features of orbital disease. Exophthalmos must be differentiated from globe enlargement which can be achieved by comparing the corneal diameter of each eye (normal horizontal corneal diameter = 16.5 ± 0.60 mm). This can be done by using callipers or a Schirmer tear test strip. With globe enlargement, but not exophthalmos, corneal diameter will be increased on the affected side. Observation from above, comparing the relative position of the anterior aspect of the globes, is also helpful in detecting subtle exophthalmos. Thorough ophthalmic examination should then be performed. Occasionally, orbital disease can result in scleral indentation which may be apparent on funduscopy or diagnostic imaging. Tonometry should be performed if possible as any external pressure on the globe is likely to result in elevated intraocular pressure (IOP). Intraoral inspection is another important step in the examination of a patient with suspected orbital disease. The pterygopalatine fossa (caudal to the last upper molar tooth) may be swollen, bruised or fistulated. There may also be evidence of dental disease which can extend to involve the orbit, as the molar tooth roots are separated from the orbit by a relatively thin layer of alveolar bone. Furthermore, opening the jaw may elicit pain as the vertical ramus of the mandible impinges on the orbital soft tissues.

Clinical signs of orbital disease

➔ Exophthalmos (commonly)
➔ Enophthalmos (rarely)
➔ Strabismus (globe deviation)
➔ Nictitans protrusion
➔ Periocular swelling
➔ Chemosis and conjunctival hyperaemia
➔ Ocular discharge
➔ Lagophthalmos (incomplete eyelid closure)
➔ Pain/difficulty on opening jaw/inappetence
➔ Swelling/fistulation of pterygopalatine fossa
➔ Restriction to globe retropulsion
➔ IOP elevation
➔ Scleral indentation

→ Exophthalmos, globe deviation (strabismus) and protrusion of the nictitans are hallmark features of orbital disease.

Ancillary diagnostic tests

Diagnostic imaging techniques are used to confirm orbital disease and yield information as to the most likely aetiology. Conventional radiography can be used to assess for orbital fractures, radiopaque foreign bodies such as gun-shot pellets and dental abscesses. Ultrasonography is extremely useful in examining the orbital soft tissues. It is readily available, relatively inexpensive and can usually be performed in the conscious patient. It should be possible to differentiate soft tissue masses from areas of abscessation and cysts, and can be used to guide biopsy sampling. Collected samples may be submitted for culture and susceptibility testing and, depending on whether an aspirate or portion of tissue is collected, cytology and histology respectively. Ultrasonography has limited value in diagnosis of disease processes involving the orbital apex or bony orbit, however. MRI and CT have much superior diagnostic value for examination of these regions and in detecting extension of disease beyond the orbit (which is a useful indicator of tumour malignancy). CT is also valuable for screening for thoracic metastasis, being more sensitive than conventional radiography.

Congenital anomalies of the globe and orbit

Anophthalmos and microphthalmos

True, primary anophthalmos (the congenital complete absence of an eye) is exceedingly rare as some discernible ocular tissue is almost invariably present. Microphthalmos (a congenitally small eye) is much more common, varying in severity from a slightly smaller than normal eye with apparent normal function to extreme microphthalmos associated with multiple ocular defects and blindness (Figs. 5 and 6). Accompanying ocular anomalies may include colobomatous defects of the eyelid, iris, optic nerve, choroid and sclera, persistent pupillary membranes and retinal dysplasia. Abnormalities of globe size and structure may have an inherited basis or result from infectious or toxic insult to the developing kitten *in utero*. The cat is particularly sensitive to the teratogenic effects of the fungistatic agent griseofulvin when given during the first half of gestation. Ocular defects include anophthalmia, cyclopia and optic nerve aplasia.

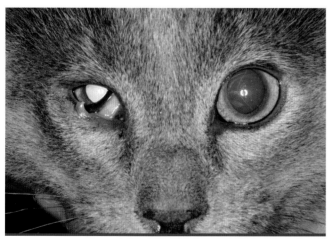

Figure 5. Microphthalmos of the right eye in a 6-month-old Domestic shorthair. Note the passive protrusion of the nictitans and retention of ocular discharge. The eye retained vision.

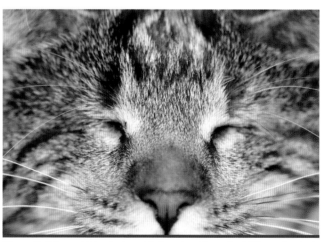

Figure 6. Extreme bilateral microphthalmos in a 6-month-old Domestic shorthair.

Hydrophthalmos

Hydrophthalmos (a congenitally large globe) occurs with congenital glaucoma or very early life ocular disease (Figs. 7-9). Congenital glaucoma may be seen sporadically in any breed and may be associated with multiple ocular defects including pectinate ligament dysplasia, ectopia lentis, spherophakia and uveal cysts. It is also reported to occur as an inherited autosomal recessive trait in the Siamese in which it is associated with gradually progressive globe enlargement, elongated ciliary processes and spherophakia (McLellan et al., 2004).

Breed-related exophthalmos

Brachycephalic breeds demonstrate exophthalmos as a result of relatively shallow orbits (Fig. 10). The clinical relevance of the exophthalmos mainly relates to the resultant lagophthalmos (incomplete blinking) and predisposition to corneal dessication and ulceration. Furthermore, brachycephalic breeds are at an increased risk of traumatic globe proptosis.

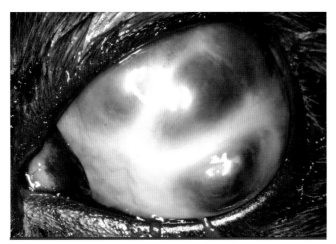

Figure 7. Hydrophthalmos in a 14-week-old Domestic shorthair. The eye was congenitally enlarged and cystic. The cornea also demonstrates fibrosis.

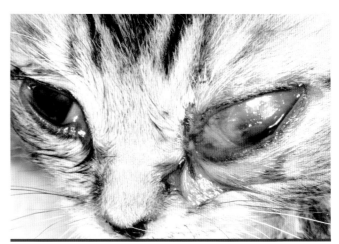

Figure 8. Bilateral congenital glaucoma in a 6-week-old Domestic shorthair. The left globe is enlarged (hydrophthalmic) and there is secondary ocular surface disease. Note the corneal oedema, vascularisation and mucoid discharge.

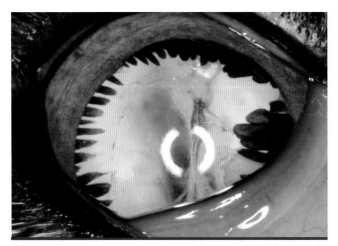

Figure 9. Congenital glaucoma in an 8-month-old Domestic shorthair. Note the elongated ciliary processes and secondary cataract formation.

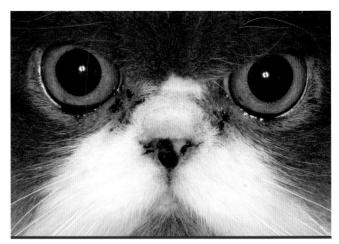

Figure 10. Breed-related exophthalmos in a 1-year-old Exotic shorthair.

Acquired anomalies of the globe and orbit

Buphthalmos

Buphthalmos (acquired globe enlargement) occurs as a result of globe stretching in glaucoma. Although glaucoma may be primary (without evidence of any antecedent intraocular disease), it is most commonly secondary in nature in the cat, occurring as a sequel of chronic uveitis (Figs. 11 and 12).

Phthisis bulbi

Phthisis bulbi refers to a shrunken, blind globe. Phthisis occurs as an end-stage response to severe intraocular disease and results from destruction of the ciliary epithelium and hence aqueous humour production ceases. In cats, it most commonly results from severe intraocular inflammation especially arising from traumatic injury (Fig. 13). Phthitic eyes are usually comfortable but may suffer from secondary effects including retention of discharges and entropion. If there are signs of pain, then enucleation is indicated. Cats are at a unique risk of intraocular sarcoma development after intraocular injury in particular when there has been lens damage (see Chapter 8). This risk further prompts early enucleation in blind feline eyes with severe intraocular disease.

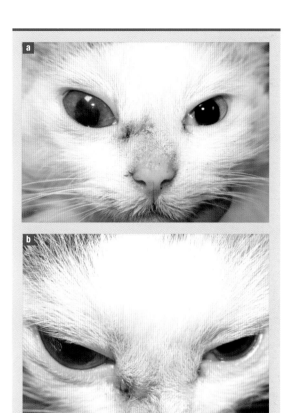

Figure 12. a) Buphthalmos in a 6-year-old Domestic shorthair with secondary glaucoma. b) When viewed from above, the eye can be seen to be enlarged rather than being exophthalmic.

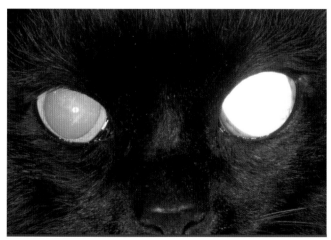

Figure 11. Buphthalmos of the left eye of a 7-year-old Domestic shorthair with secondary glaucoma as a result of chronic idiopathic anterior uveitis. Note the mydriasis.

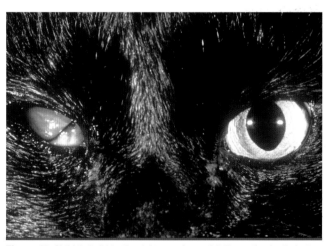

Figure 13. Phthisis bulbi in the right eye of an adult Domestic shorthair as a result of a traumatic injury. Note the small palpebral aperture, nictitans protrusion and corneal opacification. Courtesy of John Mould.

Trauma

Orbital and globe trauma most commonly occur following road traffic accidents, animal fights, malicious attacks by humans and iatrogenic injury – typically during dental procedures (Perry et al., 2015; Smith et al., 2003). The patient must be thoroughly assessed for any life-threatening injuries requiring immediate treatment before attention can be directed to any orbital or ocular damage. Chemical restraint, if safe to perform, will facilitate examination. Gentle palpation of the periocular region may reveal crepitus and/or emphysema but skull radiography or CT should be performed if fractures are suspected and will also identify any ballistic lead pellets. MRI is superior in assessing soft tissues, in particular potential central nervous system (CNS) involvement, but should not be employed if ferrous metallic foreign bodies are suspected.

Blunt and penetrating trauma

Blunt trauma to the globe often results in rupture of uveal vessels and resultant intraocular haemorrhage (Figs. 14-16). Haemorrhage often precludes complete intraocular examination and thus, ultrasonography (or even MRI if concurrent orbital or CNS disease is suspected) is useful to assess for further traumatic intraocular damage such as lens luxation, retinal detachment and scleral rupture (Figs. 17-19). Penetrating ocular injuries demand careful examination for evidence of lens capsule rupture which can lead to phacoclastic uveitis and/or endophthalmitis (Fig. 20).

Orbital fractures are usually treated conservatively although large, mobile fractures may require specialist internal fixation (Fig. 21). Treatment of ocular trauma depends on the extent of injury and prognosis for vision. Enucleation should be offered if there is severe damage to the internal eye or posterior scleral rupture as there is a significant risk of chronic uveitis, secondary glaucoma, phthisis bulbi and potential for intraocular sarcoma development (Fig. 22). Anterior corneal and scleral ruptures, which may be associated with uveal prolapse, require specialist repair (Fig. 23).

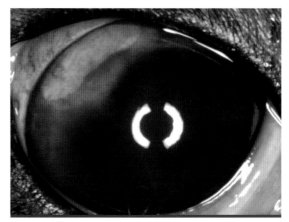

Figure 14. Hyphaema and conjunctival hyperaemia following blunt trauma.

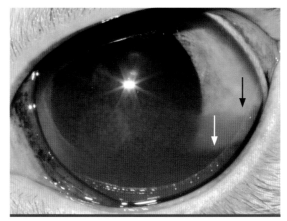

Figure 15. Hyphaema (white arrow) and fibrin (black arrow) settling ventrally following a road traffic accident.

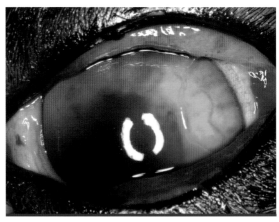

Figure 16. Conjunctival haemorrhage, chemosis, hyphaema and miosis following a road traffic accident.

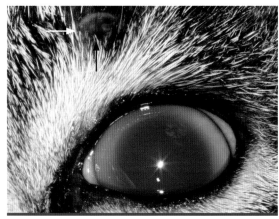

Figure 17. Ballistic lead pellet injury causing hazy hyphaema. The site of entry can be seen dorsal to the eye (arrows). The pellet was identified during conventional radiography within the orbit and there was evidence of a dorsal scleral rupture on ultrasonography.

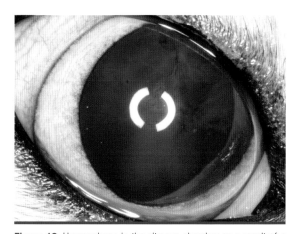

Figure 18. Haemorrhage in the vitreous chamber as a result of a gun-shot injury.

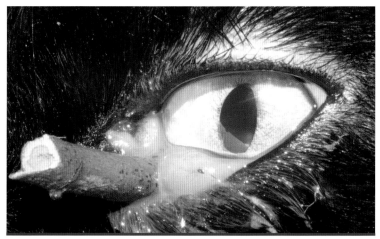

Figure 19. Orbital stick injury. MRI revealed no evidence of globe penetration or orbital fracture and the stick was successfully removed.

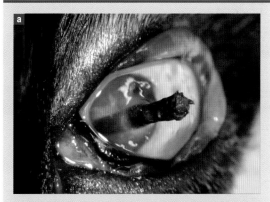

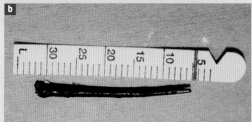

Figure 20. a) A thorn can be seen penetrating the cornea and lens. b) The 27 mm thorn had also penetrated the posterior wall of the globe causing a focal retinal detachment. The lens was extracted via phacoemulsification and the cornea repaired by direct suturing. The eye retained vision.

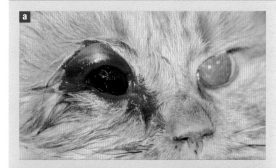

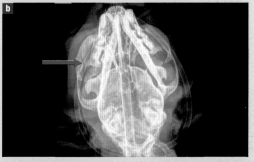

Figure 21. a) Nine-month-old Domestic shorthair after a recent road traffic accident. The right globe is affected by total hyphaema, chemosis and there was a large scleral rupture (not visible). b) Skull radiography revealed a fracture of the zygomatic arch (arrow). The fracture was treated conservatively and the eye was enucleated.

Globes which have undergone contusion without loss of corneoscleral integrity or severe intraocular damage are treated for uveitis – typically with systemic nonsteroidal antiinflammatory drugs (NSAIDs), topical corticosteroids and topical mydriatics/cycloplegics. Monitoring of IOP is required as red blood cells, inflammatory cells and fibrin may impede aqueous outflow and prompt the use of topical antiglaucoma medications. Intracameral tissue plasminogen activator injections are used to dissolve fibrin clots but should not be used within 48 hours of an intraocular bleed owing to their ability to precipitate further haemorrhage.

Globe proptosis

Globe proptosis refers to the anterior displacement of the globe beyond the orbital rim and is almost always traumatic in origin. Proptosis most commonly occurs following road traffic accidents and dog attacks, and is most common in brachycephalic breeds with shallow orbits. An incredibly significant amount of trauma is required to cause proptosis in mesaticephalic breeds which results in more severe tissue damage with an increased incidence of accompanying head and CNS trauma (Figs. 22-24). Once life-threatening injuries have been ruled out or successfully treated, attention can move to assessment of the extent of ocular damage and prognosis for vision. Prognosis for vision restoration following proptosis is even poorer (usually hopeless) in cats than dogs as tractional damage to the optic nerve tends to be more common and severe which relates to the shorter optic nerve in this species. In a study of 18 cats with traumatic proptosis, no cat regained vision in the affected eye (Gilger et al., 1995), Furthermore, accompanying corneoscleral perforation and uveal trauma with significant intraocular haemorrhage are common. For these reasons, surgical repositioning of a proptosed globe is rarely performed in the cat. If it is attempted, then a lateral canthotomy will facilitate the procedure. Following replacement, a temporary tarsorrhaphy (see Chapter 5) should be performed to maintain the globe in position until the orbital soft tissue swelling subsides and to protect the cornea from dessication. Systemic NSAIDs and antibiotics are prescribed and reassessment is performed after two to three weeks.

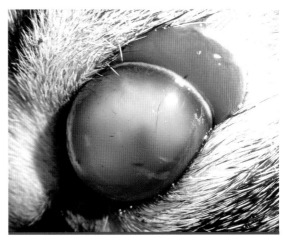

Figure 22. Large dorsolateral scleral rupture and globe proptosis in a 6-year-old Domestic shorthair following a road traffic accident. There is uveal prolapse through the rupture and the eye was enucleated.

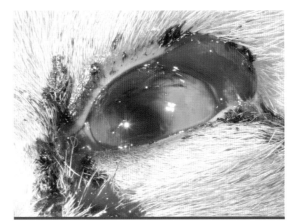

Figure 23. Dorsolateral scleral rupture caused by a dog bite. There is uveal prolapse and hyphaema. Surgery was successfully performed to replace the uveal tissue and repair the rupture.

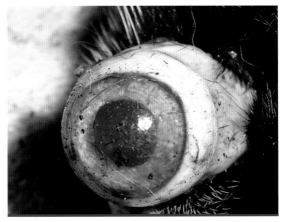

Figure 24. Globe proptosis following a road traffic accident. The cat died as a result of severe CNS trauma.

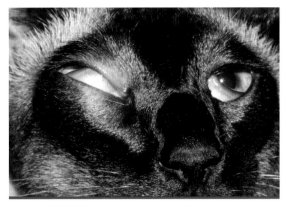

Figure 25. Right exophthalmos and nictitans protrusion in a 7-year-old Siamese with a retrobulbar abscess.

Orbital abscessation and cellulitis

Bacterial infections of the orbit are seen relatively frequently in feline practice. Bacteria may reach the orbit by a variety of routes: haematogenous dissemination, traumatic (including iatrogenic) penetrating injuries, migrating foreign bodies or spread from contiguous regions such as alveolar tooth roots, the nasal cavity or frontal sinus. A typical history is of relatively acute onset exophthalmos, globe deviation, nictitans protrusion and reluctance to eat (Figs. 25-27). On examination there is restriction to globe retropulsion and pain on jaw opening. Swelling of the pterygopalatine fossa is common (Fig. 25b). Diagnosis is usually confirmed by ultrasonography although it is important to rule out dental disease, orbital foreign bodies and extension of sino-nasal disease and additional imaging modalities, such as CT or MRI, may need to be employed to do this (Lybaert et al., 2009; Tovar et al., 2005) (Figs. 25-28).

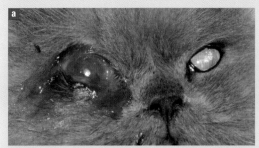

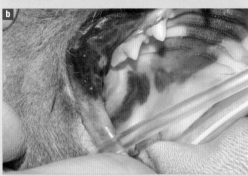

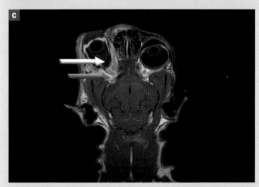

Figure 26. a) Right exophthalmos in a 5-year-old British Blue with orbital cellulitis. b) The right pterygopalatine fossa and lip commissure are bruised and swollen. c) Dorsal T1 MR image of the skull showing right retrobulbar abscessation (reduced signal intensity, white arrow) and cellulitis (increased signal intensity, red arrow).

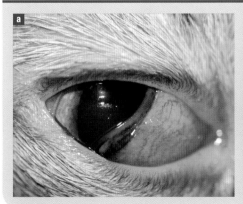

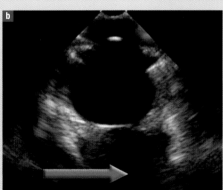

Figure 27. a) Exophthalmos and raised IOP in an 8-year-old Domestic shorthair. b) Ultrasonography revealed an oval hypoechoic abnormality (arrow) in the retrobulbar space consistent with an abscess which was drained transorally (Fig. 31).

Abscesses may be drained using ultrasound guidance and a transtemporal approach, or by a transoral approach when abscessation extends down to the pterygopalatine fossa (Fig. 30). Samples are submitted for cytology and culture and susceptibility testing with the most frequent bacterial genera identified being *Pasteurella* and *Bacteroides* (Wang et al., 2009). A protracted course of systemic antibiotics, for a minimum of four weeks, is advised to reduce the risk of recurrence along with appropriate analgesia in the form of oral NSAIDs.

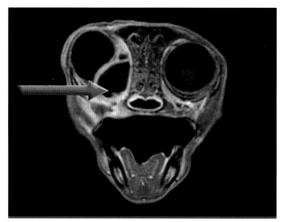

Figure 28. Transverse MR image of the skull of a 6-year-old Domestic shorthair with exophthalmos. In the right ventromedial orbit (left of the image), there is a hypointense mass effect (arrow), consistent with a retrobulbar abscess, causing scleral indentation and exophthalmos.

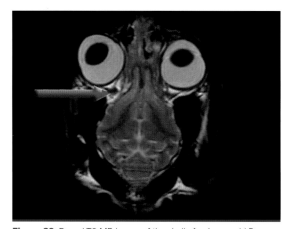

Figure 29. Dorsal T2 MR image of the skull of a 4-year-old Domestic shorthair with mild exophthalmos and nictitans protrusion. There is a hyperintense mass effect in the right retrobulbar space (left of the image, arrow) consistent with cellulitis.

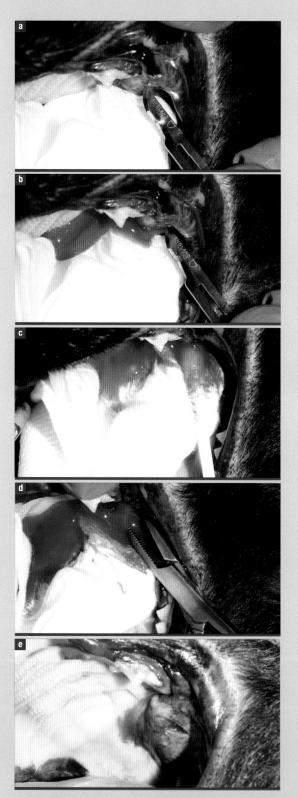

Figure 30. Transoral drainage of the retrobulbar abscess demonstrated in Fig. 28. a) A no. 15 Bard-Parker scalpel blade is used to make an incision through the mucosa of the swollen pterygopalatine fossa. b) There is immediate drainage of haemorrhagic-purulent discharge. c) A sample is collected for bacterial culture and susceptibility testing (*Pasteurella multocida* was cultured). d) Closed haemostat forceps are carefully introduced for 1 cm and opened to increase drainage. e) Following gentle globe massage via closed eyelids, the abscess is completely drained.

Less commonly, and varying with geographical location, other infectious agents may invade the feline orbit. There are several reports of fungal organisms causing orbital infections, usually as a result of extension of sino-nasal infection, with *Aspergillus* spp. being most commonly implicated (Barrs et al., 2014; Kano et al., 2011). Treatment usually involves orbital exenteration and systemic antifungal therapy but prognosis is extremely guarded.

Senile enophthalmos

Gradual sinking of the globe caudally into the orbit (enophthalmos) occurs in many geriatric cats as a result of loss of orbital adipose tissue. If this is marked then complications such as retention of ocular discharge and entropion develop. The entropion will require surgical correction if there are signs of ocular surface disease (Fig. 31).

Orbital cystic disease

Cystic anomalies of the feline orbit are rare but may arise in the glandular structures of the orbit or periorbital tissues. They may occur congenitally or following trauma, inflammation or neoplasia. Orbital conjunctival inclusion cysts result when there has been intraorbital displacement of conjunctival tissue, most commonly iatrogenically when conjunctival tissue is inadvertently left behind following enucleation (Groskopf et al., 2010). The zygomatic salivary gland, which is located ventrally within the orbit, may also undergo cystic change to form a mucocoele (Fig. 32). Reported presenting signs include swelling ventral to the eye and in the caudal vestibule of the oral cavity (Speakman et al., 1997). An orbito-nasal cyst, of undetermined origin, has been reported in a young European shorthaired cat (Zemljič et al., 2011). Orbital cysts are treated by complete resection which, depending on the location, may require an orbitotomy.

Orbital neoplasia

Orbital neoplasia is usually malignant and carries a poor prognosis in the cat (Attali-Soussay et al., 2001). In contrast to the dog, feline orbital tumours are usually secondary either resulting from local extension of sino-nasal disease or metastatic spread. Squamous cell

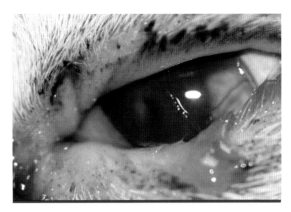

Figure 31. Enophthalmos as a result of loss of orbital adipose tissue with secondary lower eyelid entropion in a 14-year-old Domestic shorthair. There is corneal vascularisation laterally and a developing sequestrum medially.

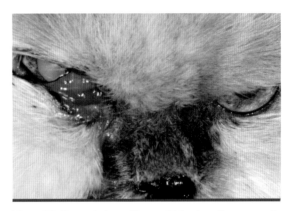

Figure 32. Chemosis in an 18-year-old Persian with a zygomatic mucocoele. Diagnosis was made on MRI.

carcinoma is the most common secondary tumour but fibrosarcomas and osteosarcomas are also encountered with reasonable frequency (Attali-Soussay et al., 2001; Groskopf et al., 2010) (Figs. 33 and 34). Lymphoma is the most common metastatic tumour (Fig. 35). MRI and/or CT are excellent imaging modalities for the investigation of orbital neoplasia and bony lysis is considered an important indicator of tumour malignancy (Lederer et al., 2014; Armour et al., 2004; Dennis, 2000) (Figs. 33-35).

Restrictive orbital myofibroblastic sarcoma

Restrictive orbital myofibroblastic sarcoma describes an unusual condition of progressive orbital sclerosis. The condition was originally termed orbital sclerosing

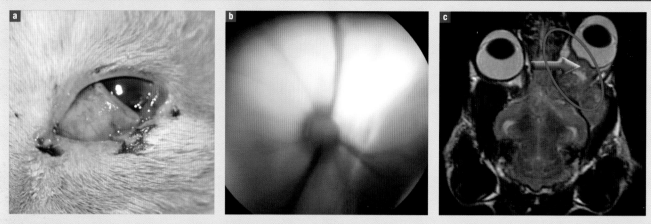

Figure 33. a) Exophthalmos, nictitans protrusion and chemosis in a 12-year-old Domestic shorthair with orbital squamous cell carcinoma. b) Funduscopy revealed an indented sclera. c) Dorsal T2 MR image of the skull. Note the large orbital mass causing scleral indentation (arrow) and exophthalmos (circled).

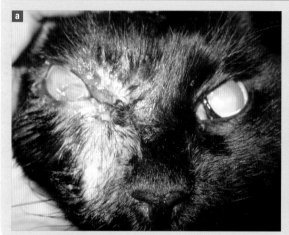
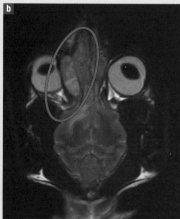

Figure 34. a) Exophthalmos, skin ulceration at the medial canthus, exposure keratitis and lateral deviation of the right globe. b) Dorsal T2 MR image of the skull revealed increased signal intensity of the right nasal sinus and orbit and medial globe compression (left of the image, circled). The evident bony destruction was suggestive of a carcinoma.

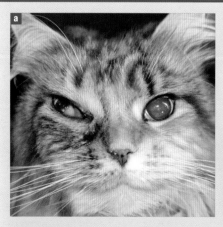
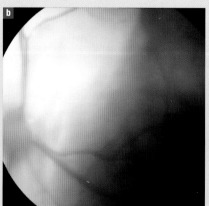
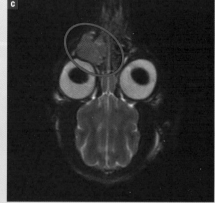

Figure 35. a) Swelling ventral to the right globe and nictitans protrusion in a 14-year-old Domestic longhair with orbital lymphoma. b) Funduscopy revealed scleral indentation. c) Dorsal T2 MR image of the skull revealed a right sino-orbital mass (left of the image, circled).

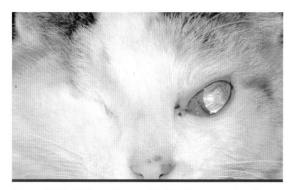

Figure 36. Restrictive orbital myofibroblastic sarcoma in a 6-year-old Domestic shorthair. The right eye was removed 6 months previously and the left orbit is now affected with neoplastic invasion causing exophthalmos and lateral strabismus. Courtesy of John Mould.

Surgery tip

Enucleation must be performed with real caution in the cat as there is a particular risk of iatrogenic tractional injury to the optic chiasm and contralateral blindness.

pseudotumour owing to similarities with the human condition although there is an argument that the feline disease represents a true neoplastic process. Middle-aged to old cats are affected with an insidious progression of signs over weeks to months. The condition begins unilaterally with the orbital tissues and eyelids becoming progressively fixed in place by fibrous tissue but bilateral disease almost always ensues (Fig. 36). Exposure keratitis is common as a result of inability to blink (lagophthalmos). Diagnosis is by histopathological examination of biopsy specimens which reveals infiltration of affected tissues by neoplastic spindle cells (Bell et al., 2011). This condition is poorly responsive to therapy with systemic antiinflammatory and immunosuppressive medications. Orbital exenteration may be performed but most affected cats are euthanased.

Globe removal techniques

Enucleation

Enucleation must be performed with particular caution in the cat as there is a real risk of iatrogenic traumatic injury of the optic chiasm and contralateral blindness (Donaldson et al., 2014). The feline optic nerve is relatively short owing to a less pronounced 'S' shape than the canine. This means that even minimally applied traction to the optic nerve can cause damage to the chiasm. The use of retrobulbar injection of local anaesthetic agents prior to enucleation and the surgical instrumentation required are discussed in Chapter 2.

The two main surgical approaches to enucleation are the transpalpebral and the transconjunctival (Figs. 37 and 38). The transconjunctival approach is generally advised in the cat as it facilitates identification of orbital tissues for resection minimising traction on the orbital soft tissues and optic nerve. The transconjunctival approach, however, is contraindicated in the presence of known ocular surface neoplasia or infection. In this situation, the transpalpebral approach is employed. The placement of a silicone intraorbital prosthesis immediately before skin closure will prevent skin cavitation providing an enhanced cosmetic outcome (Fig. 39).

Orbital evisceration and intraocular prosthesis

Evisceration refers to the removal of the intraocular contents via a large (170°-180°) dorsal scleral incision. The corneo-scleral shell is left in place and an intraocular prosthesis is inserted before closure of the overlying sclera and conjunctiva. The main indication for the procedure in cats is glaucoma as a result of noninfectious and nonneoplastic aetiology. The procedure, however, is rarely performed in the cat owing to the risk of posttraumatic intraocular sarcoma development.

Orbital exenteration

Orbital exenteration is aimed at local control of disease which is potentially fatal or relentlessly progressive. The globe is removed followed by resection of some or all of the orbital soft tissues. In the cat, the main indications are orbital neoplasia (including restrictive orbital myofibroblastic sarcoma) and mycosis. Often, the amount of periocular skin that needs to be removed prevents routine skin closure and, in this situation, a caudal auricular axial flap may be used (Fig. 40).

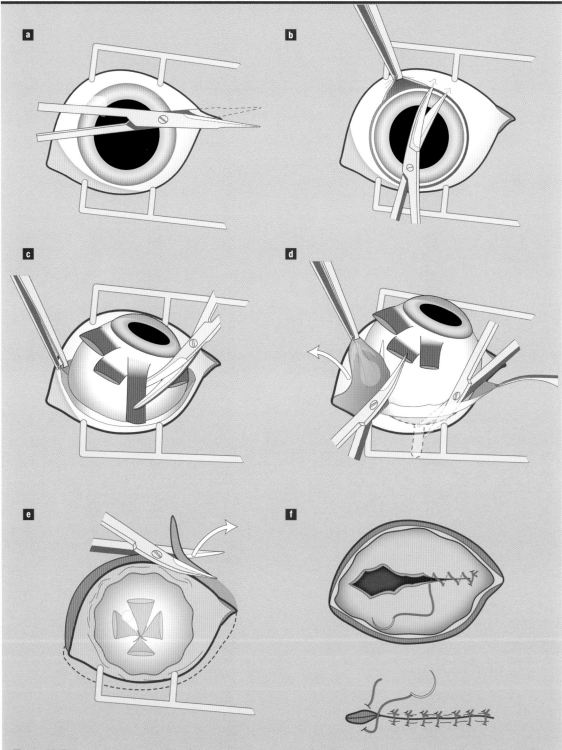

Figure 37. Transconjunctival enucleation. a) A lateral canthotomy, extending 10 mm from the canthus, is performed with tenotomy scissors to increase exposure. b) Starting a few mm behind the limbus, curved tenotomy scissors are used to incise the conjunctiva and Tenon's capsule for 360°. c) Blunt-sharp dissection is used to excise the insertions of the extraocular muscles. d) Without traction on the globe, curved tenotomy scissors are used to incise the optic nerve and any remaining fascial attachments. e) The eyelids, nictitans and all associated conjunctiva are excised. f) 3/0 – 4/0 absorbable suture, in a simple continuous pattern, is then used to close the deep fascia followed by subcutaneous closure. If required, the eyelid skin is then apposed using 4/0 nonabsorbable monofilament suture material.

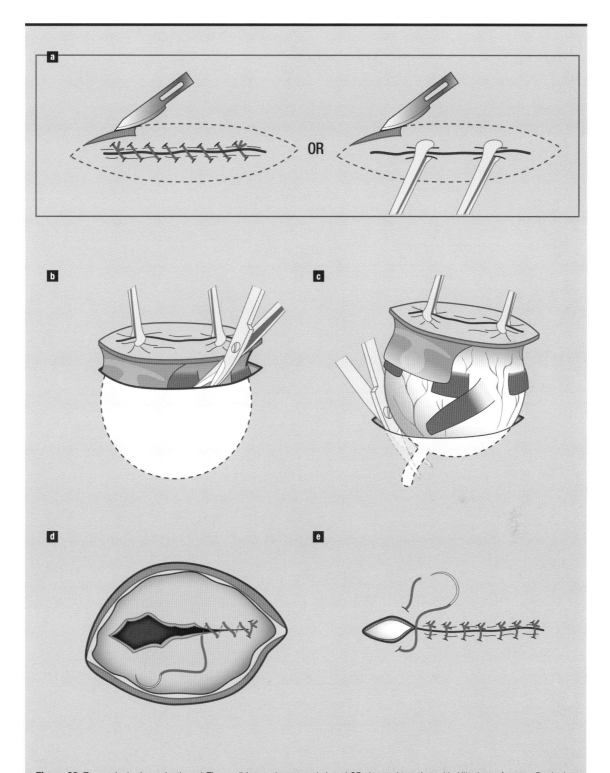

Figure 38. Transpalpebral enucleation. a) The eyelids may be sutured closed OR clamped together with Allis tissue forceps. Beginning approximately 5 mm from the eyelid margin, a surgical blade is used to incise the periocular skin. b) With tenotomy scissors, blunt dissection is performed towards the globe but taking care not to penetrate the conjunctival sac. Beyond the conjunctival fornices, the extraocular muscle attachments around the globe are transected. Medially, dissection external to the nictitans is performed. In all other planes, dissection is performed as close to the sclera as possible. c) The optic nerve is then transected along with any remaining fascial attachments. d and e) The globe, eyelids and nictitans are removed en bloc before wound closure as for the transconjunctival technique.

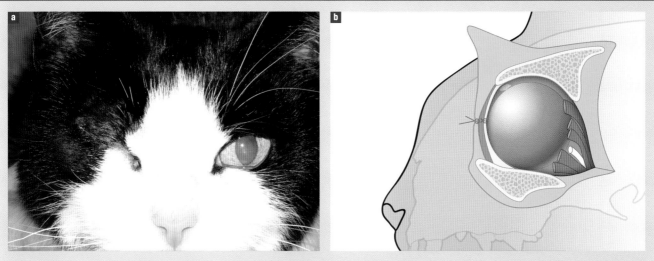

Figure 39. a) A silicone intraorbital prosthesis may be placed in the orbit following enucleation to improve cosmesis. b) Illustration depicting sagittal view of intraorbital prosthesis placement.

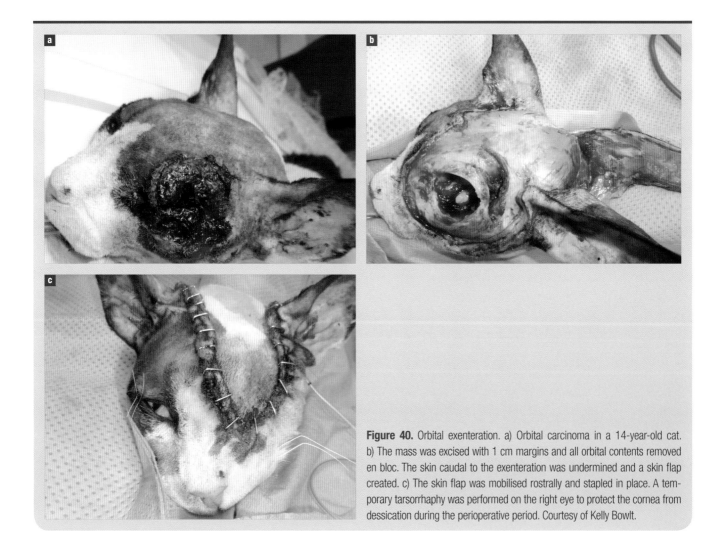

Figure 40. Orbital exenteration. a) Orbital carcinoma in a 14-year-old cat. b) The mass was excised with 1 cm margins and all orbital contents removed en bloc. The skin caudal to the exenteration was undermined and a skin flap created. c) The skin flap was mobilised rostrally and stapled in place. A temporary tarsorrhaphy was performed on the right eye to protect the cornea from dessication during the perioperative period. Courtesy of Kelly Bowlt.

References

ARMOUR MD, BROOME M, DELL'ANNA G et al. (2011). A review of orbital and intracranial magnetic resonance imaging in 79 canine and 13 feline patients (2004-2010). *Veterinary Ophthalmology*; 14:215-226.

ATTALI-SOUSSAY K, JEGOU JP, CLERC B (2001). Retrobulbar tumors in dogs and cats: 25 cases. *Veterinary Ophthalmology*; 4:19-27.

BARRS VR, BEATTY JA, DHAND NK et al. (2014). Computed tomographic features of feline sino-nasal and sino-orbital aspergillosis. *The Veterinary Journal*; 201:215-222.

BELL CM, SCHWARZ T, DUBIELZIG RR (2011). Diagnostic features of feline restrictive orbital myofibroblastic sarcoma. *Veterinary Pathology*; 48:742-750.

DENNIS R (2000). Use of magnetic resonance imaging for the investigation of orbital disease in small animals. *Journal of Small Animal Practice*; 41:145-155.

DONALDSON D, MATAS RIERA M, HOLLOWAY A et al. (2014). Contralateral optic neuropathy and retinopathy associated with visual and afferent pupillomotor dysfunction following enucleation in cats. *Veterinary Ophthalmology*; 17:373-384.

GILGER BC, HAMILTON HL, WILKIE DA et al. (1995). Traumatic ocular proptoses in dogs and cats: 84 cases (1980-1993). *Journal of the American Veterinary Medical Association*; 206:1186-1190.

GROSKOPF BS, DUBIELZIG RR, BEAUMONT SL (2010). Orbital extraskeletal osteosarcoma following enucleation in a cat: a case report. *Veterinary Ophthalmology*; 13:179-183.

KANO R, SHIBAHASHI A, FUJINO Y et al. (2013). Two cases of feline orbital aspergillosis due to *Aspergillus udagawae* and *A. viridinutans*. *Journal of Veterinary Medical Sciences*; 75:7-10.

LEDERER K, LUDEWIG E, HECHINGER H et al. (2014). Differentiation between inflammatory and neoplastic orbital conditions based on computed tomographic signs. *Veterinary Ophthalmology*; DOI: 10.1111/vop.12197.

LYBAERT P, DELBECKE I, COHEN-SOLAL A (2009). Diagnosis and management of a wooden foreign body in the orbit of a cat. *Journal of Feline Medicine and Surgery*; 11:219-221.

MCLELLAN GJ, BETTS D, SIGLE K et al. (2004). Congenital glaucoma in the Siamese cat – a new spontaneously occurring animal model for glaucoma research. (abstract). *35th Annual Meeting of the American College of Veterinary Ophthalmologists*, Washington, DC.

PERRY R, MOORE D, SCURRELL E (2015). Globe penetration in a cat following maxillary nerve block for dental surgery. *Journal of Feline Medicine and Surgery*; 17:66-72.

SMITH MM, SMITH EM, LA CROIX N et al. (2003). Orbital penetration associated with tooth extraction. *Journal of Veterinary Dentistry*; 20:8-17.

SPEAKMAN AJ, BAINES SJ, WILLIAMS JM et al. (1997). Zygomatic salivary cyst with mucocele formation in a cat. *Journal of Small Animal Practice*; 38:468-470.

TOVAR MC, HUGUET E, GOMEZI MA (2005). Orbital cellulitis and intraocular abscess caused by migrating grass in a cat. *Veterinary Ophthalmology*; 8:353-356.

WANG AL, LEDBETTER EC, KERN TJ (2009). Orbital abscess bacterial isolates and in vitro antimicrobial susceptibility patterns in dogs and cats. *Veterinary Ophthalmology*; 12:91-96.

ZEMLJIČ T, MATHEIS FL, VENZIN C et al. (2011). Orbito-nasal cyst in a young European short-haired cat. *Veterinary Ophthalmology*; 14Suppl(1):122-129.

5

The eyelids, nictitans and lacrimal system

Anatomy and function

The eyelids develop from surface ectoderm and join to fuse along the future palpebral fissure. They remain fused until 10-14 days after birth. In the adult cat, the palpebral fissure measures approximately 28 mm in length, although there is some variation with brachycephalic cats tending to have slightly longer eyelids. The eyelids are composed of an outer layer of skin, a supportive tarsal plate, smooth and striated muscle and an inner conjunctival lining (Fig. 1). The upper and lower eyelid of the cat lack true cilia (eyelashes) but, in the upper eyelid, the first row of hairs fulfils much the same function. The tarsal plate of each eyelid contains approximately 30 lipid-secreting meibomian glands whose openings form a distinct groove along the eyelid margin (also referred to as the 'grey line'). The relatively thin, striated orbicularis oculi muscle is closely attached to the overlying skin and completely encircles the palpebral fissure. This muscle is responsible for eyelid closure and is innervated by the palpebral branch of the facial nerve (CN VII). As with most mammals, the upper eyelid of the cat is more mobile than the lower. The main elevator of the upper eyelid is the striated levator palpebrae superioris muscle, which is innervated by the oculomotor nerve (CN III), and the smooth Müller's muscle, which is sympathetically innervated. Lower eyelid depression is performed by the malaris muscle which is innervated by the dorsal buccal branch of the facial nerve. The main function of the eyelids is to protect and maintain the health of the ocular surface. To do this effectively they need to be in close apposition with the cornea and to be able to meet completely during blinking.

The nictitans (syn. nictitating membrane, third eyelid) consists of a T-shaped cartilage covered on both the palpebral and bulbar surfaces with conjunctiva (Fig. 2). The nictitans gland is located at the base of the cartilage and contributes significantly to tear production, producing an estimated 30-50 % of the total aqueous tear volume.

The lacrimal system has both secretory and excretory components (Fig. 3). The secretory component consists of the various glands that contribute to the preocular tear film. The tear film of the cat is approximately 7 μm thick and is made up of three layers.

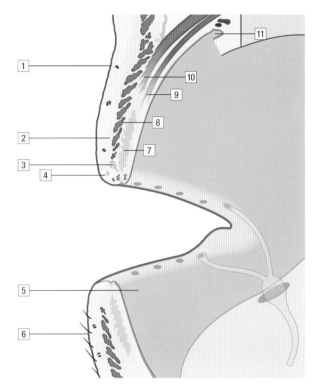

Figure 1. Eyelid anatomy.

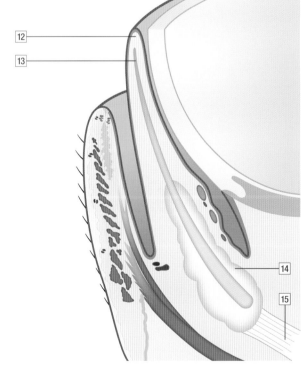

Figure 2. Nictitans anatomy.

1. Upper eyelid
2. Tarsal plate
3. Moll's glands
4. Zeis' glands
5. Palpebral conjunctiva
6. Lower eyelid
7. Meibomian glands
8. Orbicularis oculi muscle
9. Müller's muscle
10. Levator palpebrae superioris muscle
11. Fornix
12. Nictitans
13. Cartilage skeleton
    of the nictitans
14. Nictitans gland
15. Ligamentous attachment of the nictitans gland
16. Superiotemporal lacrimal gland
17. Lacrimal duct
18. Canaliculi
19. Lacrimal sac
20. Nasolacrimal duct

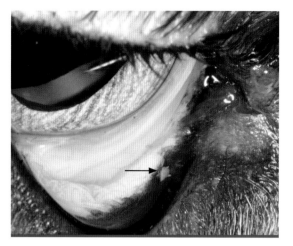

Figure 4. Lacrimal punctum (arrow) in the lower eyelid.

There is an inner mucin layer, which is produced by the conjunctival goblet cells, a middle aqueous layer produced by the lacrimal and nictitans glands and an outer lipid layer produced by the meibomian glands. The tear film is essential for ocular surface health and is evenly distributed by the nictitans and eyelids. The excretory component consists of the upper and lower lacrimal puncta, their respective canaliculi, the lacrimal sac and the nasolacrimal duct (Fig. 3). Tears are channelled towards these puncta which are located just inside the eyelid margin found in the region close to the medial canthus on the inner eyelids (Fig. 4). The tears are then drained via the canaliculi into the rudimentary lacrimal sac which is located within the lacrimal bone. From the sac, tears drain via the nasolacrimal duct into the vestibule of the nasal or oral cavity.

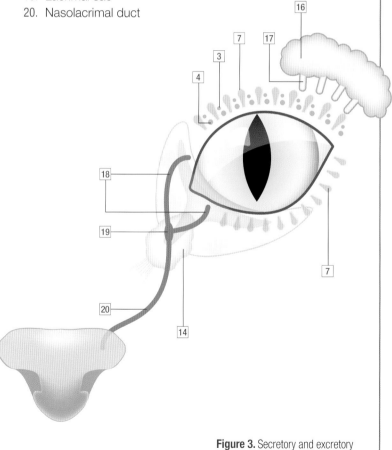

Figure 3. Secretory and excretory components of the nasolacrimal system.

→ Complete blinks are infrequent in the cat, occurring at a rate of 1 to 5 every 5 minutes.

→ The nictitans is T-shaped. The crossbar of the T takes a reverse S-form in the cat.

→ The nictitans gland contributes significantly to tear production, producing an estimated 30-50 % of the total aqueous volume.

Diseases of the eyelids

Ophthalmia neonatorum

Adhesion of the eyelid margins beyond the time of normal eyelid opening (10-14 days in the cat) is termed ankyloblepharon, which may be partial or complete (Figs. 5 and 6). Ophthalmia neonatorum occurs when an infection develops behind the eyelids and, in the cat, feline herpesvirus-1 (FHV-1) is usually implicated. There is swelling behind the eyelids and beads of pus may be seen to emanate from the medial canthus. Treatment involves separating the eyelids with tenotomy scissors, irrigation of the ocular surface and medical treatment for any viral and/or bacterial infection. Complications include corneal ulceration, symblepharon, corneal perforation and endophthalmitis (Fig. 7).

Eyelid coloboma

Eyelid coloboma (agenesis) refers to a congenital absence of all or part of the eyelid. It is usually a bilateral condition and, in cats, most commonly affects the lateral region of the upper eyelid (Figs. 8-10). Any breed of domestic cat may be affected and the condition has also been reported in large cats including leopards and cougars. Eyelid coloboma is often associated with other congenital ocular anomalies such as persistent pupillary membrane (Figs. 8 and 9), retinal dysplasia and choroidal and optic nerve head colobomas. Eyelid colobomas are usually associated with signs of ocular surface disease as a result of trichiasis, inadequate blinking and evaporative tear loss. Close ophthalmic examination is indicated which will often reveal signs of conjunctivitis, corneal vascularisation and current or previous corneal ulceration. Choice of treatment depends on the presence and extent of ocular surface disease and the size and location of the eyelid defect. Very small colobomas may require no treatment at all. However, some benefit from simple ocular lubrication, and a few cases require direct closure of the defect after surgical debridement. For more extensive defects resulting in keratitis, surgical eyelid reconstruction is advocated and several techniques have been described. The Roberts and Bistner procedure and its modifications involve the rotation of a pedicle of skin, orbicularis oculi and tarsus from the lower eyelid to the upper eyelid defect (Roberts and Bistner, 1968) (Fig. 11). Conjunctiva, either mobilised from the upper eyelid or harvested from the nictitans, is then sutured to the inside of the pedicle and eyelid margin and the lower eyelid defect is closed. With this technique there remains a risk of trichiasis as haired skin is left adjacent to the ocular surface with no attempt to create an eyelid margin. The lip-to-lid and Mustardé techniques address this potential problem (Esson, 2001; Whittaker et al., 2010) (Fig. 12).

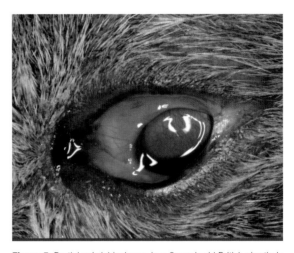

Figure 5. Partial ankyloblepharon in a 9-week-old British shorthair. The eyelids are completely fused laterally (right) and joined by a conjunctival membrane medially (left). Note the protruding nictitans.

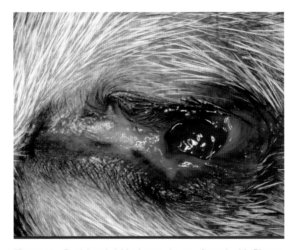

Figure 6. Partial ankyloblepharon in an 8-week-old Birman. The eyelids have only partially opened medially. There was also ophthalmia neonatorum.

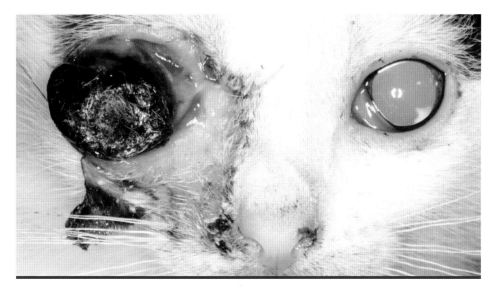

Figure 7. Globe perforation and endophthalmitis in a kitten originally presenting with advanced ophthalmia neonatorum.

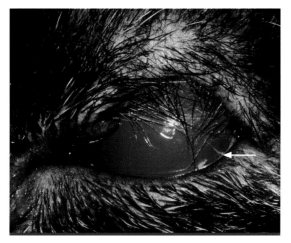

Figure 8. Agenesis of the lateral aspect of the upper eyelid in a 6-week-old Domestic shorthair. Note also the persistent pupillary membrane (arrow).

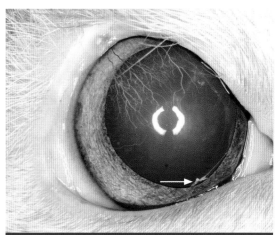

Figure 9. Agenesis of the lateral aspect of the upper eyelid in a 10-week-old Domestic shorthair. Note the persistent pupillary membrane (arrow), trichiasis and associated corneal vascularisation.

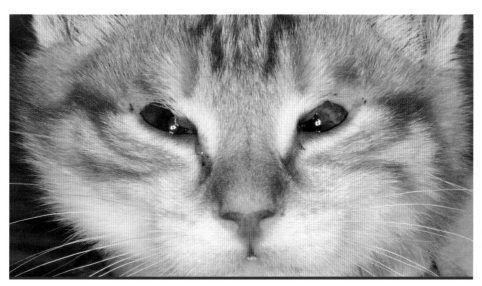

Figure 10. Bilateral agenesis of the lateral aspects of the upper eyelids in an 8-week-old Domestic longhair.

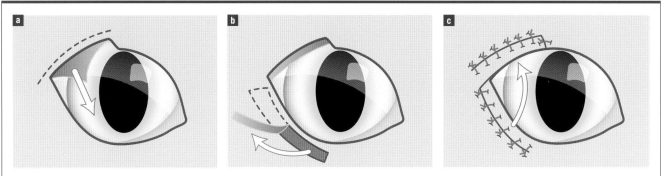

Figure 11. The Roberts and Bistner procedure for repair of eyelid agenesis. a) The recipient region is prepared by dissecting the underlying conjunctiva from the eyelid skin. b) A donor pedicle of skin and underlying orbicularis oculi muscle is harvested from the lower eyelid. c) The pedicle is transposed to the upper eyelid defect and sutured in place.

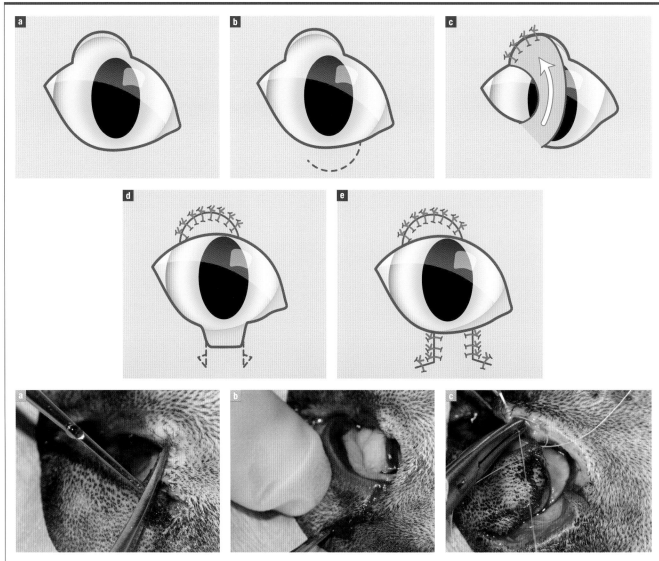

Figure 12. The Mustardé cross-lid technique for repair of eyelid agenesis. a) The margins of the recipient region of the upper eyelid are debrided with sharp dissection. b) A donor graft is constructed from the full thickness of the lower eyelid. c) The graft is transposed to the upper eyelid defect and sutured in place. d) After two weeks, the connection of the graft to the lower eyelid is sectioned. e) The lower eyelid defect is closed with an advancement sliding skin graft ('H-plasty', see Fig. 55).

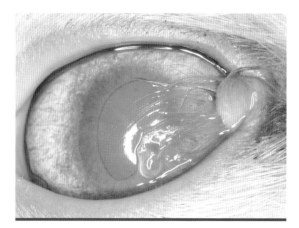

Figure 13. Dermoid in a 16-week-old Birman. The lateral canthus is affected and trichiasis is present.

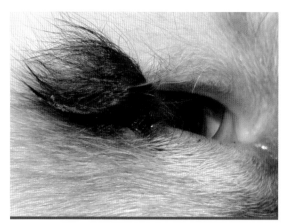

Figure 14. Dermoid in a 12-week-old Persian. The lateral canthus is affected but the numerous pigmented hairs are not contacting the cornea in this case. Courtesy of Rachael Grundon.

Dermoid

Dermoids are congenital, superficial masses which contain many of the elements of haired skin. In cats they are most commonly found in the region of the lateral canthus involving the skin and/or conjunctiva (Figs. 13 and 14). They may also be found in other locations such as on the nictitans (Fig. 15) and may also involve the cornea. Dermoids are often associated with trichiasis and, if this is accompanied with ocular surface irritation, then treatment is indicated. Treatment usually involves surgical excision, and this is curative. However, if trichiasis is mild, topical ocular lubrication could be used.

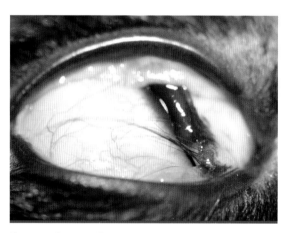

Figure 15. Dermoid affecting the anterior nictitans in this 12-week-old Domestic shorthair.

Distichiasis and ectopic cilia

Distichiasis occurs when single or multiple hairs arise from the eyelid margin, usually from the meibomian gland openings (Fig. 16). Distichiasis is a very uncommon finding in the cat but may be associated with ocular surface irritation, potentially leading to corneal ulceration and sequestrum (Fig. 17). If irritation is present, then removal of these abnormal hairs is indicated. Cryosurgery and electrolysis are the techniques of choice, although successful treatment with electrocautery has also been reported (Reinstein et al., 2011). An ectopic cilium occurs when a hair grows out of the palpebral conjunctiva. This is even rarer in the cat and treatment involves surgical excision of the hair and its follicle. Figure 18 illustrates the differences between trichiasis, distichiasis and ectopic cilium.

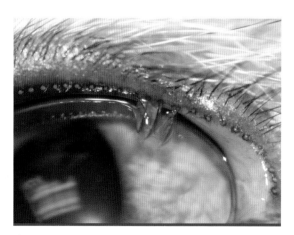

Figure 16. Distichiasis in a 6-year-old Domestic shorthair. The abnormal cilia can be seen emanating from the meibomian gland openings of the upper eyelid margin. They are causing ocular surface irritation and removal via electrolysis was later performed.

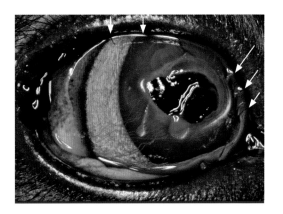

Figure 17. Distichiasis (arrows) and corneal sequestrum in a 2-year-old Burmese. The sequestrum developed following chronic ulceration thought to be caused by mechanical irritation from the abnormal hairs.

Examination tip

Application of topical anaesthetic will help determine the extent of the spastic component of the entropion and aid in surgical planning.

Surgery tip

When performing a Hotz-Celsus procedure in a cat, it is best to aim for slight over-correction of the entropion to prevent recurrence.

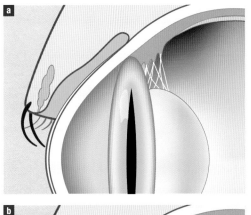

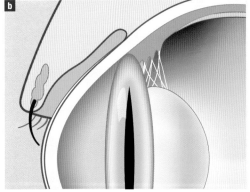

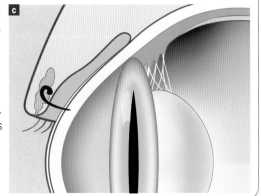

Figure 18.
a) Trichiasis – hairs arising from a normal location are inappropriately contacting the cornea.
b) Distichiasis – a hair is emerging from the meibomian gland opening.
c) Ectopic cilium – a hair is arising in the meibomian gland and emerging through the palpebral conjunctiva.

Entropion

Entropion describes inversion of an eyelid or part of it, such that skin and/or hairs come into contact with the ocular surface (Figs. 19-24). Primary anatomical entropion is most common in the Persian and other brachycephalic breeds where the medial aspect of the lower eyelids is most often affected. Older cats may develop entropion associated with loss of retrobulbar fat and resultant enophthalmos. Entropion may also occur as a blepharospastic response to ocular surface irritation. If the initial cause of the eyelid spasm is not recognised and successfully treated, then the entropion can become permanent requiring corrective surgery. A study of 50 cats with entropion found that 52 % were older cats with loss of orbital tissue volume, 32 % were young with preexisting irritative ocular surface conditions, 10 % were Persians and 6 % were young entire male Maine Coons (Williams and Kim, 2009). Most cases of feline entropion can be successfully treated with a modified Hotz-Celsus procedure (Figs. 25 and 26), although eyelid shortening is occasionally required in addition (White et al., 2012) (Fig. 27).

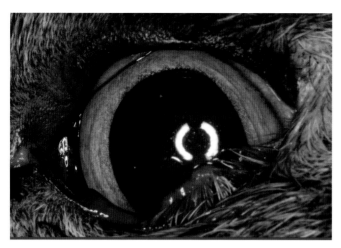

Figure 19. Primary entropion affecting the lateral aspect of the lower eyelid in a 1-year-old British Blue.

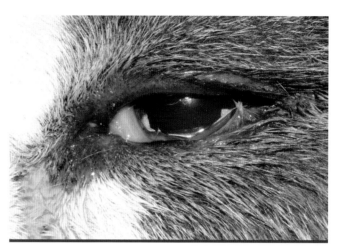

Figure 20. Entropion of the lower eyelid in an 8-year-old cat. The ocular surface is irritated causing increased lacrimation, epiphora and mild dermatitis in the region of the medial canthus.

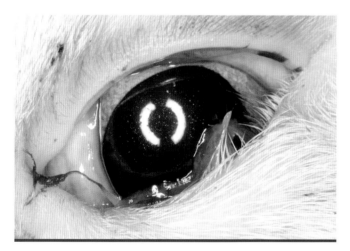

Figure 21. Entropion of the lower eyelid in an 18-month-old Maine Coon.

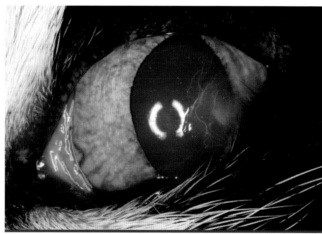

Figure 22. Entropion of the lower eyelid in the left eye of an 11-year-old Domestic shorthair. There is corneal vascularisation as a result of the chronic irritation.

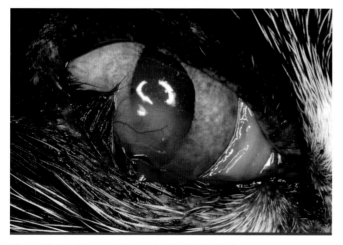

Figure 23. The right eye of the cat in Fig. 22. Similar findings are present. The cause of the entropion of both eyes was thought to be age-related loss of retrobulbar adipose tissue.

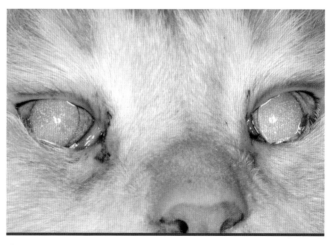

Figure 24. Bilateral primary entropion in a 1-year-old entire male Maine Coon.

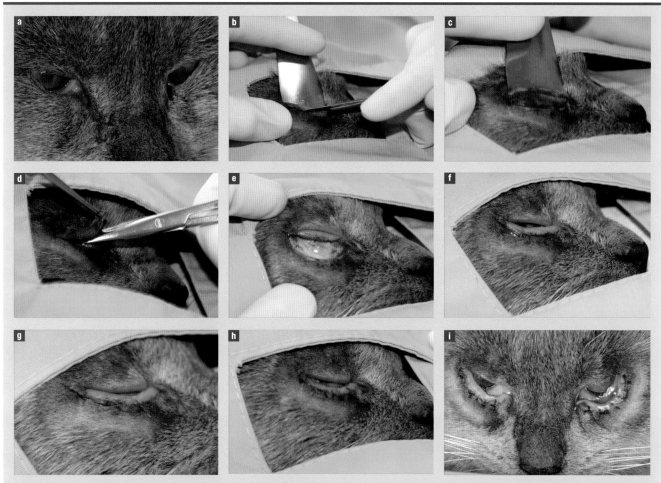

Figure 25. Hotz-Celsus procedure for entropion correction. a) Bilateral entropion and secondary keratitis in a 4-year-old entire male Domestic shorthair. b) The skin and orbicularis oculi muscle are incised using a No. 15 scalpel blade 1-2 mm from the eyelid margin, and parallel to it. A lid plate assists in stabilising the skin. c) An elliptical shape is delineated, the width determined by the degree of entropion present. d) The strip of skin and muscle are excised with a tenotomy scissors. e) The surgical wound is ready for repair. f) Using absorbable 6/0 suture material, the first suture is placed centrally. g) Because the wound margins are of unequal length, it is advisable to use the 'rule of bisection', so that each suture bisects the remaining surgical wound. h) The surgical wound is sutured along its length, with sutures 2-3 mm apart. i) Immediate postoperative appearance – it is normal to have an appearance of slight over-correction at this stage.

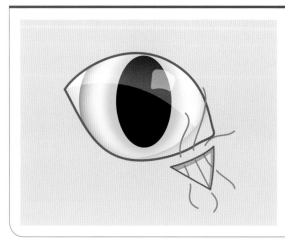

Figure 26. Modification of Hotz-Celsus technique for brachycephalic cats with entropion at the medial aspect of the lower eyelid. A triangular-shaped section of skin-orbicularis oculi muscle is excised. Care must be taken not to damage the deeper nasolacrimal duct. This procedure corrects entropion and positions the lower lacrimal punctum more ideally.

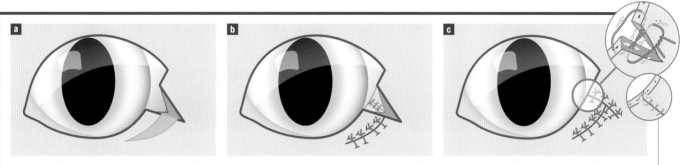

Figure 27. Entropion correction when the eyelid is over-long (e.g. in the Maine Coon), combining the Hotz-Celsus procedure with lateral eyelid wedge resection. a) An elliptical section of skin/orbicularis oculi muscle is removed, as in Fig. 25. A full thickness wedge resection is removed laterally, superimposing the Hotz-Celsus excision. b) 6/0 nonabsorbable suture material is used for closure. The Hotz-Celsus surgical wound is repaired with simple interrupted sutures. The wedge resection is repaired with a deep layer of continuous sutures. c) The eyelid margin is realigned with a figure-of-eight suture, and the remaining skin closed with simple interrupted sutures.

Blepharitis

Blepharitis (inflammation of the eyelids) may result from infectious, immune-mediated and allergic causes. Infectious causes are most common and include viral, bacterial, fungal and parasitic conditions. The eyelids are rarely affected in isolation but as part of a more generalised dermatosis of the facial skin.

Viral

Cowpox infection is fairly uncommon but usually begins by affecting the face and paws before spreading to the rest of the body. Kittens and immuno-compromised animals are most commonly affected. There is no specific treatment and most animals will recover with supportive therapy alone.

FHV-1, as well as being an important cause of feline ocular surface disease, occasionally affects the facial skin including the eyelids (Figs. 28a and b, and Fig. 29). Diagnosis is most commonly achieved by PCR or virus isolation, although typical inclusion bodies may be seen on histopathological examination of skin biopsies. Infection with FHV-1 is usually self-limiting but treatment with systemic antivirals (e.g. famciclovir) is often very effective when skin involvement is present.

→ Dermatitis caused by FHV-1 infection requires treatment with systemic antivirals such as oral famciclovir.

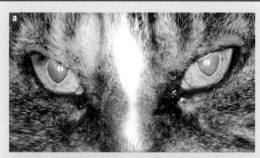
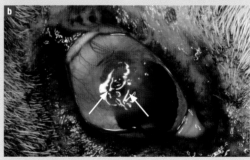

Figure 28. a) Blepharitis associated with FHV-1 infection. b) Close-up photograph of the right eye. A sequestrum is also present in the dorsolateral quadrant of the right cornea (arrows).

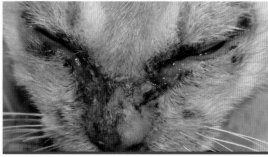

Figure 29. Facial dermatitis caused by FHV-1 infection in a 6-month-old Domestic shorthair. Courtesy of Filippo De Bellis.

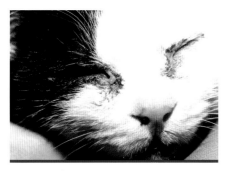

Figure 30. Six-month-old Domestic shorthair with bilateral bacterial blepharitis. Cytology revealed degenerate neutrophils and phagocytosed cocci. Complete resolution of clinical signs occurred following treatment with topical 0.5 % chloramphenicol and oral amoxycillin/clavulanate for 21 days. Courtesy of Prof Dr Jan Declercq.

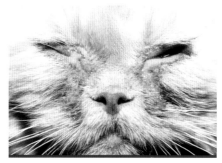

Figure 31. Four-year old Domestic shorthair with bilateral bacterial blepharitis. Cytology revealed degenerate neutrophils and phagocytosed cocci. Complete resolution of clinical signs occurred following treatment with topical 0.5 % chloramphenicol and oral amoxycillin/clavulanate for 21 days. Courtesy of Prof Dr Jan Declercq.

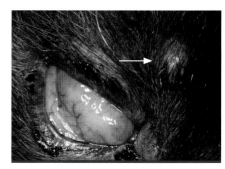

Figure 32. Mycobacterial blepharitis in a 7-year-old Domestic shorthair. The nictitans gland is thickened and protruding. Multiple skin nodules were present, the arrow points to one on the upper eyelid.

Bacterial

Bacterial infections of the eyelids usually result from cat bites and scratches (Figs. 30 and 31). Treatment involves warm compresses, drainage of large abscesses and systemic broad spectrum antibiotic therapy. Culture and susceptibility testing should be performed if there is not a prompt response to therapy. Mycobacterial blepharitis is uncommon but occasionally encountered (Fig. 32). Diagnosis is usually made on histopathological examination of biopsy specimens as culture poses problems owing to the risk of potential zoonosis.

Fungal

Feline dermatophytosis commonly affects the face and eyelids, and *Microsporum canis* is implicated most commonly (Fig. 33). Clinical signs include areas of alopecia and folliculitis, and definitive diagnosis is usually made by fungal culture. For systemic therapy, itraconazole is the drug of choice and recommended topical treatments include enilconazole or miconazole solutions (Frymus et al., 2013).

Parasitic

Feline demodecosis is uncommon but may be caused by infection with *Demodex cati*, *Demodex gatoi* and a third unnamed but morphologically distinct species of *Demodex* (Moriello et al., 2013). Localised demodecosis involving the eyelids alone is likely to be self-limiting. Treatment of choice of generalised demodecosis is 2 %

lime sulphur or amitraz dips, taking care not to allow the solution to come into contact with the globes.

Feline scabies, caused by *Notoedres cati*, is also very uncommon, and is also usually diagnosed by skin scrapes. Extra-label treatment with topical selamectin is reported to be effective (Itoh et al., 2004).

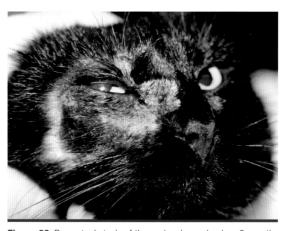

Figure 33. Dermatophytosis of the periocular region in a 6-month-old Domestic shorthair. *Microsporum canis* was cultured. Courtesy of Rachael Grundon.

➜ Care should be taken when using topical solutions around the eye; it is preferable to use systemic medication for treatment of fungal blepharitis.

Leishmaniasis is much less common in cats than in dogs, but cases are sporadically reported world-wide. As with dogs, disease is caused by infection with *Leishmania infantum,* with sandflies acting as vectors. Nodular or ulcerative skin lesions are the most frequent clinical manifestation typically affecting the head and neck. Diagnosis may be achieved by cytological examination of fine needle aspirates, PCR and serology. Treatment with allopurinol may be effective (Pennisi et al., 2013).

Immune-mediated

Immune-mediated dermatoses are fairly uncommon in cats and, in one retrospective study, accounted for only 5.5 % of all feline dermatoses (Scott et al., 2013). In this study, cutaneous adverse drug reaction (Fig. 34) was the most common cause of immune-mediated skin disease followed by pemphigus foliaceus (Figs. 35 and 36) and alopecia areata. Erythema multiforme (Fig. 37), toxic epidermal necrolysis (Fig. 38) and other rare immune-mediated dermatoses (Fig. 39) are also occasionally reported. For all of these conditions, the periocular region is affected only as part of a more

➜ Leishmaniasis is much less common in cats than in dogs, but cases are sporadically reported world-wide.

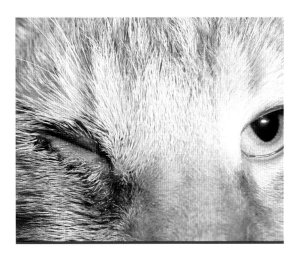

Figure 34. Blepharitis of the right eye as a result of an adverse reaction to topical tetracycline.

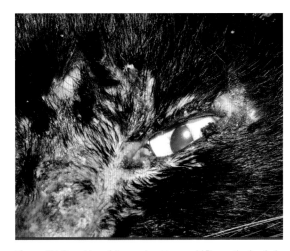

Figure 35. Pemphigus foliaceus in a 5-year-old Domestic shorthair.

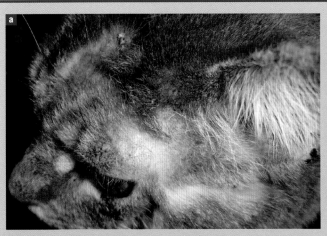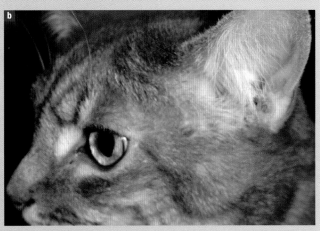

Figure 36. a) Pemphigus foliaceus affecting the eyelids, nasal planum, forehead and ear tips of a 7-year-old Domestic shorthair. b) There was a good response to systemic immunosuppressive corticosteroid treatment. Courtesy of Jane Coatesworth.

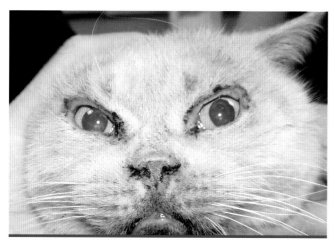

Figure 37. Erythema multiforme with opportunistic infection with *Malassezia* sp. in a 9-year-old Domestic shorthair. Courtesy of Filippo De Bellis.

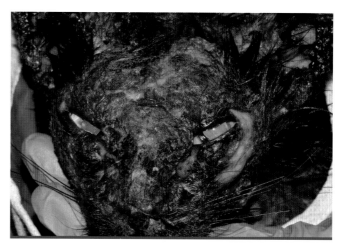

Figure 38. Toxic epidermal necrolysis in a 5-year-old Domestic shorthair, with epidermal detachment on the face as well as over other regions of the body.

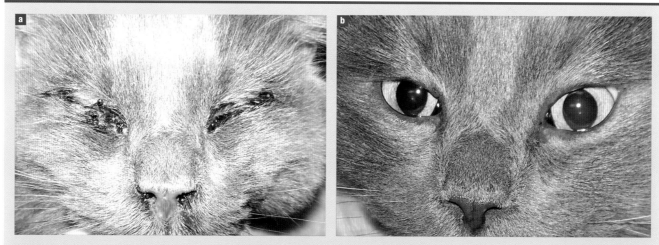

Figure 39. a) Immune-mediated ulcerative blepharitis in a 4-year-old British Blue. The mucocutaneous junctions of the nares are also affected. b) A definitive diagnosis was not achieved but the cat made a full recovery following a course of systemic immunosuppressive corticosteroids. Courtesy of Filippo De Bellis.

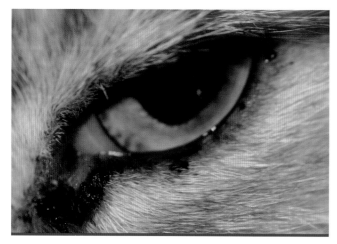

Figure 40. Medial canthal erosion in a 6-year-old Domestic shorthair.

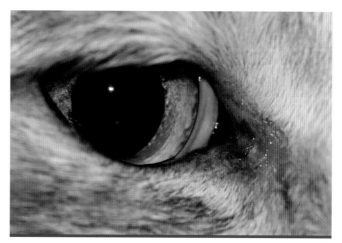

Figure 41. Medial canthal erosion in a 5-year-old Domestic shorthair.

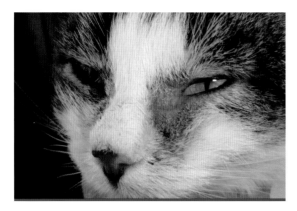

Figure 42. Atopic dermatitis with secondary *Malassezia* sp. infection in a 3-year-old Domestic shorthair. Courtesy of Jane Coatesworth.

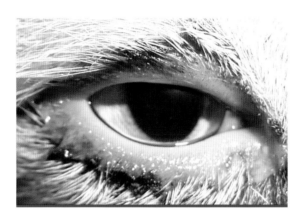

Figure 43. Blepharitis thought to be the result of a food allergy.

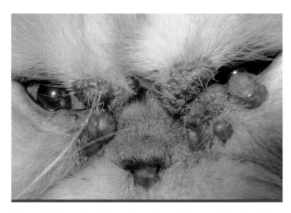

Figure 44. Apocrine hidrocystomas in a 10-year-old Persian. Courtesy of Filip Nachtegaele.

→ Eyelid neoplasms affect cats less commonly than dogs but tend to be more malignant.

generalised dermatosis, and opportunistic bacterial and yeast infections are common. The reader is directed to current dermatology texts for details of treatment of these immune-mediated dermatoses. Medial canthal erosion is more common in dogs than in cats but is occasionally encountered. The skin of the medial canthal region becomes inflamed and ulcerates (Figs. 40 and 41). When there is no identifiable cause (e.g. FHV-1, nasolacrimal obstruction, breed-related epiphora), an immune-mediated aetiology is suspected. Treatment with topical dexamethasone ophthalmic ointment is usually effective.

Allergic

Atopic dermatitis (Fig. 42), flea-bite allergy and food allergy (Fig. 43) are the most common allergic dermatoses in cats and the eyelid skin may be affected as part of more generalised disease (Scott et al., 2013). Definitive diagnosis and treatment of allergic dermatoses can be challenging and consultation with a dermatologist is advised.

Apocrine hidrocystomas

Sometimes referred to as cystic adenomas, apocrine hidrocystomas are smooth, round cystic lesions affecting the eyelids and associated skin (Fig. 44). They may be single or multiple and the Persian is predisposed. They were originally considered to be benign neoplasms but current research suggests that the lesions are proliferative rather than truly neoplastic (Giudice et al., 2009). Treatment can be problematic but options include drainage, surgical excision and chemical ablation with trichloroacetic acid (Yang et al., 2007).

Eyelid neoplasia

Squamous cell carcinoma is the most frequently encountered neoplasm in cats. Those with nonpigmented eyelids and white periocular hair are predisposed, as chronic exposure to UV light (more specifically, UVB radiation) has been identified as the principle cause (Newkirk and Rohback, 2009; Murphy, 2013). The neoplasm appears as a raised or ulcerative lesion on the eyelid skin and may or may not affect the eyelid margin initially (Figs. 45 and 46a). It is a locally aggressive tumour and metastasis occurs relatively late

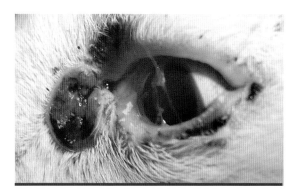

Figure 45. Squamous cell carcinoma affecting the medial canthus in an 8-year-old Domestic shorthair. Cats with nonpigmented eyelids and white periocular hair are predisposed.

in the disease. Diagnosis is best achieved by biopsy and histopathological examination; however, cytology of impression smears can also be useful. Treatment of choice is surgical excision, but as complete excision requires margins of up to 5 mm, a blepharoplastic procedure is required to treat the resultant defect (Murphy, 2013). Options include the lip-to-lid flap and various rotational and advancement skin flaps (Schmidt et al., 2005; Hunt, 2006). If adequate margins are not achieved, then recurrence is likely (Fig. 47). An alternative or adjunct to surgical excision is beta radiation with strontium-90 using an ophthalmic applicator designed for human use (Murphy, 2013). When employed as sole therapy, it is reserved for superficial lesions no deeper than 3 mm. This treatment has the advantages of sparing local tissue and being repeatable.

Mast cell tumours are probably the next most common neoplasm to affect the eyelids. Their appearance can vary from diffuse eyelid swellings to well-circumscribed ulcerative lesions (Figs. 48 and 49). Periocular feline mast cell tumours are usually histologically benign and excision is usually curative with a low risk of recurrence (Montgomery et al., 2010).

Surgery tip

The most important suture in any eyelid margin repair is the figure-of-eight suture (Fig. 27c). Take time to get this right - gentle but accurate apposition is essential to maintain normal function.

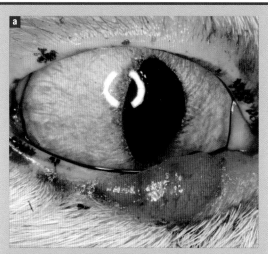

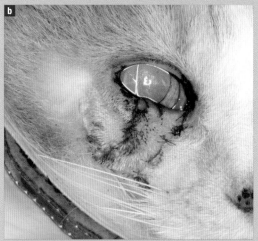

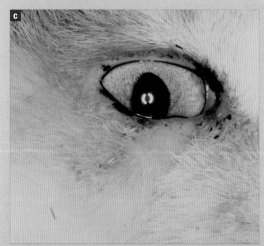

Figure 46. a) Squamous cell carcinoma affecting the nonpigmented lower eyelid of this white-haired cat. b) Immediate postoperative photograph. The tumour has been excised and the resultant eyelid defect repaired using a lip-to-lid transposition graft. c) One month following surgery. The surgical site has healed well (see Fig. 56 for illustration of the procedure).

Eyelid neoplasms in cats

(in order of decreasing frequency)

→ Squamous cell carcinoma

→ Mast cell tumour

→ Basal cell carcinoma

→ Haemangiosarcoma

→ Adenocarcinoma

→ Fibrosarcoma

→ Peripheral nerve sheath tumour

→ Lymphoma

Other tumour types reported to affect the feline eyelid margin include basal cell carcinoma, haemangiosarcoma (Fig. 50), adenocarcinoma, fibrosarcoma (Fig. 51), peripheral nerve sheath tumour and lymphoma (Figs. 52 and 53). Owing to the potential for malignancy, histopathological examination of incisional biopsy specimens is prudent to help treatment planning and assess the need for further investigations. For eyelid masses involving one third or less of the length of the eyelid and for when relatively small margins are required, treatment via excision and direct closure may be performed (Figs. 54-56).

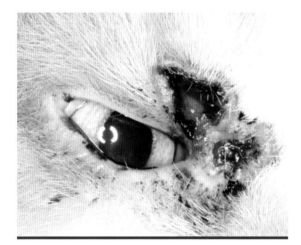

Figure 47. Squamous cell carcinoma has recurred in this cat following failure to remove adequate margins during the initial surgical excision of the neoplasm.

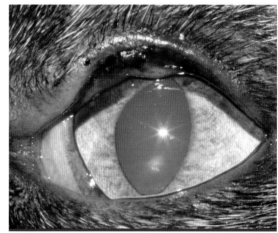

Figure 48. Mast cell tumour affecting the upper eyelid of an 8-year-old Siamese. The eyelid is diffusely thickened and the palpebral conjunctiva is hyperaemic.

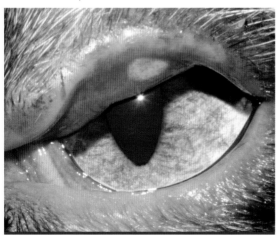

Figure 49. Mast cell tumour affecting the upper eyelid of a 7-year-old Domestic shorthair. In this case, the tumour is relatively nodular.

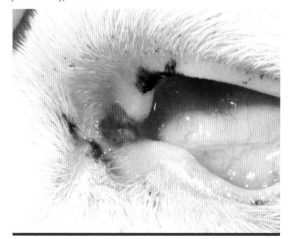

Figure 50. Haemangiosarcoma affecting the medial canthus in a 12-year-old Domestic shorthair.

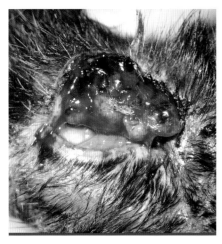

Figure 51. Fibrosarcoma affecting the upper eyelid of a 13-year-old Domestic shorthair.

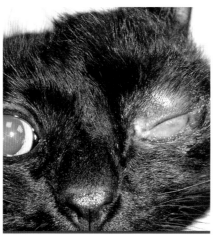

Figure 52. Cutaneous lymphoma extensively affecting the upper and lower eyelids, as well as the conjunctiva and nictitans in a 10-year-old Domestic shorthair.

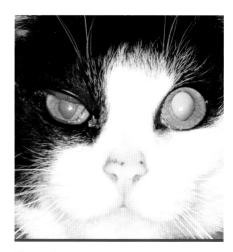

Figure 53. Lymphoma affecting the upper right eyelid in an FeLV-positive 3-year-old Domestic shorthair.

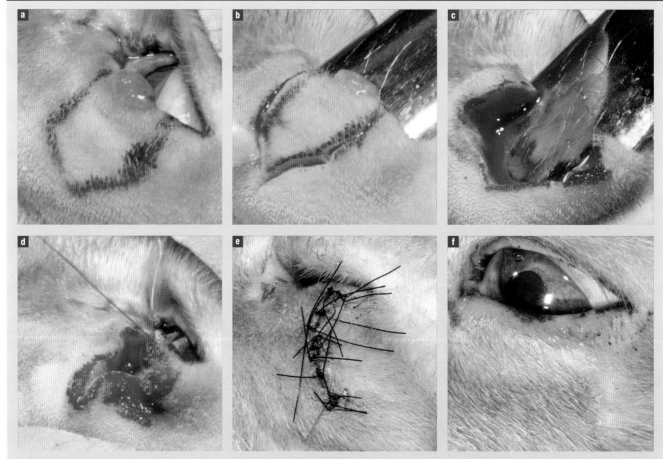

Figure 54. Eyelid mass removal. a) A surgical pen is used to delineate the area of excision including at least a 5 mm margin. An inverted house-shaped excision is planned to facilitate accurate closure of the defect. b) A No. 15 scalpel blade has been used to incise the skin using a lid plate for support. c) Full thickness excision has been completed using a tenotomy scissors. d) Closure begins with placement of a figure-of-eight suture to exactly appose the eyelid margin using 6/0 absorbable suture. e) The wound is closed in two layers. The tarsoconjunctival layer is closed with a 6/0 simple continuous absorbable suture. The skin is apposed using 4/0 simple interrupted nonabsorbable sutures. f) Appearance two weeks after suture removal.

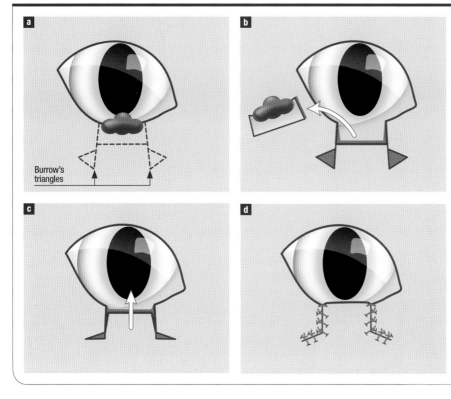

Figure 55. Advancement sliding skin graft ('H-plasty'). a) After full-thickness excision of the eyelid neoplasm, two slightly diverging vertical skin incisions are continued which should be at least twice as long as the defect, and Burrow's triangles (arrows) are created. b) Burrow's triangles are excised at the base of both of the skin incisions in order to facilitate sliding of the skin graft. c) The flap is created by mobilising the skin after subcutaneous dissection, and slid just beyond the eyelid margin to fill the defect. d) The skin flap is sutured to the eyelid margins, and then simple interrupted sutures are used to repair the skin.

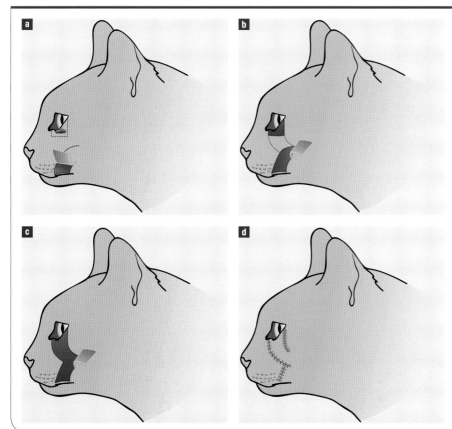

Figure 56. Mucocutaneous flap from lip to lower eyelid ('lip-to-lid' transposition graft). a) After full-thickness excision of the lower eyelid neoplasm, a full-thickness pedicle is dissected from the caudal aspect of the lip. b) Releasing skin incisions are made ventral to the lower eyelid defect to connect the two areas. c) The incised skin between the eyelid defect and the lip pedicle is excised, creating one continuous defect. The flap is dissected free and rotated into the defect. d) The pedicle is secured at the eyelid margins and then sutured into the skin defect in two layers. The donor site at the lip is also sutured (see Fig. 46 for clinical photographs).

The tarsorrhaphy

A tarsorrhaphy is the procedure in which the upper and lower eyelids are sutured together. Temporary tarsorrhaphies are occasionally used to protect the ocular surface and globe, for example following surgical repair of corneal ulceration. In this situation, the tarsorrhaphy is usually only partial, allowing for the continued application of topical therapy. Complete tarsorrhaphy is useful in the management of proptosis in which case sutures are usually left in place for a minimum of 14 days. To perform the tarsorrhaphy, sutures are passed at the level of or just anterior to the meibomian gland openings in the eyelid margin to reduce the risk of corneal irritation (Fig. 57). Either a simple interrupted or a horizontal mattress suture pattern may be employed. In the latter case, stents can be used to reduce the risk of damage to the eyelid skin.

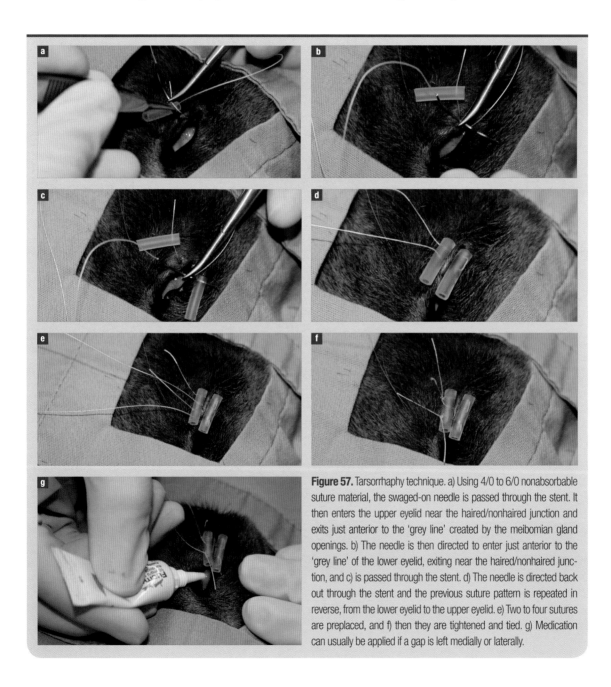

Figure 57. Tarsorrhaphy technique. a) Using 4/0 to 6/0 nonabsorbable suture material, the swaged-on needle is passed through the stent. It then enters the upper eyelid near the haired/nonhaired junction and exits just anterior to the 'grey line' created by the meibomian gland openings. b) The needle is then directed to enter just anterior to the 'grey line' of the lower eyelid, exiting near the haired/nonhaired junction, and c) is passed through the stent. d) The needle is directed back out through the stent and the previous suture pattern is repeated in reverse, from the lower eyelid to the upper eyelid. e) Two to four sutures are preplaced, and f) then they are tightened and tied. g) Medication can usually be applied if a gap is left medially or laterally.

Diseases of the nictitans

Nictitans protrusion

Protrusion of the nictitans is fairly common in cats and often occurs in conjunction with generalised systemic illness, in which case it tends to be bilateral and is occasionally referred to as Haw's syndrome (Fig. 58). Systemic conditions associated with bilateral protrusion of the nictitans include chronic diarrhoea, dysautonomia and tetanus. Unilateral protrusion may occur as a result of enophthalmos in response to anterior segment pain (Fig. 59), as part of Horner's syndrome (Fig. 60) or as a result of orbital disease (Fig. 61). The nictitans may also become fixed in a protruded position as a result of symblepharon formation (Fig. 62).

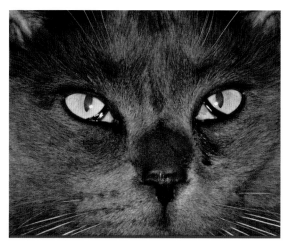

Figure 58. Bilateral protrusion of the nictitans in a cat with diarrhoea (Haw's syndrome).

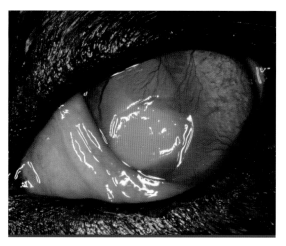

Figure 59. Unilateral protrusion of the nictitans in response to the pain caused by corneal ulceration.

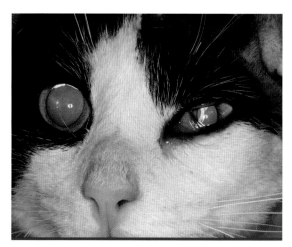

Figure 60. Protrusion of the nictitans of the left eye in a cat with Horner's syndrome. This eye also demonstrates ptosis and pupillary miosis. The cause of the Horner's syndrome was iatrogenic damage to sympathetic fibres during middle ear surgery to remove an inflammatory polyp.

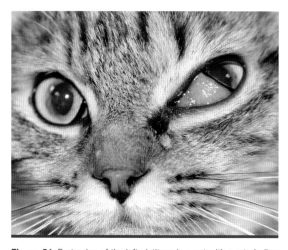

Figure 61. Protrusion of the left nictitans in a cat with a retrobulbar abscess.

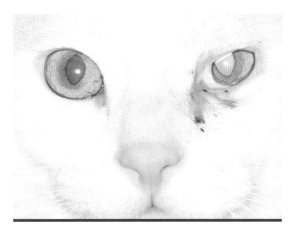

Figure 62. The nictitans of the left eye is fixed in this protruded state as a result of symblepharon formation.

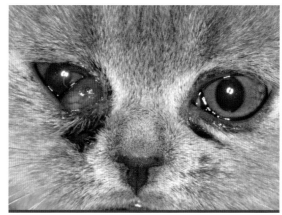

Figure 63. Prolapse of the nicitans gland ('cherry eye') in a 10-week-old British shorthair.

Prolapse of the nictitans gland

Nictitans gland prolapse is far less common in cats than in dogs but is occasionally encountered, being most common in the Burmese (Fig. 63). The condition may be unilateral or bilateral, and may occur in isolation or in conjunction with eversion of the nictitans cartilage. Unless neoplasia is present, prolapsed glands should never be excised owing to their contribution to tear production. Surgical replacement of the gland with the Morgan pocket technique is usually very effective in this species (Chahory et al., 2004).

Nictitans cartilage eversion

Eversion of the nictitans cartilage is fairly rare in the cat and is usually unilateral (Fig. 64). The condition can be successfully treated by excision of the kinked portion of the cartilage via an incision in the bulbar conjunctiva of the nictitans (Williams et al., 2012).

Neoplasia of the nictitans

Neoplasms uncommonly affect the feline nictitans but potential tumours include haemangioma, haemangiosarcoma, melanoma, fibrosarcoma, lymphoma and adenocarcinoma. Depending on the type of neoplasm and its extent, treatment usually involves surgical excision of the mass or of the entire nictitans.

The nictitans flap

The nictitans flap is occasionally useful in the management of corneal ulceration and bullous keratopathy.

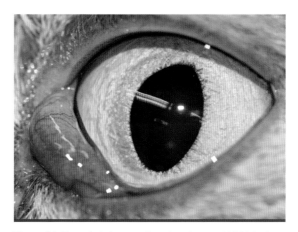

Figure 64. Everted nictitans cartilage in a 2-year-old British shorthair. Courtesy of Filip Nachtegaele.

It can offer comfort and a level of support for the healing cornea. It is not, however, a suitable alternative for direct repair of deep corneal ulceration in which more sophisticated grafting techniques are required. Disadvantages of the flap include the fact that examination of the cornea is precluded while it is in place and the flap offers no vascular supply or direct tectonic support to areas of deep ulceration. To perform the flap, two or three horizontal mattress sutures are placed through the conjunctiva on the anterior aspect of the nictitans and sutured to the dorsolateral bulbar conjunctiva or eyelid. Figure 65 (a-f) illustrates the eyelid method, while Figure 65 (g-m) illustrates episcleral fixation. Nictitans flaps are usually left in place for at least 10-14 days and topical ophthalmic solutions can still be applied during this period.

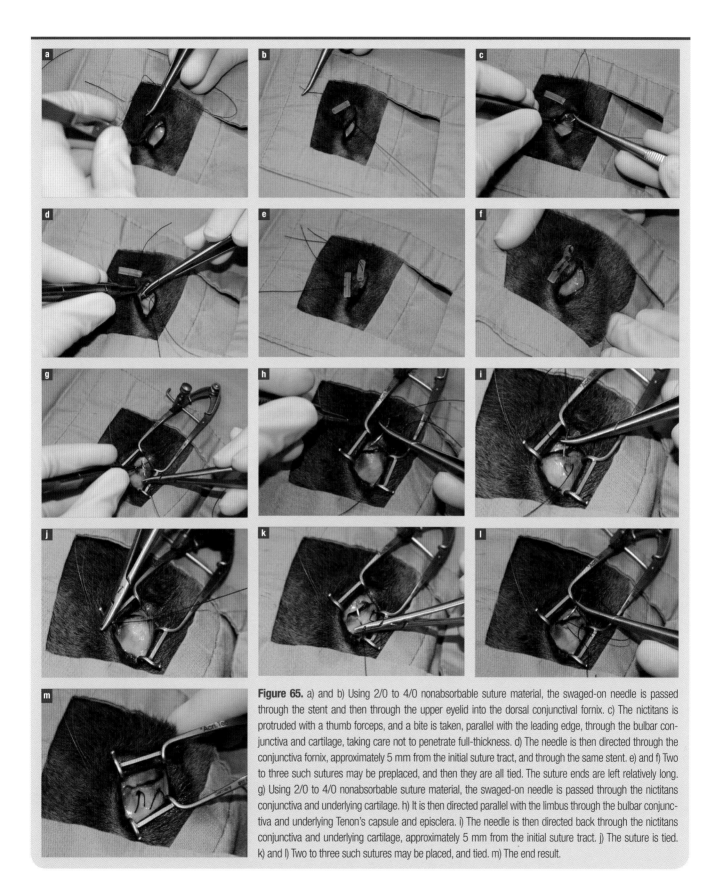

Figure 65. a) and b) Using 2/0 to 4/0 nonabsorbable suture material, the swaged-on needle is passed through the stent and then through the upper eyelid into the dorsal conjunctival fornix. c) The nictitans is protruded with a thumb forceps, and a bite is taken, parallel with the leading edge, through the bulbar conjunctiva and cartilage, taking care not to penetrate full-thickness. d) The needle is then directed through the conjunctiva fornix, approximately 5 mm from the initial suture tract, and through the same stent. e) and f) Two to three such sutures may be preplaced, and then they are all tied. The suture ends are left relatively long. g) Using 2/0 to 4/0 nonabsorbable suture material, the swaged-on needle is passed through the nictitans conjunctiva and underlying cartilage. h) It is then directed parallel with the limbus through the bulbar conjunctiva and underlying Tenon's capsule and episclera. i) The needle is then directed back through the nictitans conjunctiva and underlying cartilage, approximately 5 mm from the initial suture tract. j) The suture is tied. k) and l) Two to three such sutures may be placed, and tied. m) The end result.

Diseases of the nasolacrimal system

Epiphora

Epiphora is the most common feline nasolacrimal abnormality and is often breed-related. Computed tomography has revealed that brachycephalia is associated with dorsal displacement of the facial bones and upper canine teeth (Schlueter et al., 2009). This orientation results in the nasolacrimal duct adopting a steep V-shaped course which is thought to compromise its function in tear drainage (Fig. 66).

Nasolacrimal duct obstructions are quite unusual in cats but may be congenital in origin or associated with the presence of foreign bodies or dacryocystitis. The latter is most commonly associated with FHV-1 infection (Fig. 67). A single case report documents obstruction caused by a tooth root abscess with resultant epiphora and mucopurulent discharge (Anthony et al., 2010).

Congenital abnormalities of the nasolacrimal apparatus are rare in cats but include imperforate lacrimal puncta (Fig. 68) and lacrimal canalicular atresia (Fig. 69). Symblepharon is a common cause of punctal occlusion (Fig. 70). An imperforate punctum is usually straightforward to treat if the accompanying canaliculus is properly developed. Treatment involves resection of the conjunctiva overlying the lacrimal canaliculus (Fig. 71). There are more complex surgical procedures to create alternative drainage if epiphora remains and is problematic. These involve creating a new opening in the conjunctival sac and creating a drainage pathway to the nasal cavity (conjunctivorhinostomy), maxillary sinus (conjunctivosinusotomy) or mouth (conjunctivobuccostomy).

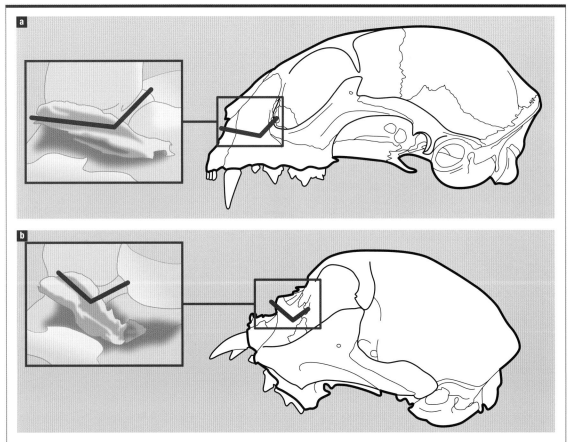

Figure 66. a) Nasolacrimal system in a mesocephalic cat. b) Nasolacrimal system in a brachycephalic cat. The facial bones and upper canine teeth are displaced dorsally leading to almost horizontally rotated upper canine teeth. This results in a steeply oriented nasolacrimal duct and potentially inefficient tear drainage.

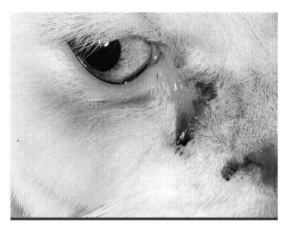

Figure 67. Epiphora of the right eye as a result of dacryocystitis in a 1-year-old Domestic shorthair. Note the mucopurulent discharge at the ipsilateral naris.

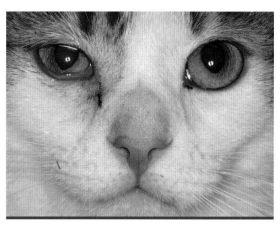

Figure 68. Imperforate upper and lower puncta of the right eye a 6-month-old Domestic shorthair. Note that, following application of fluorescein dye to each eye, the dye does not appear at the right naris (negative Jones test) but does at the left (positive Jones test).

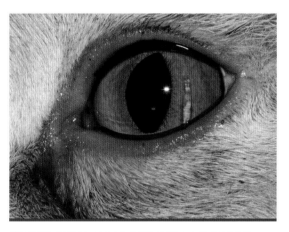

Figure 69. Epiphora as a result of lacrimal canalicular atresia.

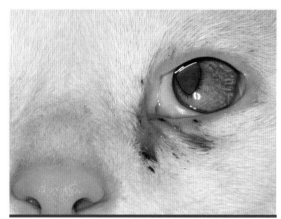

Figure 70. Epiphora as a result of symblepharon, with resulting occlusion of the nasolacrimal punctum and a permanently protruding nictitans.

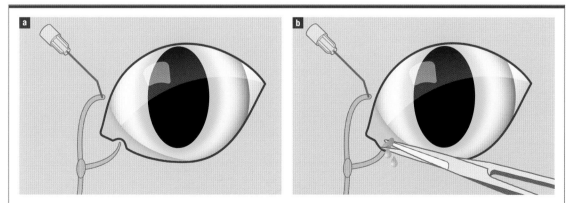

Figure 71. Surgery for imperforate lacrimal punctum. a) In the case of an imperforate lower punctum, the upper punctum is cannulated and gently but firmly flushed with sterile saline. The conjunctiva usually bulges in the region where the lower punctum should be. b) The conjunctiva adjacent to the bulge is steadied with a fine-toothed forceps, and using a sharp small tenotomy or Westcott's scissors, the conjunctiva over the bulge is excised. The canaliculus is again flushed via the upper punctum confirming patency, and several days of topical steroid-antibiotic drops are prescribed (corticosteroids may reduce the chance of new conjunctiva growing over the newly formed punctum).

Keratoconjunctivitis sicca

Keratoconjunctivitis sicca (KCS) is a relatively uncommon, but significant, condition in the cat. It occurs as a result of an inadequate production of the aqueous component of the tear film. Most cases of feline KCS occur secondary to blepharoconjunctivitis associated with FHV-1 infection. Neurogenic KCS is occasionally encountered and occurs as a result of damage to the parasympathetic supply to the lacrimal glands, for example following orbital trauma or in dysautonomia. Anaesthetic and analgesic agents are commonly associated with reduction in tear production in a number of species. In cats specifically, systemic atropine sulphate used alone or in combination with ketamine hydrochloride and acetylpromazine maleate has been shown to transiently reduce tear production (Arnett et al., 1984). Topical ophthalmic agents may also have a negative effect with 1 % tropicamide significantly reducing tear production for up to 4 hours in normal cats (Margadant et al., 2003). Clinical signs include ocular discharge, a lacklustre cornea, conjunctival hyperaemia and superficial corneal vascularisation (Fig. 72). Occasionally corneal ulceration is a feature. The diagnosis is made on the basis of a Schirmer tear test (STT) reading less than 10 mm/minute with accompanying clinical signs. Treatment involves the correction of any identifiable underlying cause if possible and tear replacement with topical lubricants. The efficacy of topical ciclosporin has not been reported in cats but, anecdotally, some cases seem to respond. In a few selected cases where medical therapy is unsuccessful or not possible, parotid duct transposition offers a surgical treatment option (Whittaker et al., 2010).

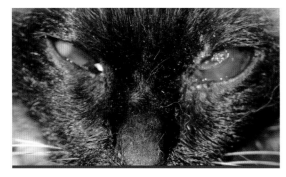

Figure 72. Bilateral keratoconjuncivitis sicca in an aged Siamese. Significant respiratory disease related to FHV-1 infection was also present. Courtesy of Filip Nachtegaele.

Trauma to the eyelids, nictitans and nasolacrimal system

Traumatic laceration to these structures usually results from cat scratches (Fig. 73). Resection of eyelid tissue should be kept to an absolute minimum and particular attention is paid to the precise reconstruction of the eyelid margin. A one or two-layer closure using absorbable 6/0 suture material is employed taking care that suture ends are not able to come into contact with the ocular surface (Fig. 74). The eyelids are very well vascularised and thus usually heal well in the absence of infection. Lacerations to the nictitans should also be repaired if possible although healing can be more problematic than that of the eyelids. Absorbable 8/0 suture is usually employed. Injuries to the canaliculi can occur in conjunction with trauma to the medial canthus. Repair can be challenging and requires microsurgical facilities and experience. The main complication encountered is canalicular stenosis with resultant epiphora. To reduce the chance of this, cannulation of the canaliculus with silastic tubing can be employed (Fig. 75). The tubing should be left in place for at least three weeks.

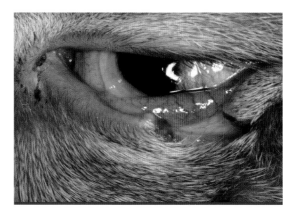

Figure 73. Full-thickness laceration of the lower eyelid as a result of a cat fight.

➔ In contrast to the dog, immune-mediated KCS has not been reported in the cat.

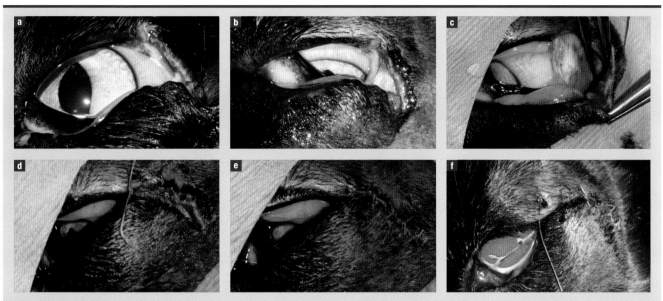

Figure 74. Surgical repair of a full thickness eyelid laceration. a) Laceration of the lateral canthus resulting in interruption of the smooth eyelid margin and a wound that prevents normal blinking. b) The hair is clipped and the area is cleaned in preparation for surgery. c) The conjunctiva is gently debrided and a small amount of contracted tissue is resected. d) The first suture placed is the figure-of-eight absorbable 6/0 suture to realign the eyelid margins. e) Four simple interrupted absorbable 6/0 sutures are placed to close the skin. The suture ends of the figure-of-eight absorbable 6/0 suture have been incorporated underneath the adjacent simple interrupted suture to prevent the ends from contacting the globe. f) A temporary tarsorrhaphy using nonabsorbable 4/0 suture is placed to reduce tension on the eyelid repair while it is healing. Courtesy of Rachael Grundon.

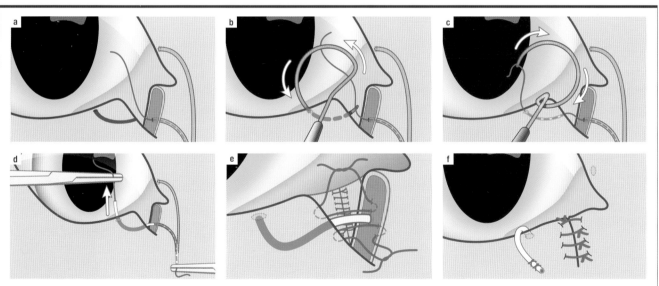

Figure 75. Surgical repair of a lower canalicular laceration. a) 3/0 nylon is passed retrograde via the nasal ostium until it emerges from the distal portion of the lacerated canaliculus. b) A pigtail probe is inserted into the inferior lacrimal punctum and rotated to emerge from the proximal end of the laceration. The suture is threaded through the eye of the probe and tied to it. c) The probe is then redirected through the proximal part of the canaliculus to emerge, with the nylon suture, from the lower punctum. d) The suture is removed from the probe and silastic tubing is threaded over the nasal end of the suture and carefully drawn up the nasolacrimal duct and though the severed canaliculus to emerge from the punctum. e) Two simple interrupted 6/0 polyglactic acid sutures are used to appose the subconjunctival tissues. f) The skin is closed as for any eyelid laceration using 6/0 polyglactic acid suture. A figure-of-eight suture is used at the eyelid margin and simple interrupted sutures are used to close the remaining defect. The tubing is sutured to the skin adjacent to the lower eyelid and left in place for 2-3 weeks while the duct heals.

References

ANTHONY JM, SANDMEYER LS, LAYCOCK AR (2010). Nasolacrimal obstruction caused by root abscess of the upper canine in a cat. *Veterinary Ophthalmology*; 13:106-109.

ARNETT BD, BRIGHTMAN AH 2ND, MUSSELMAN EE (1984). Effect of atropine sulfate on tear production in the cat when used with ketamine hydrochloride and acetylpromazine maleate. *Journal of the American Veterinary Medical Association*; 185:214-215.

CHAHORY S, CRASTA M, TRIO S et al. (2004). Three cases of prolapse of the nictitans gland in cats. *Veterinary Ophthalmology*; 7:417-419.

ESSON D (2001). A modification of the Mustardé technique for the surgical repair of a large feline eyelid coloboma. *Veterinary Ophthalmology*; 4:159-160.

FRYMUS T, GRUFFYDD-JONES T, PENNISI MG et al. (2013). Dermatophytosis in cats: ABCD guidelines on prevention and management. *Journal of Feline Medicine and Surgery*; 15:598-604.

GIUDICE C, MUSCOLO MC, RONDENA M et al. (2009). Eyelid multiple cysts of the apocrine gland of Moll in Persian cats. *Journal of Feline Medicine and Surgery*; 11:487-491.

HUNT GB (2006). Use of the lip-to-lid flap for replacement of the lower eyelid in five cats. *Veterinary Surgery*; 35:284-286.

ITOH N, MURAOKA N, AOKI M et al. (2004). Treatment of Notoedres cati infestation in cats with selamectin. *Veterinary Record*; 154:409.

MARGADANT DL, KIRKBY K, ANDREW SE et al. (2003). Effect of topical tropicamide on tear production as measured by Schirmer's tear test in normal dogs and cats. *Veterinary Ophthalmology*; 6:315-320.

MONTGOMERY KW, VAN DER WOERDT A, AQUINO SM et al. (2010). Periocular cutaneous mast cell tumors in cats: evaluation of surgical excision (33 cases). *Veterinary Ophthalmology*; 13:26-30.

MORIELLO KA, NEWBURY S, STEINBERG H (2013). Five observations of a third morphologically distinct feline Demodex mite. *Veterinary Dermatology*; 24:460-462.

MURPHY S (2013). Cutaneous Squamous Cell Carcinoma in the Cat: Current understanding and treatment approaches. *Journal of Feline Medicine and Surgery*; 15:401-407.

NEWKIRK KM, ROHRBACH BW (2009). A retrospective study of eyelid tumors from 43 cats. *Veterinary Pathology*; 46:916-927.

REINSTEIN SL, GROSS SL, KOMÁROMY AM (2011). Successful treatment of distichiasis in a cat using transconjunctival electrocautery. *Veterinary Ophthalmology* 14 Suppl; 1:130-134.

ROBERTS SR, BISTNER SI (1968). Surgical correction of eyelid agenesis. *Modern Veterinary Practice*; 49:40-43.

SCHLUETER C, BUDRAS KD, LUDEWIG E et al. (2009). Brachycephalic feline noses: CT and anatomical study of the relationship between head conformation and the nasolacrimal drainage system. *Journal of Feline Medicine and Surgery*; 11:891-900.

SCHMIDT K, BERTANI C, MARTANO M et al. (2005). Reconstruction of the lower eyelid by third eyelid lateral advancement and local transposition cutaneous flap after 'en bloc' resection of squamous cell carcinoma in 5 cats. *Veterinary Surgery*; 34:78-82.

WHITE JS, GRUNDON RA, HARDMAN C et al. (2012). Surgical management and outcome of lower eyelid entropion in 124 cats. *Veterinary Ophthalmology*; 15:231-235.

WHITTAKER CJ, WILKIE DA, SIMPSON DJ et al. (2010). Lip commissure to eyelid transposition for repair of feline eyelid agenesis. *Veterinary Ophthalmology*; 13:173-178.

WILLIAMS D, KIM J-Y (2009). Feline entropion: a case series of 50 affected animals (2003-2008). *Veterinary Ophthalmology*; 12:221-226.

WILLIAMS D, MIDDLETON S, CALDWELL A (2012). Everted third eyelid cartilage in a cat: a case report and literature review. *Veterinary Ophthalmology*; 15:123-127.

YANG SH, LIU CH, HSU CD et al. (2007). Use of chemical ablation with trichloroacetic acid to treat eyelid apocrine hidrocystomas in a cat. *Journal of the American Veterinary Medical Association*; 230:1170-1173.

6

The conjunctiva

Anatomy and function

The conjunctiva is a thin vascular mucous membrane that completely lines the inner surface of the eyelids, the inner and outer surfaces of the nictitans, and the anterior sclera. It is reflected at the dorsal and ventral fornices, creating the conjunctival sacs (Fig. 1). The palpebral conjunctiva lines the inner surfaces of the upper and lower eyelids. The bulbar conjunctiva covers the anterior aspect of the globe and connects to it at the corneoscleral limbus. It is mainly nonpigmented in the cat, although the conjunctiva at the leading edge of the nictitans tends to be pigmented in those with darker coat colours.

Histologically, the conjunctiva consists of a superficial nonkeratinised columnar epithelium and an underlying substantia propria. The epithelium forms a protective barrier from the external environment and contains goblet cells which secrete mucins which are important constituents of the preocular tear film (see Chapter 5). Directly beneath the epithelium lies the substantia propria, which is composed of two layers: a superficial adenoid layer and a deeper fibrous layer. The superficial layer contains numerous lymphoid follicles that represent conjunctiva-associated lymphoid tissue (CALT), which provides an integral immunological role in protection against infectious agents, completing the defensive role of the conjunctiva.

Much of the conjunctiva is quite mobile, but it is tightly adhered at the eyelid margins, the leading edge of the nictitans and at the limbus. This elasticity allows for ocular motility. The tear film coats the conjunctival epithelium, preventing it from desiccation and providing it with a certain level of nourishment. Abnormalities of the conjunctiva may lead to deficiencies in the mucin content of the tear film, decreased resistance to infectious agents and restriction of ocular motility.

→ Nonhaemolytic streptococci and *Staphylococcus epidermidis* are the most commonly isolated commensal organisms from the conjunctiva.

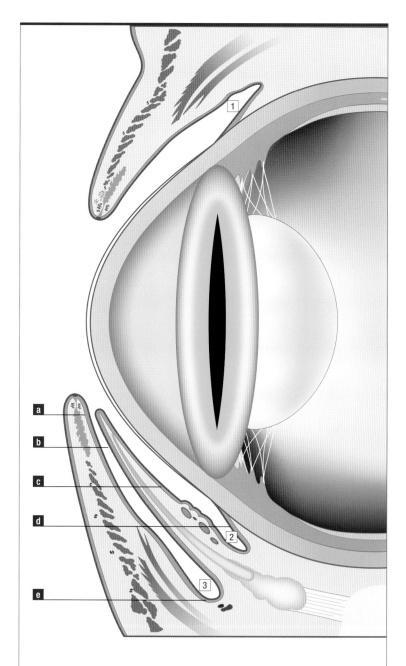

Figure 1. Regions of the conjunctiva in cross section.

a	palpebral	1	dorsal conjunctival fornix
b	anterior nictitans	2	posterior (bulbar) ventral conjunctival fornix
c	posterior nictitans		
d	bulbar	3	anterior (palpebral) ventral conjunctival fornix
e	fornix		

Congenital conditions

Dermoid

An ocular dermoid is a congenital island of normal haired skin present in an abnormal location (see Chapter 5). Dermoids are typically situated at the lateral canthus or on the lateral limbus involving the conjunctiva and cornea (Figs. 2 and 3). If the hairs make contact with the ocular surface they may induce irritation, presenting as increased lacrimation and blepharospasm. Dermoids may occur in any breed of cat, but are more common in the Birman and Burmese, in which they may be inherited. The treatment of choice is surgical removal with conjunctival resection, along with superficial lamellar keratectomy if the cornea is also involved.

Acquired conditions

Symblepharon

Symblepharon is the adhesion of the bulbar, palpebral or nictitans conjunctiva either to itself or to the cornea. In cats, it is most often a sequel to feline herpesvirus-1 (FHV-1) infection but may also occur following chemical injury to the ocular surface. Depending on severity and location, symblepharon may cause problems with ocular motility, tear production and distribution, and vision. Conjunctival fusion over the lacrimal puncta may lead to chronic epiphora and adhesions involving the conjunctiva of the nictitans may result in its fixed protrusion (Fig. 4). In its most severe form, the entire cornea may be conjunctivalised causing blindness (Figs. 5-8). Surgical management of symblepharon is extremely challenging as the conjunctival adhesions to the cornea tend to reform following their removal. This is because the limbal stem cells, which are essential for normal corneal epithelial formation, are destroyed during the initial inflammatory process.

→ Symblepharon forms as the result of destruction of stem cells at the limbus, which are essential for the maintenance of healthy functional corneal epithelium.

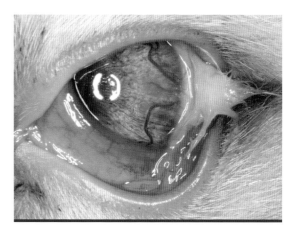

Figure 2. Conjunctival dermoid with a protruding tuft of hair causing conjunctivitis in a 3-month-old Birman.

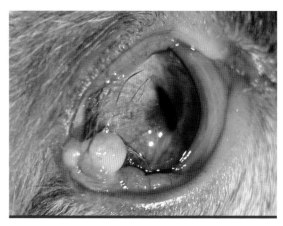

Figure 3. Conjunctival dermoid arising near the lateral limbus in a 6-month-old Birman × Burmese.

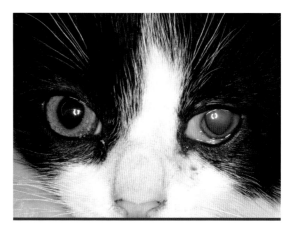

Figure 4. Symblepharon in the left eye of a Domestic shorthair kitten. The palpebral conjunctiva and the conjunctiva in the palpebral aspect of the nictitans are fused, resulting in permanent partial nictitans protrusion.

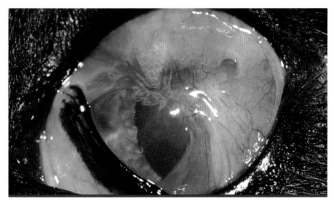

Figure 5. Symblepharon in a 2-year-old Domestic shorthair. There has been radial ingrowth of bulbar conjunctiva towards the central cornea. The cat previously had corneal ulceration associated with FHV-1 infection.

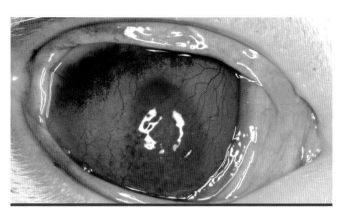

Figure 6. Symblepharon in the right eye of a 3-year-old Domestic shorthair. The entire corneal surface has been replaced with thin conjunctival epithelium. Pigment is migrating into the cornea from the dorsal limbus.

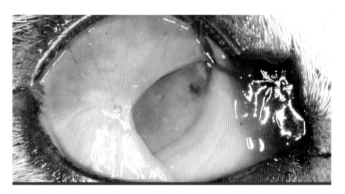

Figure 7. Extensive symblepharon with adhesion of the dorsal and ventral palpebral conjunctiva to each other, but not to the underlying cornea. The visible cornea (centrally) demonstrates pigmentation and conjunctival adhesions.

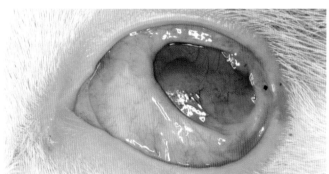

Figure 8. Extensive symblepharon. The nictitans is prominent due to ahesion to the dorsal bulbar conjunctiva. The cornea is covered with a thin layer of conjunctival epithelium. There is chemosis and conjunctival hyperaemia.

Trauma

Conjunctival trauma is commonly accompanied by injury to adjacent structures, such as the eyelids and cornea. Chemosis (conjunctival oedema) and conjunctival haemorrhage commonly occur (Fig. 9) and may interfere with assessment of intraocular structures. Examination should include close inspection of the fornices for the presence of foreign bodies and assessment for conjunctival ulceration with the aid of fluorescein dye. Treatment involves removal of any foreign body, application of a broad spectrum topical antibiotic and, where indicated, systemic nonsteroidal antiinflammatory (NSAID) drugs.

Conjunctivitis

Conjunctivitis is very common in cats. Clinical signs always include hyperaemia, but may also include ocular discharge, chemosis, thickening or ulceration, subconjunctival haemorrhage and follicle formation (Figs. 10-26).

It may be classified according to:
- Duration (acute, chronic or recurrent)
- Appearance (follicular, haemorrhagic)
- Nature of discharge present (serous, mucoid, mucopurulent, purulent)
- Cause (infectious, traumatic, secondary to keratitis, tear film abnormalities, trichiasis, uveitis or orbital disease).

→ Classification of conjunctivitis by cause is most helpful to enable appropriate treatment.

Figure 9. Subconjunctival haemorrhage and chemosis in both eyes of a cat that suffered a road traffic accident with head trauma. The left conjunctival tissue has petechial haemorrhages; the right has purpuric haemorrhages.

Neonatal conjunctivitis

Ophthalmia neonatorum is a form of conjunctivitis that develops in the neonatal period, usually as a result of delayed and/or incomplete opening of the eyelids (ankyloblepharon, see Chapter 5). This allows mucous to become trapped, with subsequent secondary infection with *Chlamydophila felis*, FHV-1 or opportunistic bacteria such as *Staphylococcus* spp. (Fig. 10). If the eyelids remain fused, they should be gently and gradually prised apart by inserting a closed forceps directed towards the closed canthus, and very gradually opening it. The ocular surface should then be irrigated with sterile saline or dilute 1:50 povidone iodine aqueous solution. The degree of conjunctivitis can then be assessed and the cornea should be checked for ulceration. On-going treatment involves ocular surface irrigation and topical broad spectrum antibiotics four times daily.

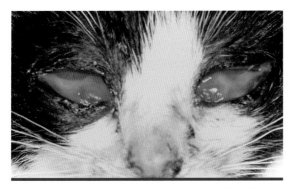

Figure 10. Ophthalmia neonatorum in a 3-week-old kitten. Bilateral ankyloblepharon resulted in severe conjunctivitis and keratitis, which persisted after the eyelids had been opened.

Infectious conjunctivitis

Infectious conjunctivitis is a very common problem in cats, particularly those in shelters or breeding establishments. The two most important causes are FHV-1 and *Chlamydophila felis*.

Viral conjunctivitis
Feline herpesvirus-1 (FHV-1)

FHV-1 is a DNA virus that infects domestic and wild feline species. It is very widespread, with an estimated 75-97 % of the world's cat population seropositive for the virus. FHV-1 invades and replicates in the epithelia of the conjunctiva and respiratory tract, with more limited replication in the corneal epithelium. FHV-1 can cause both primary and secondary conjunctivitis and keratitis. It also predisposes towards secondary bacterial infection, which can worsen the clinical signs.

Primary disease in young kittens presents as cat flu. Ocular signs include a serous to mucopurulent discharge, conjunctival hyperaemia and chemosis (Fig. 11) and, in some cases, corneal ulceration. Because FHV-1 can induce rapid lysis of susceptible cells, this predisposes towards symblepharon formation (Figs. 4-8). Corneal ulcers may be dendritic (i.e. branching) and are typically very painful (see Chapter 7). The specific cause of the pattern is not known, but it occurs with replication of the virus in the corneal epithelium. These dendritic ulcers are considered pathognomonic for FHV-1 infection, and are most common on days 3 and 12 after primary infection.

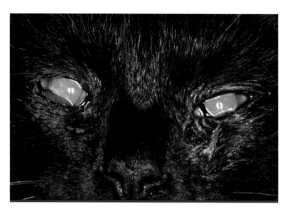

Figure 11. Herpetic conjunctivitis in a 3-month-old Domestic shorthair. The conjunctiva is hyperaemic and thickened, with epithelial erosions.

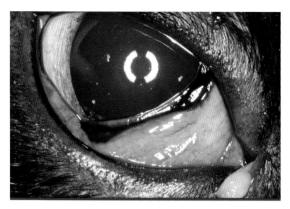

Figure 12. Conjunctivitis associated with FHV-1 infection in a cat with concurrent upper respiratory tract disease. Conjunctival hyperaemia, mild chemosis and mucopurulent discharge are present.

Rose Bengal dye may be superior for diagnosing this pattern of ulceration as the epithelium of the basement membrane often remains intact (see Chapter 1). These branching ulcers can progress and coalesce, resulting in broader geographic ulcers. Systemic signs are an important feature of primary infection and include pyrexia, lethargy, anorexia, upper respiratory tract disease (coughing, sneezing and nasal discharge) and facial dermatitis.

Following primary infection, approximately 80 % of cats become latent carriers with the virus dormant in the trigeminal ganglia. Subsequent periodic reactivation of the virus is caused by stress-related events, such as rehoming, parturition or corticosteroid treatment, and leads to recrudescent disease. The clinical signs are varied and can include a milder conjunctivitis, conjunctival hyperaemia and swelling, and dendritic or geographic corneal ulceration (Figs. 12-15). Associated syndromes include chronic stromal keratitis, corneal sequestrum, eosinophilic (proliferative) keratitis, uveitis and dermatitis.

Diagnosis of FHV-1 infection is covered in Chapter 7, and treatment is covered in Chapters 2 and 7.

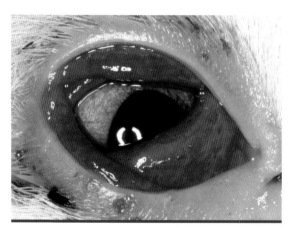

Figure 13. Conjunctivitis caused by FHV-1 infection, with chemosis, subconjunctival haemorrhage in a 14-month-old Domestic shorthair from a cat shelter. The diagnosis was made based on virus isolation from a conjunctival swab.

→ Reduction of stress and provision of good nursing care are very important aspects in control of FHV-1 associated disease.

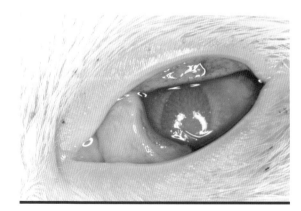

Figure 14. Conjunctivitis and keratitis caused by FHV-1 infection in a young adult Domestic shorthair. There is conjunctival hyperaemia, mild chemosis, corneal oedema and peripheral corneal neovascularisation. The diagnosis was made based on a positive PCR for FHV-1 DNA from a conjunctival swab.

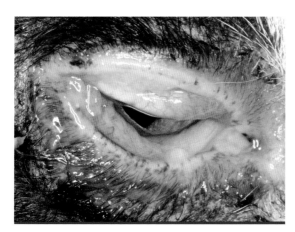

Figure 15. Severe conjunctivitis in an adult cat caused by FHV-1 infection.

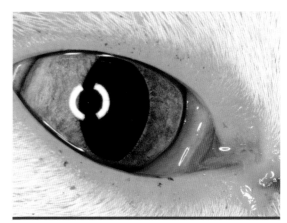

Figure 16. Mild conjunctivitis with mucopurulent ocular discharge in a young Domestic shorthair, presenting because of oral mucosal ulceration caused by feline calicivirus infection.

Feline calicivirus (FCV)

FCV is a common cause of upper respiratory disease. Typical systemic signs of infection include fever, rhinitis, oral mucosal ulcerations and chronic stomatitis. FCV was previously thought to cause only mild conjunctivitis but recent studies suggest that certain strains of FCV may cause more significant ocular surface disease (Gerriats et al., 2012). Approximately 10 % of affected cats may display mild, moderate or severe signs of conjunctivitis along with conjunctival epithelial ulceration, on occasion being so severe as to preclude visualisation of the cornea (Stiles, 2013) (Fig. 16). Laboratory diagnosis is made by virus isolation or by PCR. FCV is an RNA virus, and therefore cannot be effectively treated with antiviral medications that inhibit DNA synthesis, such as those used to treat FHV-1. The use of topical broad spectrum antibiotics is always advisable to reduce complications associated with secondary bacterial infection. Topical or systemic NSAIDs could be considered when inflammation is severe or prolonged.

Bacterial conjunctivitis
Chlamydial conjunctivitis

Chlamydiae are obligate intracellular organisms that have a tropism for mucous membranes. In cats, *Chlamydophila felis* is the pathogenic species. Prevalence of infection is higher in cats under one year of age, and presenting ocular signs include blepharospasm, serous ocular discharge, conjunctival hyperaemia and pronounced chemosis (Figs. 17-20). Initially, the condition is usually unilateral, but with time often becomes bilateral. Serous discharge is often present which may later become mucopurulent and the conjunctiva may become thickened. In chronic cases, conjunctival hyperaemia, hyperplasia and follicle formation are often found. Left untreated, a chronic carrier state can develop in the gastrointestinal and urogenital tracts.

Diagnosis is achieved through consideration of the history and clinical signs, along with PCR testing for the organism. Cytology of conjunctival epithelial scrapings or brushes may occasionally demonstrate intracytoplasmic elementary bodies and thus be diagnostic. The organism can be harboured at sites distant from the eye, such as the gastrointestinal or urogenital tracts, so systemic treatment is always required even if only ocular signs are apparent. The recommended treatment is doxycycline 10 mg/kg orally once daily for three to six weeks. Caution must be taken as oral doxycycline has been associated with oesophageal ulceration and stricture formation in cats, and therefore the medication should always be followed by a water or food swallow. Azithromycin appears to be a less effective treatment. Cats that remain infected should be assessed for systemic immunosuppression, including testing for feline leukaemia virus (FeLV) and feline immunodeficiency virus (FIV). Topical treatment should involve cleansing the ocular surfaces, and a broad spectrum topical antibiotic that has antichlamydial efficacy, such as tetracycline, if this is available.

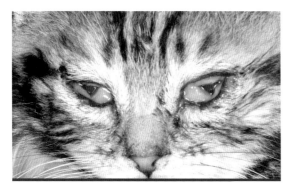

Figure 17. Conjunctivitis in a 10-week-old Domestic shorthair caused by *Chlamydophila felis* infection, with bilateral chemosis and mucopurulent ocular discharge.

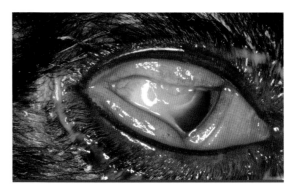

Figure 18. Conjunctivitis associated with *Chlamydophila felis* infection, presenting with purulent ocular discharge, chemosis and conjunctival hyperaemia, along with corneal ulceration and keratitis. The condition had been untreated for two weeks.

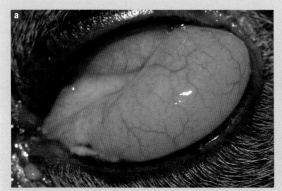
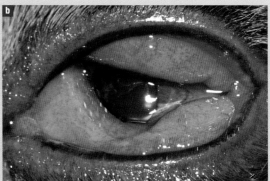

Figure 19. a) Conjunctivitis associated with *Chlamydophila felis* infection, presenting as dramatic chemosis and mucoid ocular discharge affecting the left eye of a 10-month-old Burmese. The cornea could not be seen. b) The same eye eight hours after administration of a NSAID injection. Chemosis has reduced allowing examination of the cornea and intraocular structures.

Mycoplasmal conjunctivitis

Mycoplasma spp. are not uncommonly identified in cases of conjunctivitis but their role as primary pathogens remains controversial. *Mycoplasma* spp. are often found in the presence of other conjunctival pathogens and have also been cultured in cats without conjunctivitis. Clinical signs attributed to mycoplasmal conjunctivitis include unilateral conjunctivitis with conjunctival hyperaemia and serous to purulent ocular discharge that typically becomes bilateral after a few days. Occasionally a pseudodiphtheritic membrane develops that is thought to be characteristic of the condition (Fig. 20). The disease course may be self-limiting after 30 days. Treatment is the same as for chlamydial conjunctivitis, and it typically responds well to therapy.

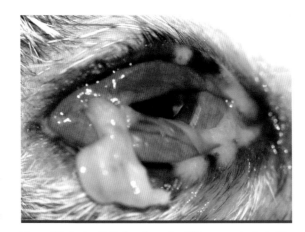

Figure 20. Conjunctivitis in a 4-month-old European shorthair. *Mycoplasma* sp. was the assumed cause due to the severe chemosis, subconjunctival haemorrhage and hyperaemia and a pseudodiphtheritic membrane. Courtesy of Filip Nachtegaele.

Lipogranulomatous conjunctivitis

Lipogranulomatous conjunctivitis is an inflammatory condition that occurs in older cats (Kerlin and Dubielzig, 1997; Read and Lucas, 2001). The meibomian glands are affected in one or both eyes. Presenting signs are of regional nonulcerative nodules visible beneath the palpebral conjunctiva (Figs. 21-24). The nodules are pale in colour, ranging from white to cream-yellow in appearance. Concurrent eyelid neoplasia occurs in many cases. Histologically, there are large cell-free lipid lakes surrounded by regions of granulomatous inflammation. Multi-nucleated macrophages are occasionally identified. Any breed of cat can be affected but there is a higher incidence in the Persian. Solar radiation is suspected to play a role in pathogenesis as it tends to occur in older animals with little periocular pigmentation. If adverse clinical signs are not apparent, monitoring alone may be sufficient. Surgical treatment is required if there is irritation, and involves curettage of the glands through the conjunctival surface. Where multiple glands are affected close to each other, a strip of conjunctiva and underlying lipogranulomas may be resected, and the defect is allowed to heal by secondary intention without any need for suturing.

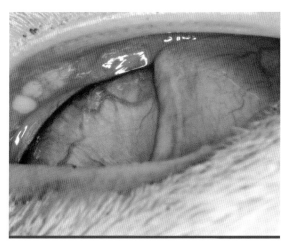

Figure 21. Lipogranulomatous conjunctivitis affecting the palpebral conjunctiva of the upper eyelid of a 17-year-old Domestic shorthair.

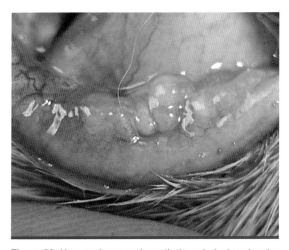

Figure 22. Lipogranulomas underneath the palpebral conjunctiva with adjacent conjunctivitis in a 14-year-old Persian.

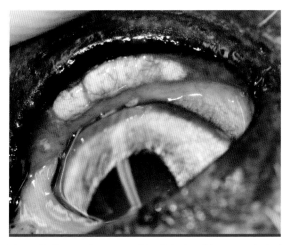

Figure 23. Lipogranulomatous nodular thickening of the upper palpebral conjunctiva in a 16-year-old Burmese. Courtesy of Filip Nachtegaele.

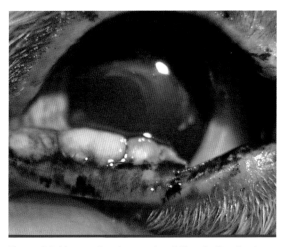

Figure 24. Lipogranulomatous conjunctivitis affecting the lower eyelid of a 17-year-old Domestic shorthair. A row of large white smooth subconjunctival nodules are present.

Eosinophilic (proliferative) conjunctivitis

There are several eosinophilic disorders that affect cats. Ocular syndromes of blepharitis, conjunctivitis and keratitis associated with eosinophilic inflammation can occur in isolation or in combination. Eosinophilic conjunctivitis is much less common than eosinophilic keratitis (see Chapter 7) and has been described in case series of five (Pentlarge, 1999) and twelve (Allgoewer et al., 2001) cats. Age at initial presentation varies, but mean age is approximately seven years. One or both eyes can be affected and clinical signs include thickening, depigmentation and erosions of the eyelid margins, blepharospasm, and swelling and redness of the conjunctiva (Figs. 25 and 26). Definitive diagnosis is made on cytological examination of conjunctival scrapings or histological examination of biopsy specimens, with eosinophils and mast cells being seen (Fig. 27). Other inflammatory cells usually found on cytology include neutrophils, lymphocytes and plasma cells. The role played by FHV-1 infection in the development of the condition remains undetermined (see Chapter 7). Treatment involves topical immunosuppressive therapy, typically a corticosteroid such as 0.1 % dexamethasone phosphate. Initial intensive treatment four times daily can be tapered to effect according to the clinical response to treatment, which is usually rapid. Topical 0.02 % ciclosporin ointment used twice daily is preferable if a diagnosis of FHV-1 infection has been made. Cats that cannot be medicated topically may be treated with oral megoestrol acetate, but there are many potential side effects to this treatment that need to be considered. Many cases require long-term treatment, and on-going monitoring for relapse is recommended.

Keratoconjunctivitis sicca

Keratoconjunctivitis sicca is a disorder of the lacrimal secretory system, and affects both the conjunctiva and cornea. It is a rare diagnosis in cats but may occur following severe FHV-1 infection or as part of feline dysautonomia. The condition is discussed in more detail in Chapters 5 and 7.

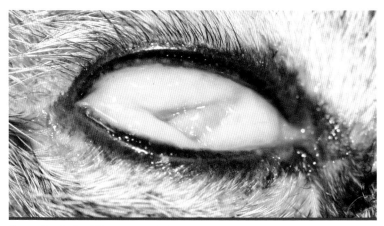

Figure 25. Eosinophilic conjunctivitis in an 11-year-old European shorthair with severe chemosis and tenacious discharge. Many eosinophils were found on conjunctival cytology. Courtesy of Filip Nachtegaele.

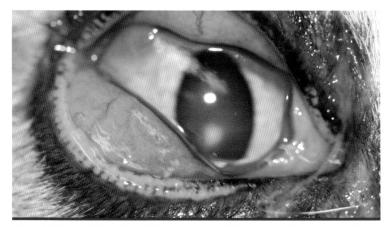

Figure 26. Eosinophilic conjunctivitis in a 14-year-old European shorthair. Conjunctivitis and chemosis were present along with mild keratitis. The diagnosis was confirmed by cytology. Courtesy of Filip Nachtegaele.

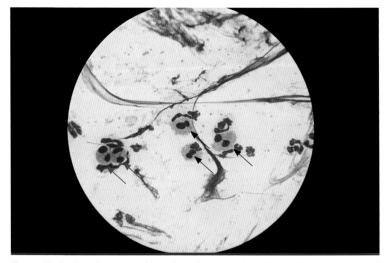

Figure 27. Cytology from a cat with eosinophilic conjunctivitis. Neutrophils (red arrows) and eosinophils (black arrows) are present.

Parasitic conjunctivitis

Thelazia nematodes are known to affect many species, including cats, humans, dogs, foxes and wolves. *T. callipaeda* has been reported in Asia and has recently become endemic in regions of southern Europe. *T. californiensis* has been reported in cats in the western United States. A vector is required to complete the lifecycle, thought to be the *Phortica variegata* fruit fly in the case of *T. callipaeda*, and *Fannia* sp. fly in the case of *T. californiensis*. The adult worms and first stage larvae (L1) reside beneath the nictitans, and may cause conjunctivitis and epiphora (Figs. 28 and 29). L1s are ingested by the vector feeding on the ocular secretions, and L3 develop within it over three weeks. Case numbers are rising, likely due to increased awareness and possibly due to the spread of vector populations and the infestation of wildlife species, including foxes.

Treatment involves mechanical removal of the adult worms and the use of parasiticides. A topical dermatological preparation containing 10 % imidacloprid and 2.5 % moxidectin has been found efficacious for disease control (Bianciardi and Otranto, 2005). Oral milbemycin oxime at 2 mg/kg has been found to have a therapeutic efficacy of 53.3 % with a single treatment, and 73.3 % with two treatments, one week apart (Motta et al., 2012). Macrocyclic lactones, such as moxidectin, have also been used topically to kill the parasites.

Neoplasia

Several forms of neoplasia have been reported to affect the feline conjunctiva and the most common of these are discussed below. It is imperative that a rapid diagnosis is achieved, as many of these tumours are malignant and require prompt treatment for the best possible outcome. A lesion that involves only the superficial layers of the conjunctiva will be easy to manipulate, and is mobile when the tissue is moved. Deeper lesions are more firmly attached and therefore do not move freely when the conjunctiva is manipulated. Clinical assessment of a conjunctival mass and of nonspecific conjunctivitis, either diffuse or nodular, is complimented by laboratory testing. The results may help to distinguish between inflammation, infection,

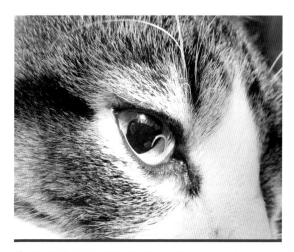

Figure 28. *Thelazia callipaeda* in the eye of a young male cat, noted incidentally at castration in Switzerland. Two adult worms are seen emerging from the ventral conjunctival sac posterior to the nictitans. Courtesy of Dr Bruna Motta.

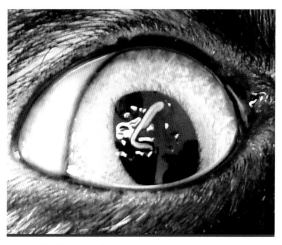

Figure 29. *Thelazia callipaeda* on the cornea of a young male cat in Switzerland. The cat was examined after a similar parasite was found in the eye of an in-contact dog. Courtesy of Dr Ülle Kell.

granuloma and neoplasia. Squamous cell carcinoma can be diagnosed by exfoliative cytology. A fine needle aspiration biopsy, incisional biopsy or excisional biopsy is required for other tumour types. Conjunctival biopsy is a relatively straight-forward procedure. Sedation or general anaesthesia is advisable for the procedure in most cats. Topical anaesthetic (e.g. 0.5 % proxymetacaine) is applied to the anticipated biopsy site with a cotton-tipped applicator for ten seconds. It is maximally effective after one minute, and the duration of maximum effect is approximately

25 minutes. The conjunctival sac should be cleansed with dilute 1:50 povidone iodine aqueous solution. Using a fine-toothed forceps, such as the Bishop-Harmon, the affected conjunctiva is raised and then sectioned with a small tenotomy scissors (Fig. 30). The sample should then be placed in 10 % formalin, with prior placement on a piece of card being useful to prevent tissue contracture and aiding histological orientation and examination. The conjunctival defect should not need to be sutured if it is less than 1 cm squared. Gentle pressure is applied to the site and the bleeding should stop in 2-3 minutes. If it does not, adrenaline (epinephrine) diluted to 1:10,000 may be applied to the area to provide vasoconstriction. A topical broad spectrum antibiotic is used for 3-5 days, pending the laboratory results.

Neoplastic involvement of the deeper conjunctival layers may result in extension into the orbit. B-mode ultrasonography may therefore be useful in preoperative clinical assessment, although advanced diagnostic imaging such as magnetic resonance imaging (MRI) or computed tomography (CT) are preferable in assessing potential orbital invasion (see Chapter 4).

Squamous cell carcinoma

Feline squamous cell carcinoma (SCC) does not typically affect the conjunctiva alone. It is thought to arise due to exposure to excessive UVB radiation, and occurs much more frequently in cats lacking periocular and conjunctival pigmentation. It is a locally invasive tumour which can infiltrate the eyelids or the globe (Figs. 31 and 32). It is also important to consider that conjunctival SCC could represent metastasis from elsewhere in the body such as the lung or middle ear. Surface cytology or biopsies are necessary to distinguish it from inflammatory processes such as granulation tissue or eosinophilic conjunctivitis, and from other neoplastic diseases. Many treatments have been advocated and include surgical excision or debulking (including enucleation in some cases), cryotherapy, hyperthermia, immunotherapy, radiation and photodynamic therapy. The prognosis is guarded unless complete excision with adequate margins can be achieved, which can be a challenge in the ocular area.

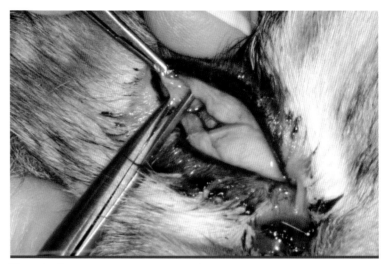

Figure 30. Conjunctival biopsy. A fine-toothed forceps is used to gently tent the conjunctiva, which is removed with a small tenotomy scissors. Suturing is not usually required.

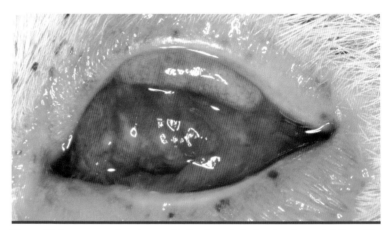

Figure 31. Squamous cell carcinoma affecting the palpebral conjunctiva and nictitans. The globe could not be seen but there was intraocular extension.

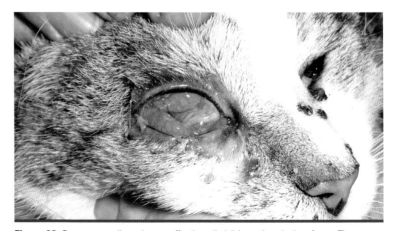

Figure 32. Squamous cell carcinoma affecting all visible conjunctival surfaces. The cornea was also affected.

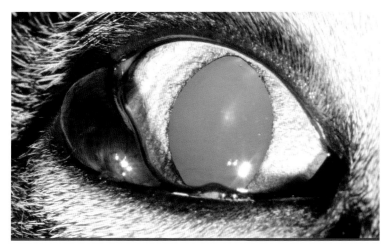

Figure 33. Conjunctival melanoma. A large darkly-pigmented mass is bulging over the lateral canthus in a 12-year-old Domestic shorthair.

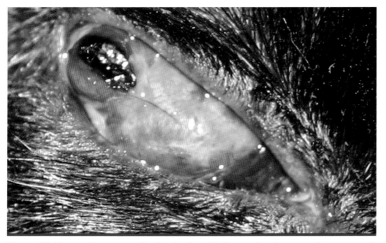

Figure 34. Haemangiosarcoma affecting the dorsal bulbar conjunctiva presenting as a rough dark red fleshy mass with necrosis in a 15-year-old Domestic shorthair.

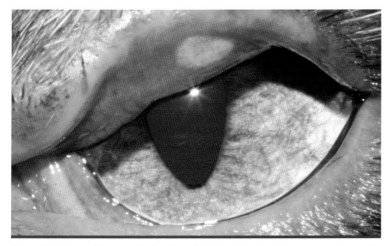

Figure 35. Mast cell tumour affecting the palpebral conjunctiva. The upper eyelid was distorted with the swelling, and a chalazion is also present. The diagnosis was confirmed by cytological examination of a fine needle aspirate sample.

Melanoma

Feline conjunctival melanoma is a relatively uncommon condition. The histological findings from 21 cases have been reported (Schobert et al., 2010). The tumour is most commonly located in the bulbar conjunctiva (Fig. 33) and the degree of pigmentation is very variable with some examples being amelanotic. Feline conjunctival melanomas are locally aggressive, may metastasise and carry a poorer long-term prognosis compared with the same neoplasm in dogs. Exenteration of the globe is usually required in order to achieve the best margins of excision and increase the chance of a favourable outcome.

Vascular conjunctival tumours

Feline vascular conjunctival tumours are rare. As the conjunctiva is a highly vascular tissue, it is susceptible to developing haemangiomas and haemangiosarcomas, and both types have been reported in a study involving eight cats (Pirie and Dubielzig, 2006). Affected cats tend to be aged and have a history of high UV-light exposure. Typical presentation is a superficial red or brown focal conjunctival nodule, arising in regions with reduced epithelial pigmentation (Fig. 34). Diagnosis is achieved by histological examination of incisional or excisional biopsy specimens. Early surgical excision is recommended and may be curative, but recurrence is possible and therefore monitoring is advised.

Other neoplastic conditions affecting the conjunctiva

Other primary conjunctival tumours are considered rare, and those reported include conjunctival mucoepidermoid carcinoma, lymphosarcoma, fibrosarcoma and mast cell tumours (Fig. 35).

References

ALLGOEWER I, SCHÄFFER E, STOCKHAUS C et al. (2001). Feline eosinophilic conjunctivitis. *Veterinary Ophthalmology*; 4:69-74.

BIANCIARDI P, OTRANTO D (2005). Treatment of dog thelaziosis caused by *Thelazia callipaeda* (Spirurida, Thelaziidae) using a topical formulation of imidacloprid 10 % and moxidectin 2.5 %. *Veterinary Parasitology*; 129:89-93.

FONTENELLE JP, POWELL CC, VEIR JK et al. (2008). Effect of topical ophthalmic application of cidofovir on experimentally induced primary ocular feline herpesvirus-1 infection in cats. *American Journal of Veterinary Research*; 69:289-293.

GASKELL RM, POVEY RC (1977). Experimental induction of feline viral rhinotracheitis virus re-excretion in FVR recovered cats. *Veterinary Record*; 100:128-133.

GERRIETS W, JOY N, HUEBNER-GUTHARDT J et al. (2012). Feline calicivirus: a neglected cause of feline ocular surface infections? *Veterinary Ophthalmology*; 15:172-179.

GOULD D (2011). Feline herpesvirus-1: Ocular manifestations, diagnosis and treatment options. *Journal of Feline Medicine and Surgery*; 13:333-346.

KAUFMAN HE, VARNELL ED, THOMPSON HW (1998). Trifluridine, cidofovir, and penciclovir in the treatment of experimental herpetic keratitis. *Archives of Ophthalmology*; 116:777-780.

KERLIN RL, DUBIELZIG RR (1997). Lipogranulomatous conjunctivitis in cats. *Veterinary and Comparative Ophthalmology*; 7:177-179.

MAGGS DJ, CLARKE HE (2004). *In vitro* efficacy of ganciclovir, cidofovir, penciclovir, foscarnet, idoxuridine, and acyclovir against feline herpesvirus type-1. *American Journal of Veterinary Research*; 65:399-403.

MOTTA B, SCHNYDER M, BASANO F et al. (2012). Therapeutic efficacy of milbemycin oxime / praziquantel oral formulation (Milbemax) against *Thelazia callipaeda* in naturally infested dogs and cats. *Parasit Vectors* 5:85.

NASISSE MP (1990). Feline herpesvirus ocular disease. *Veterinary Clinics of North America, Small Animal Practice*; 20:667-680.

PENTLARGE V (1991). Eosinophilic conjunctivitis in five cats. *Journal of the American Veterinary Medicine Association*; 27:21-28.

PIRIE CG, DUBIELZIG RR (2006). Feline conjunctival hemangioma and hemangiosarcoma: a retrospective evaluation of eight cases (1993-2004). *Veterinary Ophthalmology*; 9:227-231.

READ RA, LUCAS J (2001). Lipogranulomatous conjunctivitis: clinical findings from 21 eyes in 13 cats. *Veterinary Ophthalmology*; 4:93-98.

SCHOBERT CS, LABELLE P, DUBIELZIG RR (2010). Feline conjunctival melanoma: histopathological characteristics and clinical outcomes. *Veterinary Ophthalmology*; 13:43-46.

SLACK JM, STILES J, LEUTENEGGER CM et al. (2013). Effects of topical ocular administration of high doses of human recombinant interferon alpha-2b and feline recombinant interferon omega on naturally occurring viral keratoconjunctivitis in cats. *American Journal of Veterinary Research*; 74:281-289.

STILES J (2013). Ocular manifestations of feline viral diseases. *The Veterinary Journal*; 201:166-73.

THOMASY SM, COVERT JC, STANLEY SD et al. (2012). Pharmacokinetics of famciclovir and penciclovir in tears following oral administration of famciclovir to cats: a pilot study. *Veterinary Ophthalmology*; 15:299-306.

THOMASY SM, LIM CC, REILLY CM et al. (2011). Evaluation of orally administered famciclovir in cats experimentally infected with feline herpesvirus 1. *American Journal of Veterinary Research*; 72:85-95.

WILLIAMS DL, FITZMAURICE T, LAY L et al. (2004). Efficacy of antiviral agents in feline herpetic keratitis: results of an *in vitro* study. *Current Eye Research*; 29:215-218.

7

The cornea

Anatomy and function

The cornea and sclera together comprise the dense fibrous tunic of the globe. The cornea is composed of four layers (Fig. 1): an outer stratified squamous epithelium with a basement membrane, a thick stromal layer, Descemet's membrane and an inner cuboidal epithelium (corneal 'endothelium').

The corneal epithelium is 5-11 cells thick. The surface cells project numerous microvillae and microplicae that are coated with a glycocalyx which functions to stabilise the tear film. The stroma makes up approximately 90 % of the cornea and consists of multiple parallel lamellae of collagen fibres that extend across the entire diameter of the cornea from limbus to limbus. The fibres are supported by glycosaminoglycans, which control stromal hydration and assist in maintaining the exact parallel arrangement of the collagen lamellae necessary for corneal transparency. Multiple tiny keratocytes are scattered within the collagen bundles, and these quiescent cells are involved in corneal wound healing as they can be stimulated to transform into fibroblasts and myofibroblasts in response to corneal damage. Descemet's membrane is the exaggerated basal lamina of the inner epithelium, which is more commonly known as the corneal endothelium. The endothelium consists of a single layer of metabolically active hexagonal cells. The function of the endothelial cells is to pump ions from the stroma into the aqueous humour. These ions are followed by water, keeping the stroma in a relative state of dehydration further contributing to corneal transparency. The endothelial cells are postmitotic, so have limited ability to regenerate after injury, although adjacent viable endothelial cells can slide over to cover any defect. Loss of function of the endothelial cells leads to diffuse corneal oedema.

Structurally the sclera is similar to the cornea, but it is not transparent because the scleral collagen fibres differ in diameter and shape, are not regularly spaced, and are orientated in different directions throughout the tissue. The two structures merge in a transitional zone: the corneoscleral limbus. It is usually clearly defined as a narrow pigmented region (Fig. 2). The limbus contains the pluripotent epithelial stem cells, which are essential to the health of the ocular surface as they

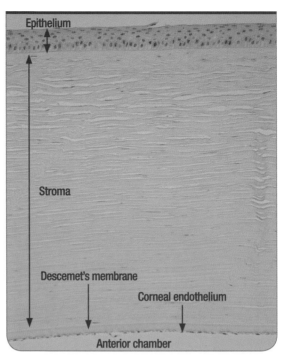

Figure 1. Histopathologic section of normal cornea. Courtesy of Karen Dunn, Focus-EyePathLab.

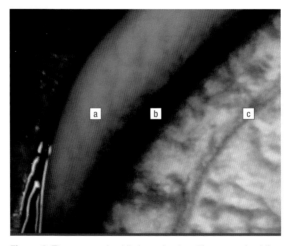

Figure 2. The corneoscleral limbus. a) sclera, b) corneoscleral limbus, c) major arterial circle of the iris.

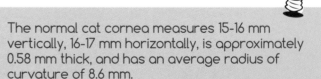
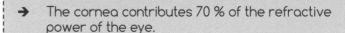

→ The normal cat cornea measures 15-16 mm vertically, 16-17 mm horizontally, is approximately 0.58 mm thick, and has an average radius of curvature of 8.6 mm.

→ The cornea contributes 70 % of the refractive power of the eye.

amplify, proliferate and differentiate into corneal epithelium. They also act as a physiological barrier to the ingress of conjunctival cells across the cornea. Dysfunction (e.g. in some cases of multiple ocular defects) or destruction (e.g. from chemical, thermal or inflammatory insults) can lead to invasion and fusion of the conjunctival epithelium onto the denuded corneal stroma resulting in symblepharon (see Chapter 6).

Cats have relatively large corneas which may help with night vision by permitting more light to enter the eye. The cornea and sclera are rigid, providing resistance to intraocular fluid pressure and maintaining the spherical shape of the globe.

Congenital and developmental conditions

Dermoid

A dermoid is a congenital displacement of skin tissue. It uncommonly affects the cornea in cats, but more usually affects the eyelids (see Chapter 5) and the conjunctiva (see Chapter 6). The hairs tend to cause irritation presenting as excessive lacrimation, and can potentially cause corneal ulceration. If the dermoid extends over the limbus to affect the cornea (Fig. 3), surgical removal by superficial lamellar keratectomy and conjunctival resection is generally required. As the cornea is only 0.5-0.6 mm thick, the use of an operating microscope and microsurgical instrumentation is necessary.

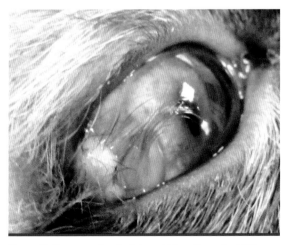

Figure 3. Corneo-conjunctival dermoid in a 5-month-old Birman. Courtesy of Filip Nachtegaele.

Microcornea and megalocornea

Microcornea occurs with microphthalmos – a congenitally small eye. There is wide variation in both the severity of the condition and in the presence of accompanying defects such as cataracts and persistent pupillary membrane remnants. Microcornea and microphthalmos have been associated with the teratogenic anomalies that can arise from medication of a pregnant queen during the first half of gestation with the fungistatic agent griseofulvin. Megalocornea, a larger than normal corneal diameter, is rare. Both conditions are congenital, bilateral and nonprogressive, and treatment is unwarranted.

Leukoma associated with persistent pupillary membranes

In most cases, persistent pupillary membranes (PPM, see Chapter 8) do not affect the cornea. However, PPM strands occasionally extend from the iris colarette anteriorly to the cornea. This results in an adherent leukoma, visible as a focal white or pigmented corneal opacity (Figs. 4 and 5). This congenital condition is nonprogressive and no treatment is usually undertaken.

Lysosomal storage disease

Lysosomal storage diseases are rare in cats. They have received a disproportionate level of interest because they potentially provide useful animal models for investigating similar conditions in people. These inherited inborn errors of metabolism result in the accumulation of by-products of metabolism within lysosomes due to the lack of a specific enzyme. They are classified according to the accumulated product. The diseases that can affect the eyes in cats include mucopolysaccharidosis types I and VI, α-mannosidosis, globoid cell leukodystrophy, and GM1 and GM2 gangliosidoses. The most common ocular manifestation is progressive bilateral diffuse corneal clouding due to structural alterations within the stroma (Fig. 6). Other systemic signs may be present depending on the type and severity of disorder, including neurological signs, skeletal abnormalities and stunted growth. The prognosis is poor. There is no treatment for storage diseases.

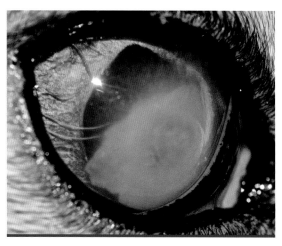

Figure 4. Adherent leukoma in a young adult Domestic shorthair due to multiple fine strands of iris tissue (persistent pupillary membrane) extending from the iris surface to attach to the inner corneal endothelium.

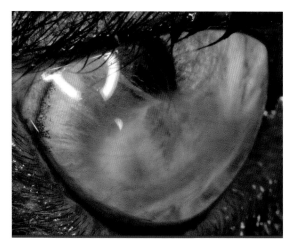

Figure 5. Adherent leukoma resulting from adhesions of multiple strands arising from the surface of the iris (persistent pupillary membrane) with the posterior cornea.

Corneal dystrophy

Corneal dystrophy is a primary inherited condition that manifests in early life. It is typically bilateral in presentation, and a breed-related or familial predisposition is suspected. Stromal corneal dystrophy occurs in the Manx cat, presenting as progressive stromal oedema that can lead to bullous keratopathy (see later). The only potentially effective treatment for advanced stromal dystrophy is penetrating keratoplasty.

Acquired conditions of the cornea

Herpetic keratitis

Feline herpesvirus-1 (FHV-1) infection is very common and has several ocular manifestations including conjunctivitis, symblepharon and ophthalmia neonatorum. FHV-1 is also a primary corneal pathogen and can directly cause corneal ulceration and stromal keratitis. Two different types of corneal ulceration occur as a result of FHV-1. The classical type is the dendritic ulcer which is considered pathognomonic for FHV-1 infection (Fig. 7). Dendritic ulcers occur during primary infection as the virus replicates in the corneal epithelium. They have a linear branching pattern, seen with fluorescein or rose bengal ophthalmic dyes (see Chapter 1). The second type is the superficial geographic epithelial ulcer, which can become chronic.

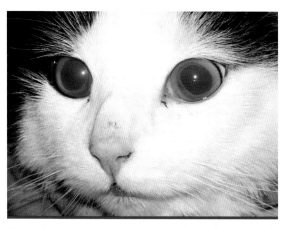

Figure 6. Suspected lysosomal storage disease in a 2-year-old Domestic shorthair with slowly progressive bilateral corneal opacity in the absence of other ocular abnormalities.

They are typically painful, and induce a superficial vascularisation response (Figs. 8 and 9). Chronic corneal ulceration, whatever the aetiology, can lead to corneal sequestrum formation (see later). Stromal keratitis occurs as a result of an immune-mediated reaction to the presence of the viral components sequestered in the epithelium or stroma. It presents as stromal oedema and cellular infiltration, along with deep stromal vascularisation (Figs. 10 and 11). It can result in significant corneal scarring. Topical immunosuppressive drugs (corticosteroids or ciclosporin) may be used with caution to treat the condition, but the use of concurrent antiviral therapy is recommended.

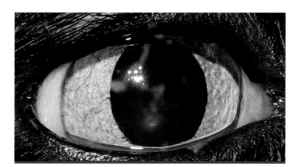

Figure 7. Herpetic keratitis in a 5-month-old Domestic shorthair with fluorescein-positive dendritic ulceration.

Diagnosis of FHV-1 is often made on the basis of the classical ocular and, occasionally, systemic clinical signs. There are some difficulties in interpreting the results of laboratory tests that are currently available to diagnose the presence of the virus. Cytology is not very useful for FHV-1 identification; while intranuclear inclusions may occur during primary infection, they are not commonly found in clinical cases. Serology has limited value, because it cannot distinguish between wild-type virus and vaccine strains, and because seropositivity does not necessarily indicate current infection. Virus isolation is considered the gold standard test, but because of logistical difficulties in preserving the virus during transport and because it can be positive in clinically normal cats, it is mainly used for research purposes rather than in clinical cases. Polymerase chain reaction (PCR) assays are a very useful diagnostic test, although there is a high prevalence of FHV-1 infection in the general feline population. Therefore, diagnosis of FHV-1 infections is best made following a careful appraisal of the history and clinical signs.

Treatment of ocular FHV-1 infections is not straightforward. In fact, there are several different opinions and options. Uncomplicated viral infection is self-limiting, running a 10-14 day course. Therefore, a practical initial approach should involve providing comfort, nursing care and a stress-free environment, along with control of any secondary bacterial infection with topical antibiotics. Corticosteroids, by any route, are generally contraindicated during active infection. If corneal ulcers are present, a topical broad spectrum antibiotic such as chloramphenicol

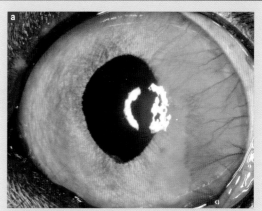

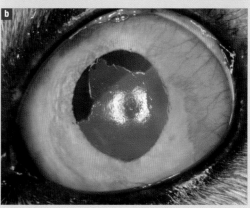

Figure 8. Herpetic keratitis in a 9-year-old Persian. a) Superficial corneal vascularisation laterally. There is interruption of the flash reflection due to irregularity of the corneal surface. b) Fluorescein staining after epithelial debridement shows the extent of the superficial geographic corneal ulcer.

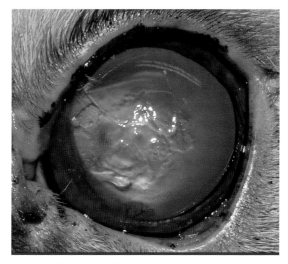

Figure 9. Chronic superficial corneal ulceration with oedema, neovascularisation and rough nonadherent epithelium, caused by FHV-1 infection.

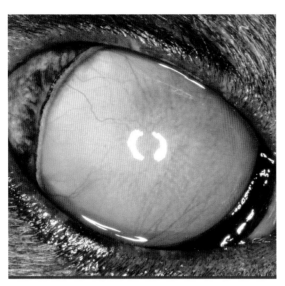

Figure 10. Stromal keratitis associated with chronic FHV-1 infection. Note the corneal oedema and neovascularisation.

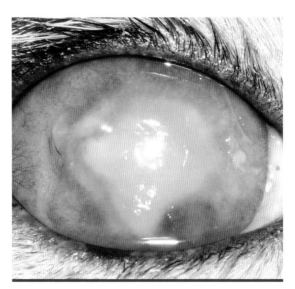

Figure 11. Chronic stromal keratitis with dense corneal neovascularisation, oedema and cellular infiltration.

or chloramphenicol, fusidic acid or 'triple' (neomycin/polymyxin B/gramicidin) antibiotic is required. Geographic ulcers with epithelial under-running may also benefit from treatment with epithelial debridement (see Fig. 8).

Antiviral medications are licensed for use in human patients, and for many of them there is a lack of convincing published evidence of safety and efficacy in cats. The necessary frequency of application of topical therapy may cause stress, which can be counterproductive. Some topical agents used, in deceasing order of reported efficacy, include idoxuridine, vidarabine, trifluorothymidine (trifluridine) and aciclovir (Maggs and Clarke, 2004; Williams, 2004). Topical cidofovir used twice daily has been found to be as effective as topical trifluorothymidine used 4-9 times daily, but safety studies have not yet been published (Fontenelle et al., 2008; Kaufman et al., 1998). Topical 0.15 % ganciclovir gel used q4-6h for 21 days has been advocated as a promising treatment option, but results of clinical trials have not been published (Gould, 2011). Systemic famciclovir has been found to be effective against FHV-1 at a dose rate of 90 mg/kg three times daily for 21 days in cats experimentally infected with FHV-1 (Thomasy et al., 2011). Subsequently 40 mg/kg three times daily for 2-3 weeks has been found to be

both safe and effective in client-owned cats (Thomasy et al., 2012), and these much lower dose rates also appear to improve clinical signs. Anecdotally, clinical improvement has been seen with dose rates of famciclovir 62.5-125 mg/cat, one to three times daily for two weeks.

Interferon is sometimes used but does not appear to be effective in controlling the clinical disease (Slack et al., 2013). Oral lysine has been found to be safe, but results of its efficacy have been conflicting. Lysine competes with arginine and therefore reduces viral replication *in vitro*. A suggested dose of 500 mg lysine given as a bolus twice daily may reduce viral shedding in latently infected cats, and may reduce the clinical signs in cats with primary FHV-1 infection. However, it should not be used as mono-therapy, but rather as part of an overall control strategy if deemed appropriate.

➜ Corneal disease syndromes that have been associated with FHV-1 infection include stromal keratitis, eosinophilic (proliferative) keratitis, corneal sequestration and keratoconjunctivitis sicca (KCS).

Eosinophilic (proliferative) keratitis

Feline eosinophilic keratitis is relatively common. Presentation is unilateral in approximately 75 % of cases, but the condition can also occur bilaterally (Dean and Meunier, 2013). The average age at presentation is five years. The disease is characterised by inflammation extending across the limbus (affecting both the conjunctiva and cornea) and the dorsolateral quadrant is most commonly involved. Typically, there is vascularisation associated with superficial white corneal plaques with a very irregular surface (Figs. 12-16). There is a suspected association with FHV-1 infection; however, a consistent relationship between the two conditions has not yet been shown. It is thought that cats that develop corneal ulceration due to FHV-1 infection may subsequently develop eosinophilic keratitis (Dean and Meunier, 2013). It could also be considered that both corneal inflammation and the stress associated with eosinophilic keratitis could be responsible for recrudescent FHV-1 disease in latently affected cats.

Diagnosis is suggested by the typical clinical appearance, and is confirmed by cytological examination of surface scrapings or brushings. Eosinophils and mast cells, along with lymphoplasmacytic inflammatory cells, are the predominant cell types found. Treatment with topical immunosuppressive agents is usually successful in controlling the disease. Topical corticosteroids, such as 0.1 % dexamethasone phosphate are effective, but it is prudent to use them concurrently with topical or systemic antiviral drugs, pending results of FHV-1 testing. Topical 1.5 % ciclosporin solution has been reported to be effective, used twice or three times daily, but no commercially available product exists (Spiess et al., 2009). If the response to treatment is not adequate or if the cat will not tolerate topical treatment, oral megestrol acetate (5 mg daily for one week, then 2.5-5 mg per week) has been used successfully. However, the potential complications of diabetes mellitus and mammary hyperplasia/neoplasia need to be considered. Relapses are possible, and so on-going monitoring is recommended, and lifelong therapy may be required.

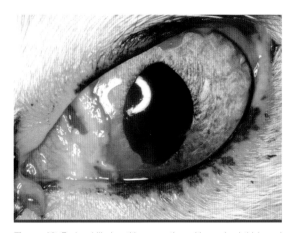

Figure 12. Eosinophilic keratitis presenting with a raised thickened white plaque on the medial cornea in a 1-year-old Domestic shorthair.

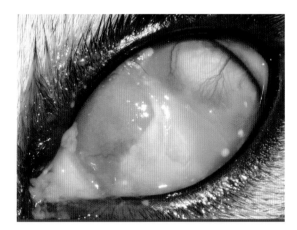

Figure 13. Eosinophilic keratitis. There are extensive proliferative white deposits within and on the cornea, along with neovascularisation.

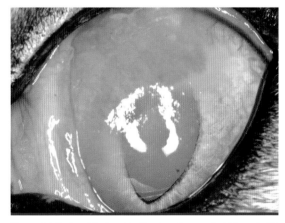

Figure 14. Eosinophilic keratitis. The dorsal cornea is thickened with fibrovascular and cellular infiltrate. Cytology confirmed the diagnosis and FHV-1 DNA was present on PCR.

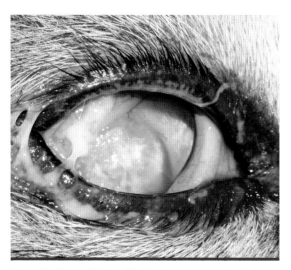

Figure 15. Eosinophilic keratitis. Note the caseous ocular discharge, upper eyelid margin depigmentation and a dense elevated rough plaque affecting the cornea.

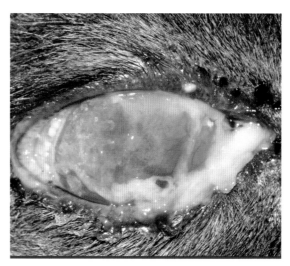

Figure 16. Eosinophilic keratitis. Note the caseous ocular discharge, multiple white plaques on the lateral conjunctiva and a densely neo-vascularised cornea with a rough epithelial surface.

Corneal sequestrum

Corneal sequestration is a relatively common condition that occurs mainly in the cat. A sequestrum is a focal area of stromal collagen necrosis associated with accumulation of pigment. Cats of any breed may be affected, although there is a breed predisposition in the Persian, Himalayan, Siamese, Burmese and Exotic shorthair. There may be an association between chronic FHV-1 infection and corneal sequestration, but FHV-1 is not known to be causative. The link is most likely due to the fact that FHV-1 infection commonly leads to corneal ulceration, and sequestrum development appears to be a nonspecific response to chronic stromal injury.

The condition is most commonly unilateral, but it can be bilateral. Clinical signs always include a characteristic focal amber, brown or black oval to circular corneal plaque (Figs. 17-26). It can be located in the central or paracentral cornea. Often, there is a surrounding corneal reaction with oedema and stromal vascularisation. The lesion itself does not uptake fluorescein because it is necrotic, dehydrated tissue, but the cornea immediately surrounding the lesion may be ulcerated (Figs. 24 and 25). The level of discomfort, manifested as blepharospasm and excess lacrimation, is variable. The diagnosis is straightforward as the lesion can be easily seen, although it must be distinguished from a corneal foreign body or iris prolapse. The depth of the necrotic tissue within the stroma varies – it most commonly affects the anterior third of the stroma but may progress to Descemet's membrane and potentially lead to corneal perforation.

Sequestra may be treated medically or surgically. The decision as to whether to opt for medical or surgical treatment is based on the current comfort of the patient, apparent risk of deepening disease with potential rupture and finances available. Conservative

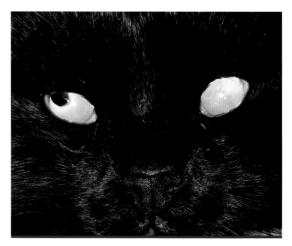

Figure 17. Corneal sequestrum as seen by distant direct ophthalmoscopy. The right eye has a focal circumscribed black opacity on the dorsolateral cornea. Closer inspection revealed a corneal sequestrum.

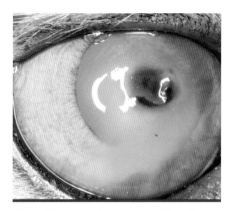

Figure 18. A corneal sequestrum at the site of a chronic nonhealing corneal ulcer. Note the deep corneal neovascularisation medially.

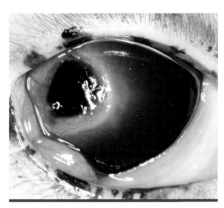

Figure 19. A dense darkly-pigmented sequestrum is present in the lateral cornea and is associated with keratitis and conjunctivitis.

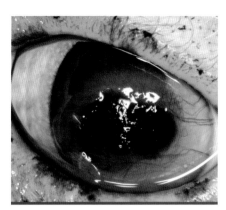

Figure 20. Paracentral corneal sequestrum with corneal neovascularisation and a rim of nonadherent epithelium ventrally.

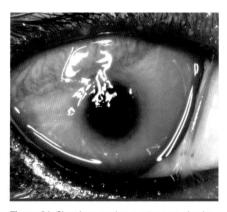

Figure 21. Chronic corneal sequestrum causing keratitis with neovascularisation and oedema.

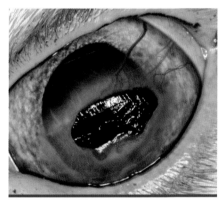

Figure 22. Central corneal sequestrum that developed less than one week after a grid keratotomy procedure on a superficial corneal ulcer.

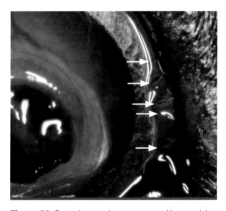

Figure 23. Central corneal sequestrum with organising fibrovascular reaction beneath it. Distichia are present on the medial upper eyelid (arrows), and are likely the cause of the sequestrum.

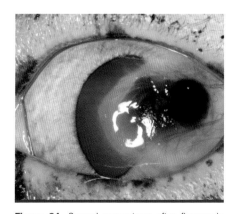

Figure 24. Corneal sequestrum after fluorescein staining. There is under-running of the fluorescein beneath the epithelium surrounding the sequestrum.

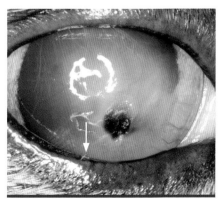

Figure 25. Corneal sequestrum after fluorescein staining. There is under-running of fluorescein dorsal and ventral to the sequestrum. The sequestrum may have developed due to irritation from a lower eyelid distichium (arrow).

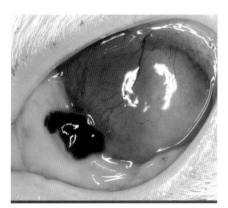

Figure 26. A partially extruded sequestrum in an eye with chronic problems associated with FHV-1 infection, including symblepharon. The nictitans is beneath the loose section of the sequestrum, which is still partly adhered to the cornea.

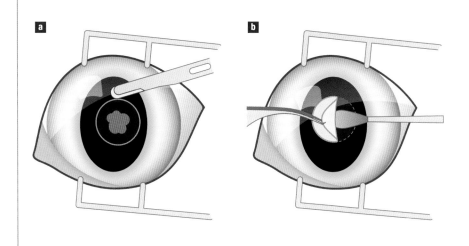

Figure 27. a) Using a No. 64 Beaver or similar blade, an incision is made around the lesion to be removed to a depth of approximately 0.15-0.25 mm (one third of corneal thickness). All of the diseased tissue needs to be removed, so a deeper incision can be made if required. b) The edge of the corneal tissue to be excised is grasped to steady it. The superficial cornea is dissected with the blade or a crescent knife. The tissue plane of excision is maintained between the corneal lamellae. The dissected tissue is excised leaving a stromal defect. A decision is made at this point as to whether a graft is required.

Keratectomy

→ Surgical excision of the corneal epithelium and variable depth of underlying stroma.

→ The aim is to resect diseased tissue to speed healing, reduce scarring and improve vision.

→ The most common indication in cats is removal of a corneal sequestrum, although it may also be used in the case of corneal dermoid, stromal abscess, superficial foreign body or chronic nonhealing superficial ulcer.

→ The procedure is outlined in Fig. 27.

→ The depth of the sequestrum can be difficult to determine preoperatively, and the surgeon should be prepared to do a grafting procedure (e.g. conjunctival pedicle graft or corneo-conjunctival transposition procedure, see later) if resection of greater than one third of the corneal depth is required to entirely remove all diseased tissue.

management of the condition involves the use of topical broad spectrum antibiotics and lubrication in the hope that the sequestrum will naturally loosen and then slough off. However, this process can take weeks or months to occur (Fig. 26), and there is a risk of progression of the corneal necrosis to more severe corneal disease or even perforation. Surgery is usually recommended as it lessens the time course of the condition and lessens the risk of complications. A keratectomy is performed to completely excise the affected cornea. If the sequestrum is more than one third depth of the cornea, a graft is required, such as a conjunctival pedicle graft, porcine small intestinal submucosal graft (Goulle et al., 2012; Featherstone et al., 2001), a corneo-conjunctival transposition (Andrew et al., 2001) or a corneal graft (Peña et al., 1998). In one study, 20 % of cases

had recurrence of the condition after both medical and surgical treatment, and it was concluded that conjunctival pedicle grafts should not be transected (Featherstone et al., 2004). On-going monitoring for recurrence will be required.

Keratoconjunctivitis sicca

Deficiency of the aqueous layer of the precorneal tear film leads to drying of the ocular surfaces, resulting in both conjunctivitis and keratitis (Fig. 28). Keratoconjunctivitis sicca (KCS) is discussed in Chapter 5. In one study, experimental FHV-1 infection was associated with reduced Schirmer tear test (STT) readings (Nasisse et al., 1989). There is also evidence that FHV-1 infection can cause tear film quality abnormalities, with reduced tear film break-up time (TFBUT) and goblet cell density, persisting at least one month following infection (Lim et al., 2009). As a result, topical muci-nomimetic therapy should be considered after FHV-1 diagnosis for at least one month, and on-going monitoring of the STT and TFBUT is recommended.

Acute bullous keratopathy

Acute bullous keratopathy, also termed corneal hydrops, usually affects younger cats. This uncommon condition has a very rapid onset and is associated with rapid progression. It is characterised by pronounced corneal oedema, with dense coalescing bullae that grossly distort the contour of the cornea (Figs. 29 and 30). Typically, there is accompanying epiphora, blepharospasm and conjunctival hyperaemia. Histologically, it is associated with Descemet's membrane rupture, but little or no inflammation can be found. The cause is not known but an association with prior antiinflammatory or immunosuppressive treatment is present in some cases. Prompt treatment is required, without which rupture of the bullae with subsequent deep corneal ulceration can occur. Surgical support is required (Glover et al., 1994) which can be provided by means of a nictitans flap, 360° conjunctival graft, conjunctival pedicle graft or temporary tarsorrhaphy. The prognosis for acute bullous keratopathy treated with timely surgery is good.

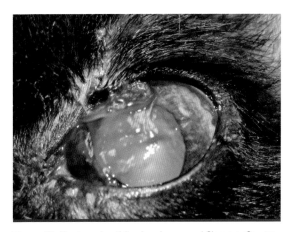

Figure 28. Keratoconjunctivits sicca in an aged Siamese. Courtesy of Rachael Grundon.

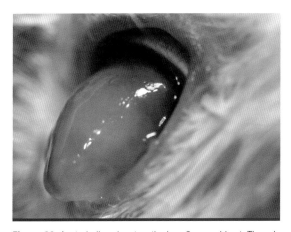

Figure 29. Acute bullous keratopathy in a 2-year-old cat. There is gross distortion of the corneal profile due to conical protrusion of the oedematous cornea. The lack of true uptake of fluorescein distinguishes it from a melting ulcer. Courtesy of Rachael Grundon.

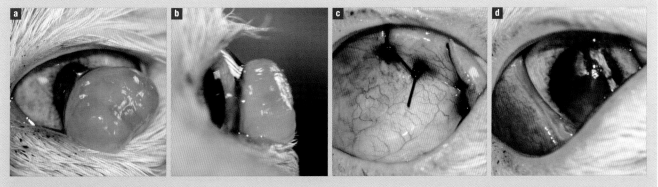

Figure 30. Acute bullous keratopathy in a 9-year-old cat that present with sudden onset corneal opacity. a) A front view of the cornea which is grossly thickened with dramatic focal oedema. b) A side view of the same eye shows the extent of the corneal protrusion. c) A nictitans flap with epibulbar conjunctival fixation was performed. d) The cornea made a good recovery, seen as the nictitans flap is released after two weeks. Courtesy of Filip Nachtegaele.

Florida keratopathy

Florida keratopathy (also known as Florida spots) is an uncommon condition affecting the corneas of cats from tropical or subtropical areas. It is nonpainful, with no evidence of inflammation. It presents as multiple small white corneal anterior stromal opacities, typically in both eyes (Fig. 31). The spots are concentrated towards the centre of the cornea, and are less numerous at the periphery. A doctoral thesis has linked similar corneal symptoms to contact injury with the Little Fire Ant (*Wasmannia auropunctata*) in French Polynesia (Theron, 2007). Otherwise, the cause is not clear, but the spots are apparently self-limiting and the condition does not respond to topical antibiotic or corticosteroid treatment.

Corneal degeneration

Corneal degeneration (Fig. 32) may occur spontaneously, secondary to corneal injury or chronic inflammation, or as a response to corneal dystrophy or lipid keratopathy. It manifests as calcium or lipid deposition within the corneal stroma. Typically, it is a unilateral condition and it is always accompanied by vascularisation. Corneal calcium and lipid can be difficult to distinguish clinically, but calcium is generally denser and thicker, while lipid has a more delicate, lacy appearance. Treatment of calcium accumulation can be attempted with topical 0.5 % EDTA eye drops two to four times daily, or surgical removal of the opacity via a keratectomy might be considered if the cat is uncomfortable. Topical antiinflammatory treatment is generally avoided, as it may promote further calcium or lipid deposition.

Corneal ulceration

Corneal ulceration is a frequently encountered problem in feline practice. It is defined as a break in continuity of the corneal epithelium, with or without loss of underlying corneal stroma. There is always some accompanying inflammation, so the term ulcerative keratitis is also used to describe the condition. There are many potential causes, including:

- Trauma e.g. cat scratch, foreign body, road traffic accident.

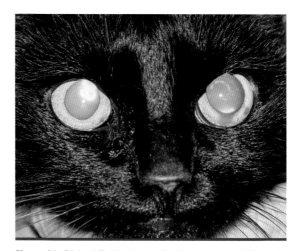

Figure 31. Bilateral Florida keratopathy in a young adult Domestic shorthair. In the left eye two focal white lesions can be seen on the ventral cornea using direct illumination. In the right eye coalescing focal white opacities are seen on the dorsal cornea using retroillumination. Courtesy of Dr Tim Cutler.

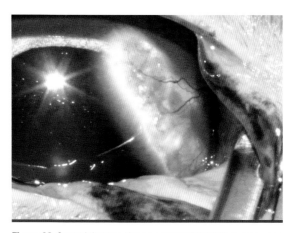

Figure 32. Corneal degeneration was present bilaterally in a 14-year-old Domestic shorthair. There is a focus of white corneal discolouration, with a lacy appearance at the periphery and a more granular appearance centrally, along with neovascularisation. No abnormalities were found on biochemistry and the cat was normolipoproteinaemic.

- Infection e.g. FHV-1, *Pseudomonas* spp., secondary bacterial infection.
- Adnexal abnormalities e.g. entropion, trichiasis, distichiasis.
- Impaired tear film distribution e.g. eyelid coloboma, mass or laceration, facial nerve paralysis, exophthalmos.
- Tear film abnormalities e.g. KCS or qualitative tear film abnormalities.

→ Topical corticosteroids are contraindicated for all types of corneal ulcer as they may potentiate collagenolysis ('melting') by destructive corneal, bacterial and inflammatory cell enzymes, or may allow reactivation of latent FHV-1.

Clinical signs of corneal ulceration include pain (blepharospasm and increased lacrimation) and focal corneal oedema due to epithelial loss. Over time, the ocular discharge may become mucopurulent or purulent, and corneal neovascularisation may occur. A basic investigation for a case of corneal ulceration should include a STT, assessment of the palpebral and corneal reflexes, careful examination of the eyelids, conjunctiva and nictitans, and staining with fluorescein. Exposed hydrophilic stroma uptakes the dye, while intact epithelium and Descemet's membrane do not. Microbiological assessment including surface cytology and bacterial culture and susceptibility testing is recommended for deep or melting corneal ulcers (see Chapter 1 for technique). A conjunctival swab for PCR for FHV-1 or *Chlamydophila felis* DNA may be required (see Chapter 6). The type of corneal ulcer is determined from its depth, location and extent, and then classified as superficial, stromal, descemetocoele, perforated or melting (see below).

Superficial corneal ulceration

Superficial corneal ulcers by definition have absent epithelium, but the underlying stroma is intact. Causes include trauma, FHV-1 infection, KCS, exposure keratitis, glaucoma and uveitis. Nonhealing chronic indolent superficial ulceration, similar to spontaneous chronic corneal epithelial defects in dogs, can also occur. Corneal neovascularisation may occur with chronicity, but is not present in every case. Uptake of fluorescein by the exposed corneal stroma clearly defines the ulcerated region (Fig. 33). There may be leakage of fluorescein underneath loose epithelium at the edges of the lesion (epithelial under-running), classifying the ulcer as a chronic nonhealing indolent ulcer.

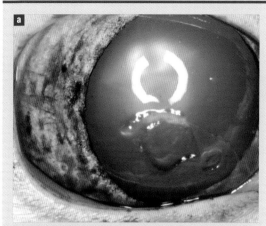

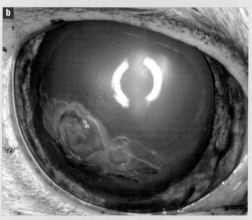

Figure 33. Superficial corneal ulcer. a) Two epithelial deficits are visible in the central cornea, with a flap of loose epithelium visible at the dorsal aspect of the larger ulcer. b) Fluorescein staining highlights the epithelial defect and the surrounding unhealthy epithelium, with under-running dye.

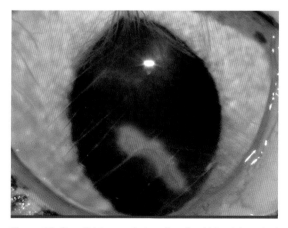

Figure 34. Superficial corneal ulceration. A grid keratotomy had been inappropriately performed and this eye is at increased risk of developing a corneal sequestrum.

→ It is CONTRAINDICATED to perform a grid keratotomy in cats, as this can lead to corneal sequestrum formation.

Treatment depends on the extent of the ulcer and on the presence or absence of complicating factors such as infection with bacteria or FHV-1, corneal sequestrum, entropion, lagophthalmos or KCS. If the underlying cause is identified and corrected, superficial corneal ulcers will heal rapidly. All superficial ulcers should be treated with a topical broad spectrum antibiotic two to four times daily to prevent infection. Chronic nonhealing ulcers may be treated with careful debridement of loose corneal epithelium from the edge of the ulcer with a dry cotton-tipped applicator. A grid keratotomy should never be considered in a cat as it may lead to corneal sequestrum formation (La Croix et al., 2001) (Figs. 22 and 34). Placement of a soft bandage contact lens supports healing. Surgical superficial keratectomy is useful for cases of prolonged nonhealing superficial corneal ulceration. A recent study found that 32.5 % of the ulcers were resolved within two weeks and 85 % within four weeks after surgery in cats (Jégou and Tromeur, 2014). The remaining cases healed with continuing appropriate medical management.

Stromal corneal ulceration

Stromal ulcers involve loss of the outer corneal epithelium along with varying degrees of the underlying stroma (Figs. 35-37). A descemetocoele occurs where there is complete focal loss of the epithelium and stroma with only Descemet's membrane and the corneal endothelium intact (Figs. 38 and 39). Fluorescein dye is used to stain the hydrophilic corneal stroma to clearly delineate the ulcerated region, staining both the walls and base of the ulcer. There may be a tendency for fluorescein to pool in the depression in the corneal surface, so excess dye

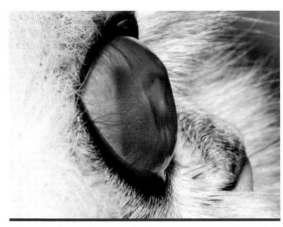

Figure 35. Side profile view of a Persian with a stromal corneal ulcer. There is corneal oedema and neovascularisation associated with a stromal corneal deficit, due to an infected corneal ulcer.

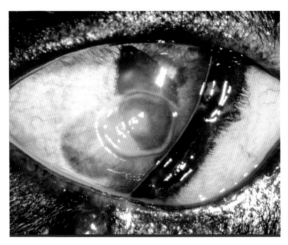

Figure 36. Stromal ulcer after fluorescein staining, associated with a central lower eyelid neoplasm.

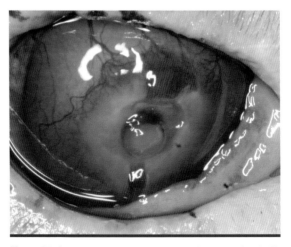

Figure 37. Chronic stromal ulcer that is very deep, associated with corneal oedema, neovascularisation and cellular infiltration.

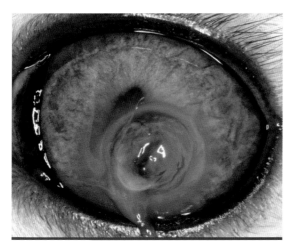

Figure 38. Descemetocoele in a 3-month-old Persian. The central cornea is clear because it is so thin, and it is bulging forwards. There is secondary iris inflammation.

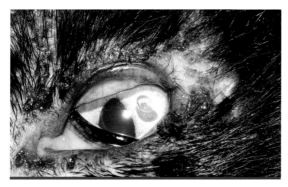

Figure 39. Descemetocoele in the left eye of a 4-year-old Domestic shorthair that was also suffering from pemphigus vulgaris, which was being treated with systemic corticosteroids.

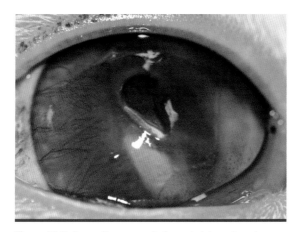

Figure 40. Reflex uveitis as a result of a central deep stromal corneal ulcer with superficial corneal vascularisation. The pupil is miotic. Small multifocal opacities are visible on the ventral aspect of the cornea especially medially, which are keratic precipitates located on the corneal endothelium.

should be gently flushed from the ocular surface with sterile saline. Fluorescein does not stain Descemet's membrane and so the absence of stain uptake at the base of a corneal ulcer should prompt a diagnosis of a descemetocoele which is a genuine surgical emergency. Any eye affected by corneal ulceration should be assessed for secondary reflex uveitis, which occurs due to stimulation of sensory nerve endings of the ophthalmic branch of the trigeminal nerve (CN V) within the cornea. Signs of reflex uveitis include miosis, aqueous flare and hypotony (Fig. 40).

Liquefactive corneal necrosis, or corneal melting, is a very serious potential complication of all forms of corneal ulceration. It occurs following liberation of collagenase enzymes (serine proteases and matrix metalloproteinases) from invading microorganisms, white blood cells, or keratocytes which cause rapid collagenolysis and loss of corneal substance. The cornea may appear white, cream or yellow due to infiltration of the corneal stroma with white blood cells and also due to corneal oedema. The smooth contour of the cornea is interrupted to a varying degree by liquefaction and the affected cornea loses rigidity and may appear to 'ooze' ventrally (Figs. 41-43). Rapid progression to corneal perforation can occur, thus this condition is an ophthalmic emergency.

Treatment depends on the extent and depth of the ulcer and on the presence or absence of complicating factors such as infection, melting or corneal sequestrum development. Deep and melting corneal ulcers require prompt and intensive treatment, and referral should be considered. If there is a risk of self-trauma, an Elizabethan collar should be fitted. An appropriate topical antibiotic is chosen, preferably based on examination of cytological specimens initially although this may need to be altered upon receipt of any pending culture and susceptibility testing (Chapter 3). The frequency of application of topical antibiotics varies according to clinical presentation and the results of laboratory testing but should initially be every 1-2 hours in cases of corneal melting. Anticollagenase medication is also essential in the case of melting ulcers, and autologous serum is most commonly used, again initially every 1-2 hours until stabilisation is achieved. Secondary

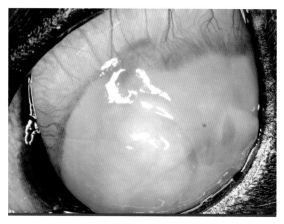

Figure 41. Melting ulcer. The dorsal cornea is vascularised and the rest of the cornea is white and has an irregular contour due to liquefactive stromal necrosis. *Pseudomonas aeruginosa* was cultured from the lesion.

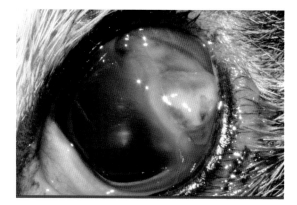

Figure 42. Melting ulcer. Focal keratomalacia is present laterally, with dense neovascularisation dorsally. *Staphylococcus* sp. was cultured from the lesion.

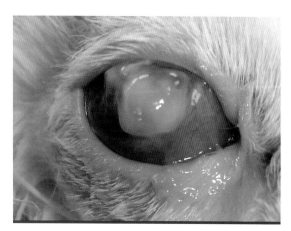

Figure 43. Melting ulcer. The cornea is densely vascularised peripherally and oedematous centrally, with keratomalacia grossly distorting the contour of the cornea. *Pseudomonas aeruginosa* was cultured from the lesion.

→ Some cats are more sensitive to topical atropine than others, and can salivate profusely. In those cats, topical 0.5 % or 1 % tropicamide could be used three times daily as an alternative.

uveitis is always present, so topical treatment with 1 % atropine is indicated to effect (to maintain relative dilatation of the pupil) but usually no more than once daily for up to three days. Topical or systemic antiviral treatment is indicated in the case of FHV-1 infection (see Chapter 6). Systemic nonsteroidal antiinflammatory drugs (NSAIDs) are useful to reduce ocular pain and help to stabilise the blood-ocular barrier. Frequent reexamination will be essential during the early stages of medical treatment to ensure the ulcer does not become deeper, get infected, or that the globe does not rupture. Surgical repair with, for example, a conjunctival pedicle or corneo-conjunctival transposition graft, should be considered for ulcers greater than one third of the stromal depth. Surgery may also be required for melting ulcers, to remove necrotic corneal tissue and stabilise the cornea. Recently, corneal collagen cross-linking has been reported as a successful treatment for infectious and noninfectious corneal melting in cats (Spiess et al., 2014). It involves using riboflavin as a photosensitiser followed by exposure to UVA light. The result is an increase in the biomechanical stability of the cornea, and also in reactive oxygen species (ROS)-induced damage to any microorganisms in the irradiated area. Availability of this treatment modality is likely to increase in the near future.

Surgical management of deep corneal ulcers

Conjunctival autografts can be used to manage deep corneal ulcers, descemetocoeles and keratectomy sites. Bulbar or palpebral conjunctiva with intact epithelium and underlying fibrous tissue, blood vessels and lymphatics is sutured into the defect, in order to provide tectonic support and promote healing.

Several different types of conjunctival grafts may be used to reinforce a weakened cornea including the conjunctival island, 360° conjunctival, conjunctival hood, conjunctival bridge, conjunctival pedicle and corneo-conjunctival transposition (CCT) grafts. The most useful in cats are the conjunctival pedicle and the CCT grafts. Technical expertise, microsurgical instrumentation and magnification, preferably with an operating microscope, are required (see Chapter 2).

Conjunctival pedicle graft

The rotational conjunctival pedicle graft is the most commonly performed surgical repair technique for deep or melting corneal ulcers. A thin strip of conjunctiva of sufficient length and width to reach and cover the corneal defect is freed from the underlying attached Tenon's capsule, and sutured into the edges of the corneal defect. For very deep ulcers, biomaterials such as those made from porcine small intestine or bladder or bovine pericardium, can first be sutured into the corneal defect to provide a scaffold for tissue regeneration before placement of a conjunctival pedicle graft (Goulle et al., 2012; Featherstone et al., 2001; Bussieres et al., 2004; Vanore et al., 2007). There are many advantages of the conjunctival pedicle graft over other procedures. It provides mechanical support, active fibroblasts and a continuous supply of serum containing growth factors and anticollagenases. It is also technically simpler to perform than a CCT. It offers the potential to save vision, allow monitoring of healing and direct application of topical medications (Figs. 44-46).

The disadvantages are significant scarring, insufficient tectonic support when used alone for full-thickness corneal defects and potential for corneal sequestrum recurrence if the pedicle is transected. The technique for conjunctival pedicle graft surgery is illustrated in Figure 47.

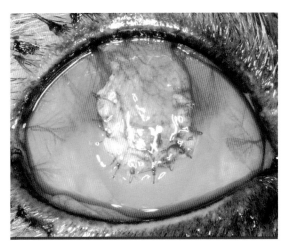

Figure 44. Conjunctival pedicle graft, one day after surgical removal of an axial corneal sequestrum. The graft is relatively thin and is well vascularised. Simple interrupted sutures hold the graft in place.

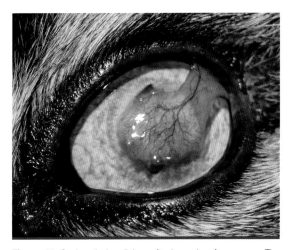

Figure 45. Conjunctival pedicle graft, six weeks after surgery. The graft is well vascularised and incorporated into the cornea.

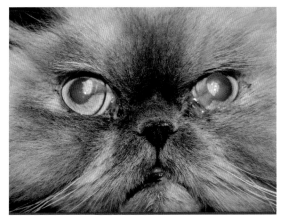

Figure 46. Bilateral conjunctival pedicle grafts, seven weeks after surgery to remove bilateral corneal sequestra. The conjunctival grafts are thin so they are not completely opaque.

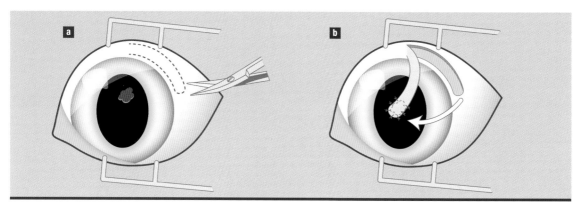

Figure 47. Conjunctival pedicle graft surgery. a) The rotational conjunctival graft is prepared by incising the (usually dorsolateral) bulbar conjunctiva with a Westcott's scissors and then undermining a thin graft parallel with the limbus using blunt dissection between the conjunctival mucosa and Tenon's capsule. The aim is to create a graft 1-2 mm wider than the corneal defect to allow for easier suturing and compensate for graft shrinkage. The graft should be 1-2 mm longer than necessary to prevent any tension on the globe when it is mobile postoperatively. b) The graft is anchored to the exposed corneal epithelium and stroma, ensuring good apposition between the conjunctival and corneal epithelia, using simple interrupted 8/0-9/0 absorbable sutures.

Corneo-conjunctival transposition

A corneo-conjunctival transposition (CCT) is a sliding advancement graft, used to repair a deep corneal stromal defect. It is comprised of partial thickness (usually half-thickness) cornea, the limbus and attached adjacent conjunctiva (Figs. 48 and 49). The advantage of this graft is that it transposes clear cornea into the area of the defect, allowing for transparency in this region (which is often central or within the visual axis) after healing. The transposed tissue is also stronger than conjunctiva alone and thus provides more mechanical support than a thinner conjunctival graft, and it is suitable to use for a focal full-thickness corneal defect. If there is uncontrolled bacterial or fungal infection, or progressive melting, the use of this type of graft should be delayed until the disease process has been stabilised. The surgical technique is outlined in Figure 50.

Surgery tip

A subconjunctival injection of saline may facilitate conjunctival dissection from the underlying Tenon's capsule.

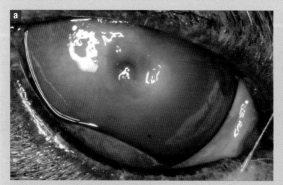
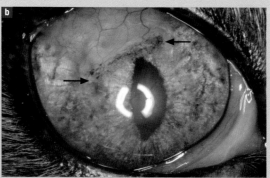

Figure 48. a) Right eye with an infected corneal stromal abscess that failed to respond to medical treatment and was starting to develop a sequestrum. b) The same eye four months after corneo-conjunctival transposition surgery. The transposed limbus can be seen (arrows), and thin vascularisation dorsal to this is from the conjunctival portion of the graft.

Surgery tip

When harvesting conjunctival autografts, care should be taken to remove as much of Tenon's capsule as possible to reduce the likelihood of tissue contraction and subsequent graft dehiscence.

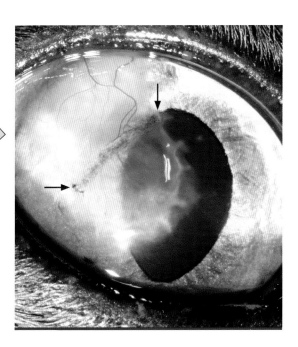

Figure 49. Two months after a corneo-conjunctival transposition surgery after removal of a deep corneal sequestrum. The corneal portion of the graft is slightly opaque but has healed well. The conjunctival portion is vascularised as expected, and the transposed limbus is visible (arrows).

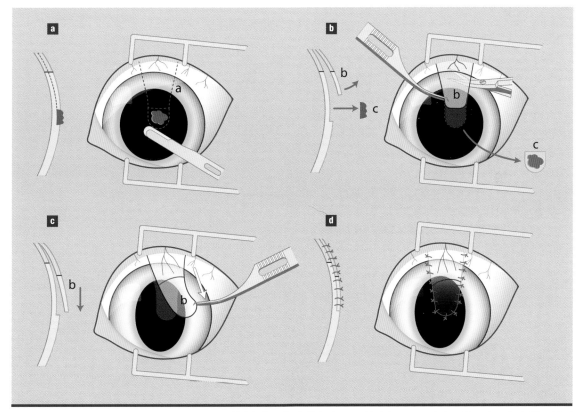

Figure 50. Corneo-conjunctival transposition surgery. a) Slightly diverging half-depth corneal incisions are made from the outer extent of the defect out to the limbus. b) The conjunctival epithelium is incised and a thin but wide conjunctival graft is prepared by dissecting the mucosa from Tenon's capsule with a Westcott's scissors. c) The cornea is gently grasped with Colibri forceps next to the defect and half-depth lamellar dissection is continued out to the limbus. The graft is mobilised by incising beneath the limbus at the junction between the corneal and conjunctival aspects of the graft. The corneal lesion is prepared by dissecting any necrotic tissue or replacement of any prolapsed iris. d) The graft is then sutured into place with simple interrupted sutures, a continuous suture, or combinations of both.

Exposure keratitis

Exposure keratitis occurs due to incomplete eyelid blinking (lagophthalmos) and premature evaporation of the precorneal tear film. Lagophthalmos may be breed-related, in which it is associated with brachycephalia, or relate to conditions such as eyelid coloboma, exophthalmos (associated with retrobulbar space-occupying lesions), hydrophthalmos (associated with glaucoma), orbital fractures and facial (CN VII) or trigeminal (CN V) nerve paralysis (Fig. 51). Treatment of exposure keratitis involves correction of the underlying problem and the use of ocular lubrication. A temporary tarsorrhaphy or permanent canthoplasty may also be indicated in certain situations (see Chapter 5).

Corneal laceration

Corneal lacerations usually result from cat claw injuries. Full thickness (penetrating) injuries may be associated with hyphaema, iris prolapse, fibrinous uveitis, hypopyon, anterior chamber collapse and lens rupture (Fig. 52). Careful examination is required to assess the depth of penetration, the limits of the laceration (i.e. does it extend beyond the limbus?) and the presence of any lens involvement. The depth of the laceration is most easily assessed using slit-lamp biomicroscopy if available (see Chapter 1). Fluorescein should be applied to assess corneal integrity by way of the Seidel test (see Chapter 1). Extension of the laceration beyond the limbus and into the sclera may be associated with damage to the underlying ciliary body, which can lead to retinal detachment. If iris prolapse is not present, the pupil should be dilated with 0.5 % tropicamide or 1 % atropine to allow examination of the lens. Rupture of the anterior lens capsule can result in severe and progressive phacoclastic uveitis that requires urgent and aggressive treatment in order to save the eye. Intraocular bacterial infection can also result in delayed septic implantation endophthalmitis. If the lens has been damaged, prompt referral should be recommended, as surgical lendectomy may be required.

Superficial corneal lacerations are treated similarly to an uncomplicated ulcer, and tend to heal well. If there is a loose flap of epithelium and anterior stroma, this can be sharply resected to aid healing (Fig. 53). Deeper

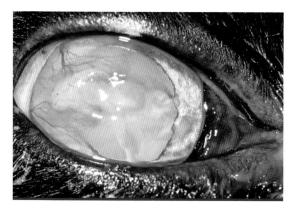

Figure 51. Exposure keratitis which occurred as a result of exophthalmos, the cause of which was retrobulbar squamous cell carcinoma. There is corneal neovascularisation and the central cornea is roughened and dull, due to the presence of a horizontally aligned stromal corneal ulcer.

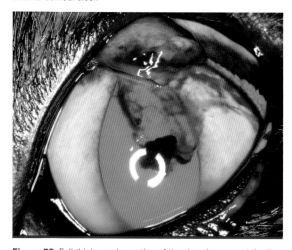

Figure 52. Full thickness laceration of the dorsal cornea at the limbus has resulted in iris prolapse. The pupil appears elongated and there is some hyphaema.

lacerations that result in gaping of the wound edges resulting in poor corneal apposition require corneal suturing with 8/0 or 9/0 absorbable suture (Fig. 54). Uveal prolapse or continued loss of aqueous from the anterior chamber are further indications for corneal suturing (Fig. 55). The length of the lens capsule tear is sometimes used as a prognostic factor to determine whether medical or surgical treatment is appropriate. However, this can be difficult to determine if there is hyphaema or fibrinous uveitis. Early prophylactic lens removal to prevent vision-threatening complications such as glaucoma and endophthalmitis has been recommended when there is substantial disruption of the lens cortex, or for lens capsule tears of 1.5 mm or greater.

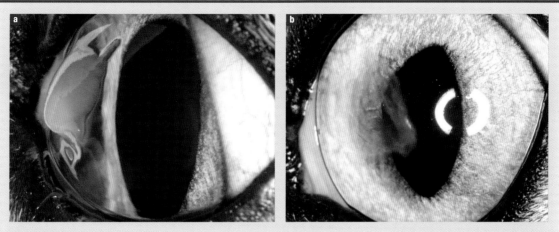

Figure 53. Corneal laceration, partial thickness. a) Side profile view of a partial thickness corneal laceration injury, with a thickened protruding oedematous flap of cornea. b) Five days after sharp excision of the flap without suturing; the defect is healing well.

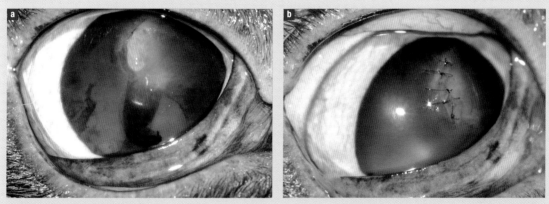

Figure 54. Corneal laceration, full thickness. a) Cat claw injury to the dorsal cornea is sealed with a thick clot of fibrin and aqueous. Hyphaema is present, and the pupil has been pharmacologically dilated to check the integrity of the anterior lens capsule. b) Seven days after direct corneal suturing with five simple interrupted 8/0 polyglactin 910 sutures, corneal oedema remains but the wound is healing well.

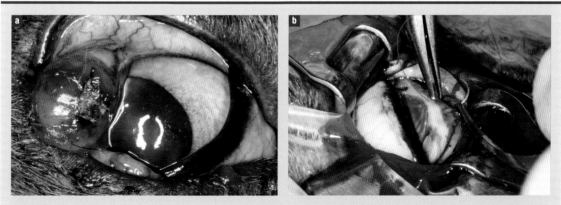

Figure 55. Full thickness corneal laceration injury as the result of a cat claw injury. a) There is a large peripheral corneal wound through which the iris has prolapsed, resulting in dyscoria (a deformed pupil shape). There is a protruding brown aqueous clot. b) Corneal repair under general anaesthesia involves replacing the prolapsed iris and direct suturing of the corneal laceration.

However, it has been found that fibrinous uveitis associated with lens capsule disruption can lead to subsequent fibrous metaplasia of the anterior lens capsule with sufficient repair to avoid the need for surgery in some cases. Medical management with topical antibiotics, NSAIDs and mydriatics in addition to systemic broad spectrum antibiotics and NSAIDs has been associated with a favourable outcome (Paulsen and Kass, 2012).

Corneal foreign body

Superficial foreign bodies (e.g. flakes of paint, husks of plant seeds) initially adhere to the tear film with surface tension (Fig. 56), but with time they can become embedded within the corneal epithelium and superficial stroma (Fig. 57). They may be difficult to see if they induce chemosis, or are located either behind the nictitans or deep within the conjunctival fornices. Superficial corneal foreign bodies can often be removed under topical anaesthesia alone by flushing or by gentle debridement with a cotton-tipped swab a 23-25 G needle.

Foreign bodies that are more deeply embedded within the cornea require more cautious removal under general anaesthesia, as they may be penetrating (with an entry wound) or perforating (with both an entry and exit wound, i.e. full thickness) (Figs. 58 and 59). A Seidel test is used to assess for aqueous leakage (see Chapter 1) and the pupil should be dilated to determine if there is damage to the anterior lens capsule. A foreign body may injure the cornea but not be present at the time of examination, and usually a tract is visible along the course of entry/exit, with resulting inflammation (Fig. 60). The techniques appropriate for removal depend on several factors, and are illustrated in Figure 61. Splinters and thorns may be removed by incising any overlying cornea using a microsurgical scalpel blade, and then carefully dislodging them with a fine needle. Corneal suturing or graft placement may be required depending on the size and depth of any resultant stromal defect. Penetrating foreign bodies may be approached externally by impaling them with two needles and removing them, followed by suturing of the corneal wound. However, in the case of a barbed thorn or when the majority of the foreign

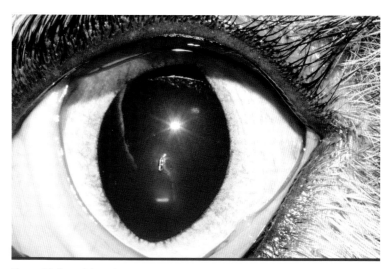

Figure 56. A small thorn foreign body is visible proud of, but adhered to, the central cornea. It was removed with a flush of sterile saline.

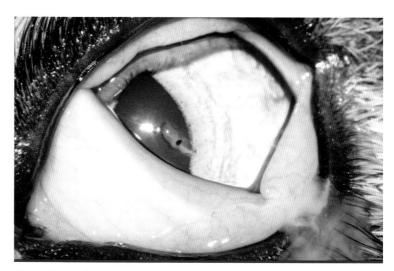

Figure 57. A small thorn was deeply embedded within the central cornea, causing some aqueous leakage. The thorn was removed under general anaesthesia, carefully using two needles to impale and prise out the thorn. The tiny wound sealed quickly and suturing was not required.

body is already within the anterior chamber, removal via a remote corneal incision may be necessary. After inserting viscoelastic through a 3 mm corneo-limbal incision, a forceps is inserted into the anterior chamber to gently pull the foreign body deeper into the eye, until it is free and can be removed through the surgical incision. Both the wound created by the foreign body and surgical incision in the peripheral cornea will require surgical repair. Postoperative management with topical antibiotics and mydriatics and systemic NSAIDs is indicated. Penetrating corneal injuries should also be treated with systemic antibiotics.

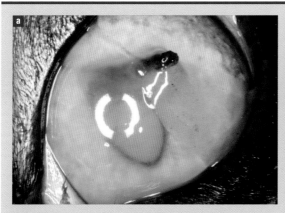 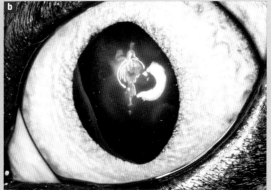

Figure 58. Thorn penetrating the cornea and entering the anterior chamber. a) A small section of the thorn is present outside the cornea but the majority is in the anterior chamber. The pupil is small but the lens escaped damage. Under general anaesthesia, a peripheral limbal incision was made to remove the thorn from the anterior chamber, and both that incision and the central corneal wound were sutured. b) The central corneal wound is visible healing well seven days after surgery; the peripheral surgical wound is at the ten o'clock position and is not visible.

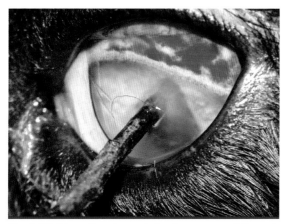 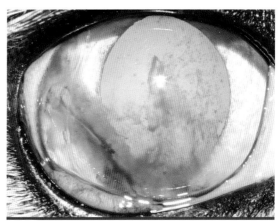

Figure 59. A large thorn is penetrating the cornea, and also penetrated through the lens into the vitreous. The eye was enucleated.

Figure 60. Foreign body penetration tract, with the entry point at the lateral cornea. There is fibrin and cellular material in the anterior chamber. The tract of the foreign body (presumed thorn) is visible but the thorn itself was not present at the time of examination. The pupil has been pharmacologically dilated.

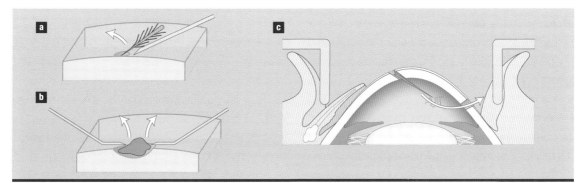

Figure 61. Removal of corneal foreign bodies. a) A superficial foreign body is dislodged with a 23-25 G sterile needle by lifting the edge away from the cornea. b) Two needles are used to impale a thorn penetrating deeply into the cornea, and the direction of pull is illustrated. c) A thorn broken at the corneal surface is removed via a remote perilimbal corneal incision, after which both wounds need to be sutured with 8/0 or 9/0 absorbable suture.

Corneal epithelial inclusion cyst

Epithelial inclusion cysts are uncommon but are an important differential diagnosis when a mass lesion is present within the cornea. They typically arise after a corneal injury or after corneal surgery (e.g. at the site of sutures) as a result of epithelial downgrowth into the corneal stroma with associated epithelial proliferation and cyst formation. The eye is usually comfortable. A superficial smooth white-cream focal mass with variable vascularisation is present, with no uptake of fluorescein (Fig. 62). Diagnosis is usually made by examination although definitive diagnosis may be made following histopathological examination of an excisional biopsy harvested by superficial keratectomy (which is usually curative). Histopathologic findings are of a nonkeratinised squamous epithelial lining within the corneal stroma, containing a lumen that is filled with keratin or mucin and abundant neutrophils.

Neoplasia

Neoplasia of the cornea or sclera is very rare in cats. Limbal melanocytomas are the most common primary tumour to affect both the cornea and sclera. They initially develop in the superficial sclera, and grow slowly, with minimal invasion, towards the limbus (Fig. 63). Treatment of choice is surgical resection with or without adjunctive cryotherapy, laser photocoagulation or strontium plesiotherapy, followed by conjunctival grafting. Feline limbal melanocytomas are generally benign, although there is a single report of a three-year-old cat that presented with suspected metastatic disease 31 months following after surgical removal of a limbal melanocytoma (Betton

et al., 1999). Squamous cell carcinoma can occasionally invade the cornea and sclera as an extension of conjunctival, eyelid or orbital disease. Corneal haemangiomas and haemangiosarcomas are very rare, and are most likely to arise after chronic corneal neovascularisation (Fig. 64). There has been a single case report of a fibrous histiocytoma in a cat (Smith et al., 1976).

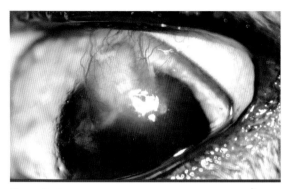

Figure 62. Corneal epithelial inclusion cyst in a cat with a history of a corneal ulcer a year previously. There is a cream-coloured vascularised thickening of the dorsal cornea.

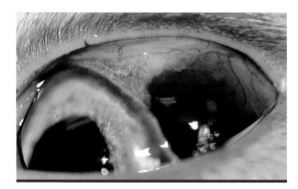

Figure 63. Epibulbar melanoma. A focal pigmented mass is visible on the sclera beneath the conjunctiva. Courtesy of Neil Wilson.

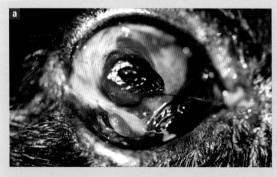
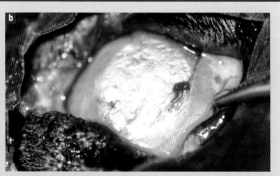

Figure 64. Corneal haemangiosarcoma. a) Chronic corneal ulceration had resulted in a corneal sequestrum and vascularisation. b) Intraoperative appearance of the cornea immediately after successful keratectomy of the diseased cornea.

References

ANDREW SE, TOU S, BROOKS DE (2001). Corneoconjunctival transposition for the treatment of feline corneal sequestra: a retrospective study of 17 cases (1990-1998). *Veterinary Ophthalmology*; 4:107-111.

BETTON A, HEALY LN, ENGLISH RV et al. (1999). Atypical limbal melanoma in a cat. *Journal of Veterinary Internal Medicine*; 13:379-381.

BUSSIERES M, KROHNE SG, STILES J et al. (2004). The use of porcine small intestinal submucosa for the repair of full-thickness corneal defects in dogs, cats and horses. *Veterinary Ophthalmology*; 7:352-359.

DEAN E, MEUNIER V (2013). Feline eosinophilic keratoconjunctivitis: A retrospective study of 45 cases (56 eyes). *Journal of Feline Medicine and Surgery*; 15:661-666.

FEATHERSTONE HJ, SANSOM J (2004). Feline corneal sequestra: a review of 64 cases (80 eyes) from 1993 to 2000. *Veterinary Ophthalmology*; 7:213-227.

FEATHERSTONE HJ, SANSOM J, HEINRICH CL (2001). The use of porcine small intestinal submucosa in ten cases of feline corneal disease. *Veterinary Ophthalmology*; 4:147-153.

FONTENELLE JP, POWELL CC, VEIR JK et al. (2008). Effect of topical ophthalmic application of cidofovir on experimentally induced primary ocular feline herpesvirus-1 infection in cats. *American Journal of Veterinary Research*; 69:289-293.

GLOVER TL, NASISSE MP, DAVIDSON MG (1994). Acute bullous keratopathy in the cat. *Veterinary and Comparative Ophthalmology*; 4:66-70.

GOULLE F (2012). Use of porcine small intestinal submucosa for corneal reconstruction in dogs and cats: 106 cases. *Journal of Small Animal Practice*; 53:34-43.

JÉGOU JP, TROMEUR F (2014). Superficial keratectomy for chronic corneal ulcers refractory to medical treatment in 36 cats. *Veterinary Ophthalmology*; DOI: 10.1111/vop.12153.

KAUFMAN HE, VARNELL ED, THOMPSON HW (1998). Trifluridine, cidofovir, and penciclovir in the treatment of experimental herpetic keratitis. *Archives of Ophthalmology*; 116:777-780.

LA CROIX NC, VAN DER WOERDT A, OLIVERO DK (2001). Nonhealing corneal ulcers in cats: 29 cases (1991-1999). *Journal of the American Veterinary Medical Association*; 218:733-735.

LIM CC, REILLY CM, THOMASY SM et al. (2009). Effects of feline herpesvirus type 1 on tear film break-up time, Schirmer tear test results, and conjunctival goblet cell density in experimentally infected cats. *American Journal of Veterinary Research*; 70:394-403.

MAGGS DJ, CLARKE HE (2004). *In vitro* efficacy of ganciclovir, cidofovir, penciclovir, foscarnet, idoxuridine, and acyclovir against feline herpesvirus type 1. *American Journal of Veterinary Research*; 65:399-403.

NASISSE MP, GUY JS, DAVIDSON MG et al. (1989). Experimental ocular herpesvirus infection in the cat. Sites of viral replication, clinical features and effects of corticosteroid administration. *Investigative Ophthalmology and Visual Science*; 30:1758-1768.

PAULSEN ME, KASS PH (2012). Traumatic corneal laceration with associated lens capsule disruption: a retrospective study of 77 clinical cases from 1999 to 2009. *Veterinary Ophthalmology*; 15:355-368.

PEÑA GIMÉNEZ MTP, FARIÑA IM (1998). Lamellar keratoplasty for the treatment of feline corneal sequestrum. *Veterinary Ophthalmology*; 1:163-166.

SMITH JS, BISTNER S, RIIS R (1976). Infiltrative corneal lesions resembling fibrous histiocytoma: clinical and pathologic findings in six dogs and one cat. *Journal of the American Veterinary Medical Association*; 169:722-726.

SPIESS AK, SAPIENZA JS, MAYORDOMO A (2009). Treatment of proliferative feline eosinophilic keratitis with topical 1.5% cyclosporine: 35 cases. *Veterinary Ophthalmology*; 12:132-137.

SPIESS BM, POT SA, FLORIN M et al. (2014). Corneal collagen cross-linking (CXL) for the treatment of melting keratitis in cats and dogs: a pilot study. *Veterinary Ophthalmology*; 17:1-11.

STILES J (2013). Feline ophthalmology. In: Gelatt KN, Gilger BC, Kern TJ (Eds) *Veterinary Ophthalmology* 5th Ed. John Wiley and Sons, Ames, Iowa, USA, 1477-1559.

THERON L (2007). *The Wasmannia auropunctata* linked keratopathy (WALK) hypothesis – the Polynesian case. http://hdl.handle.net/2268/652

THOMASY SM, COVERT JC, STANLEY SD et al. (2012). Pharmacokinetics of famciclovir and penciclovir in tears following oral administration of famciclovir to cats: A pilot study. *Veterinary Ophthalmology*; 15:299-306.

THOMASY SM, LIM CC, REILLY CM et al. (2011) Evaulation of orally administered famciclovir in cats experimentally infected with feline herpesvirus 1. *American Journal of Veterinary Research*; 72:85-95.

VANORE M, CHAHORY S, PAYEN G et al. (2007). Surgical repair of deep melting ulcers with porcine small intestinal submucosa (SIS) graft in dogs and cats. *Veterinary Ophthalmology*; 10:93-99.

WILLIAMS DL, FITZMAURICE T, LAY L et al. (2004). Efficacy of antiviral agents in feline herpetic keratitis: results of an *in vitro* study. *Current Eye Research*; 29:215-218.

8

The uveal tract

Anatomy and function

The uveal tract is the middle vascular layer of the globe. The anterior uvea consists of the iris and ciliary body, and the posterior uvea is the choroid (Fig. 1).

The iris

The iris functions to control the amount of light entering the eye by varying the size of the pupil. Histologically, it is made up of three layers; the anterior border layer, the stroma (containing the sphincter muscle) and the posterior epithelium (containing the dilator muscle). The anterior border layer is made up of fibroblasts and melanocytes. It has no epithelial surface and therefore interacts directly with the aqueous humour of the anterior chamber. The iris stroma consists of loose connective tissue containing fibroblasts, melanocytes and nonfenestrated capillaries. The anterior uvea receives a rich blood supply from the lateral and medial long posterior ciliary arteries and veins, which enter the iris near its root and form the major arterial circle. There are no lymphatic vessels. The iridal sphincter muscle is located within the posterior stroma near the pupil margin and is made up of smooth muscle fibres which interlace dorsally

and ventrally (Fig. 2). This arrangement gives rise to the vertical slit-shaped pupil when constricted. It is innervated primarily by parasympathetic fibres of just two short nerves arising from the ciliary ganglion – the malar and nasal short ciliary nerves. The posterior iris is made up of the posterior iridal pigmented epithelium and the iridal dilator muscle. The heavily pigmented posterior epithelium of the iris is continuous posteriorly with the inner, nonpigmented epithelium of the ciliary body. The iridal dilator muscle is composed of radially oriented smooth muscle fibres extending from the iris root towards the pupillary margin. Innervation is primarily by sympathetic fibres. The iris rests on the anterior lens surface. When this support is lost, as occurs with lens subluxation or luxation, the iris can appear to tremble with globe movement, a phenomenon called 'iridodonesis'.

The ciliary body

The ciliary body is continuous anteriorly with the base of the iris and posteriorly with the choroid. The ciliary body has an approximately triangular outline in sagittal cross-section, and is comprised of the anterior pars plicata and the posterior pars plana. The pars plicata contains numerous folds, termed ciliary processes, which are the

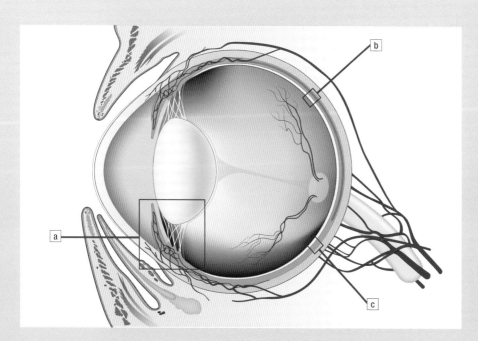

Figure 1. Schematic cross-sectional anatomy diagram and photomicrograph of the uveal tract.
a. Anterior segment of the eye, showing the iris and ciliary body.
  AC = anterior chamber
  I = iris
  PC = posterior chamber
  CC = ciliary cleft
  CB = ciliary body
  TM = corneoscleral trabecular meshwork
  S = sclera
b. Tapetal fundus region.
  RPE = Retinal Pigment Epithelium
c. Nontapetal fundus region.
  Photomicrographs courtesy of Karen Dunn, FOCUS-EyePathLab.

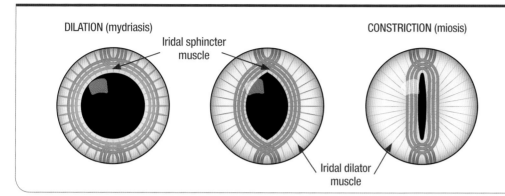

Figure 2. Position of the interlacing sphincter muscle (under parasympathetic control) and radially-orientated dilator muscle (under sympathetic control) during dilation, resting and during constriction in the vertically-orientated slit-shaped feline pupil.

primary source of aqueous humor formation. The pars plana is flat in comparison, and extends from the ciliary processes to the periphery of the retina, terminating at the ora ciliaris retinae. Histologically the ciliary processes consist of two layers of epithelium and a core of stroma which is rich in blood vessels and smooth muscle fibres. The inner nonpigmented epithelium is confluent with both the innermost layer of the posterior iris epithelium and with the neurosensory retina. The outer heavily-pigmented metabolically-active layer lies directly under the nonpigmented layer and is continuous with retinal epithelium and with the outermost layer of the posterior iris epithelium. In addition to secreting

aqueous humour, the bilayered ciliary epithelium also secretes extracellular matrix proteins that develop into the lens zonular ligaments, and hyaluronic acid which is a component of the vitreous. The stroma also contains the meridionally arranged ciliary smooth muscle, which is involved in accommodation. Aqueous humour production occurs within the ciliary body stroma by means of ultrafiltration from the capillaries. There is a potential space between the sclera and ciliary body termed the supraciliary space. Together with the more posteriorly located suprachoroidal space, these areas play a role in the uveoscleral ('unconventional') pathway of aqueous outflow.

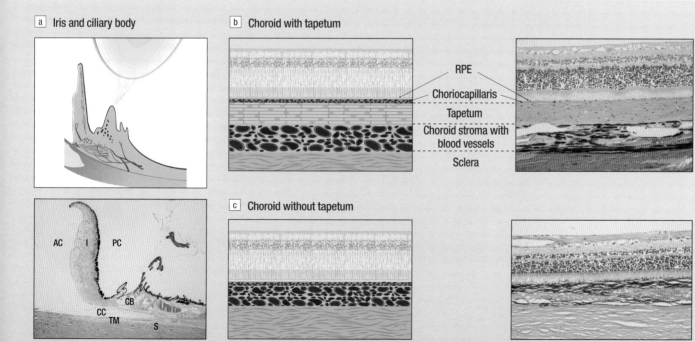

a Iris and ciliary body

b Choroid with tapetum

RPE
Choriocapillaris
Tapetum
Choroid stroma with blood vessels
Sclera

c Choroid without tapetum

AC   I   PC
CC
CB
TM   S

The choroid

The choroid is located between the retina and the sclera. Histologically it consists of five layers; Bruch's membrane (adjacent to the retinal pigment epithelium), the choriocapillaris, a cellular tapetum lucidum, the stroma (which contains large vessels) and the suprachoroid. The retina is highly metabolically active and relies on the choroid to remain functional. The choriocapillaris is a greatly fenestrated capillary bed supplying nutrition to the outer retina. The tapetum lucidum is a highly reflective layer made up of regularly arranged cells containing riboflavin-zinc rodlets.

The blood-ocular barrier

The blood-ocular barrier functions to separate the systemic circulation from the intraocular environment in order to regulate the composition of aqueous humour and nutrition of intraocular tissues. It is a physiological semi-permeable barrier that is made up of the blood-aqueous and blood-retinal barriers. The blood-aqueous barrier is formed by tight junctions between cells of the inner nonpigmented ciliary body epithelium and by nonfenestrated iridal blood vessels (Fig. 3). The blood-retinal barrier is formed by tight junctions in the retinal pigment epithelium and nonfenestrated retinal vessels. The blood-aqueous

> → The ciliary body is the principal source of aqueous humor production (by active secretion and ultrafiltration), controls accommodation and is important in the control of intraocular pressure (IOP).

barrier prevents most large molecules and cells from entering the eye and limits the immune response against the internal eye thus making it an immune-privileged site. Breakdown of the blood-aqueous barrier (as occurs with uveitis) results in modification of the composition of aqueous humour, vitreous or sub-retinal space, primarily by increased quantities of protein, cells or blood.

Congenital conditions
Congenital disorders of pigmentation

The degree of pigmentation in the normal uvea varies and, as a result, the colour of the iris and the appearance of the fundus can differ as part of normal variation. However, some congenital defects of ocular development are related to colour dilution in the uveal tract.

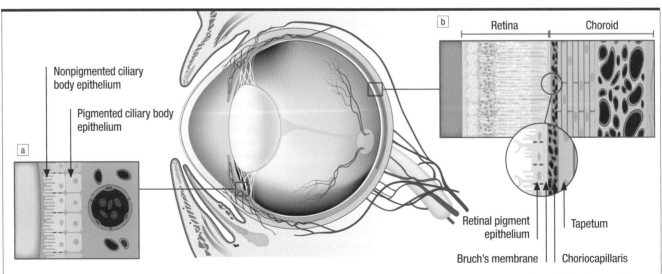

Figure 3. The blood-ocular barrier. a) The blood-aqueous barrier is comprised of an epithelial barrier located in the nonpigmented layer of the ciliary epithelium and in the posterior iridial epithelium, and by the endothelium of the iridal vessels. b) The blood-retinal barrier is comprised of an outer barrier in the retinal pigment epithelium and an inner barrier in the endothelium of the retinal vessels.

Albinism

Albinism is a congenital absence of melanin pigment. True albinism (complete absence of pigment) is very rare. Partial albinism (subalbinism) is much more common, and refers to a reduction in ocular pigmentation. Subalbinotic cats have blue irides because of the relative lack of melanin within the iris stroma (Fig. 4) and many affected cats have a white coat. Waardenburg syndrome occurs in some blue-eyed white cats, and consists of deafness, heterochromia irides (see below) and a white coat color. It is inherited as a dominant trait with complete penetrance for the white coat and blue irides. Chédiak-Higashi syndrome is inherited as an autosomal recessive trait and has been reported in Persians with a blue-smoke coat colour and pale irides. Affected cats have platelet function defects and may develop nuclear cataracts, tapetal degeneration and nontapetal fundus hypopigmentation.

Iris heterochromia

Heterochromia iridum (or irides) refers to a difference in iris coloration between the two eyes (Fig. 4), while heterochromia iridis refers to a difference in coloration of different regions of the iris of the same eye (Fig. 5). Chronic inflammation and uveal neoplasms can also lead to iris colour changes (see later).

Incomplete iris development

A wide range of congenital developmental defects can affect the uveal tract. These range in severity from complete lack of uveal tissue (aniridia - very rare) to lack of development of a segment of the uveal tract (coloboma - also very uncommon) or incomplete iris development (iris hypoplasia - uncommon).

Iris coloboma

Congenital absence of some or all iris tissue is termed an iris coloboma. So-called 'typical' colobomas arise in the area of the optic fissure (approximately 6 to 7 o'clock position) and arise due to its incomplete closure during embryological development. 'Atypical' colobomas arise in other areas of the eye. A variety of defects can occur including dyscoria (a misshapen pupil), an eccentric pupil or aniridia.

Iris hypoplasia

Iris hypoplasia arises due to defective differentiation of the neural crest. Compared with coloboma, it represents the milder end of the spectrum of incomplete expansion of the optic cup. The iris stromal tissue of lighter-coloured irides is more often affected, but pigmented irides may also be hypoplastic (Fig. 6).

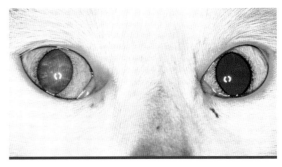

Figure 4. Heterochromia irides in a white cat. The right iris is pale yellow in colour and there is a green tapetal reflex. The left iris is blue and the fundic reflection is red, indicating a lack of posterior uveal pigmentation and tapetal development.

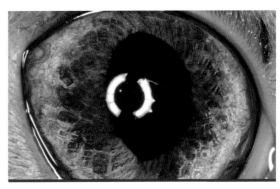

Figure 5. Heterochromia iridis in a ginger cat. Two distinct colours can be seen in the iris, with tan-brown and blue regions.

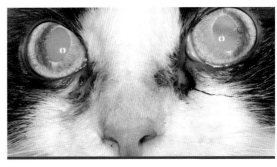

Figure 6. Bilateral iris hypoplasia in a 6-month-old cat. The periphery of the iris is blue in colour. The pupillary zone of the iris is so thin that the tapetal reflex can be seen through it.

Persistent pupillary membrane

Persistent pupillary membrane (PPM) is the most common form of anterior segment dysgenesis. It arises due to incomplete regression of embryonal tissues, which normally disappear by six weeks of age. They appear as thin strands of iridal tissue arising from the iris collarette (Figs. 7 and 8). They occasionally span the pupil and may be attached to other PPMs (Fig. 9), to the anterior lens capsule, or to the posterior cornea (Figs. 10 and 11). In the latter instance, they appear similar to acquired synechial adhesions (Fig. 12). The distinction can usually be made by determining whether the uveal tissue arises from the iris collarette (PPM) or the pupil margin (synechiae). PPMs are sometimes associated with upper eyelid agenesis (see Chapter 5).

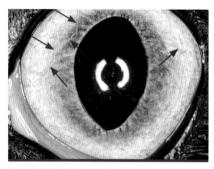

Figure 7. Persistent pupillary membrane (arrows), retaining the colour of the adjacent iris, coursing along the iris collarette dorso-medially, with a smaller remnant dorso-laterally.

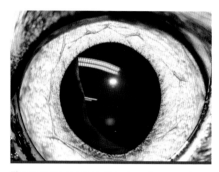

Figure 8. Iris-to-iris persistent pupillary membrane remnants along the iris collarette. Courtesy of Filip Nachtegaele.

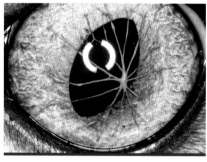

Figure 9. Persistent pupillary membrane remnants arising from the iris collarette and forming a network that meets centrally in the anterior chamber.

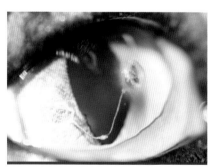

Figure 10. A single persistent pupillary membrane remnant arises from the iris collarette and extends forwards to attach to the cornea, resulting in a focal corneal opacity (leukoma).

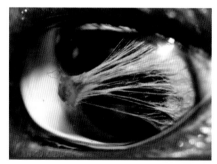

Figure 11. Multiple fine persistent pupillary membrane remnants arising from the surface of the lateral iris extend forwards to attach to the cornea, resulting in a focal corneal opacity (leukoma). Courtesy of Filip Nachtegaele.

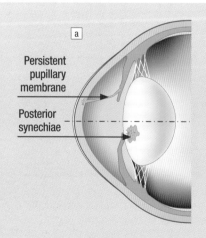

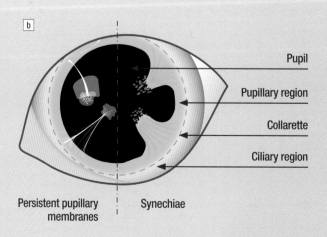

Figure 12. Persistent pupillary membranes and synechiae.
a) Cross section of an eye with a persistent pupillary membrane dorsally and posterior synechiae ventrally.
b) Persistent pupillary membranes arise from the iris collarette. Synechiae involve the pupil margin.

Acquired conditions

Ectropion uveae

The normal pigmented ruff at the pupil margin is an extension of the heavily pigmented posterior iris epithelium and is occasionally visible in colour-dilute eyes, i.e. those with a blue iris. Ectropion uveae is the term used to describe abnormal eversion of the pigmented ruff around the pupillary margin (Fig. 13). It may be congenital but is most commonly seen after previous iris inflammation often arising as a result of the formation of preiridal fibrovascular membranes (PIFM, see later).

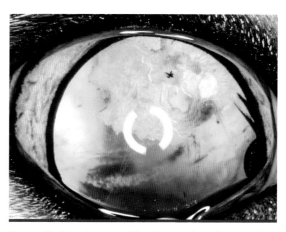

Figure 13. Ectropion uveae. The pigmented pupillary margin is everted in an eye with multiple congenital ocular defects including cataract and a uveal cyst.

Uveal cysts

Uveal cysts are not very common in cats. They can be congenital, and arise from incomplete fusion between the two layers of neuroectoderm which go on to form the bilayered iris and ciliary epithelia. They are more commonly acquired, in which case the pigmented epithelium of the iris or the inner epithelium of the ciliary body undergo spontaneous cystic hyperplasia. Clinically, they usually present as multiple, smooth, dark brown or black masses at the periphery of the pupil remaining attached to posterior iris (Figs. 14 and 15). Occasionally they may cause anterior displacement of the iris resulting in shallowing of the anterior chamber, potentially leading to increased intraocular pressure (IOP) (Gemensky-Metzler and Wilkie, 2004). The main differential diagnosis for iris cysts is uveal melanoma. Although useful in dogs, transillumination is less useful in distinguishing the two conditions in cats as the cysts tend to be more heavily pigmented. Ultrasonography, however, is a useful diagnostic tool. Treatment using the diode laser to deflate and coagulate the cysts has been reported (Gemensky-Metzler and Wilkie, 2004), although treatment is only required if they obstruct vision or cause pathological elevation of IOP.

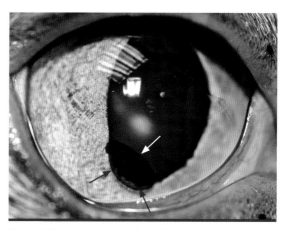

Figure 14. Uveal cyst. A pigmented, partly translucent smooth mass in the anterior chamber, attached at the pupil border (arrows).

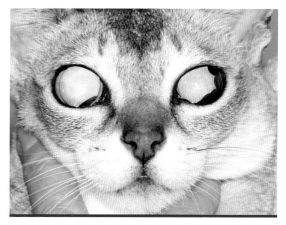

Figure 15. Bilateral uveal cysts. Multiple darkly-pigmented uveal cysts are visible behind the pupil. Vision was unaffected in the 12-year-old Singapura.

Examination tip

Pharmacological pupil dilation aids visualisation of uveal cysts which usually remain attached to the posterior iris rather than being free-floating.

Iris pigmentation

As discussed previously, the iris can vary in the degree of pigmentation at birth. Acquired changes in pigmentation may also arise due to age, metabolic factors (e.g. portosystemic shunt), inflammation or neoplasia.

Iridal melanosis

Acquired pigmentation of the iris can be a benign change resulting either from an increase in melanin content of melanocytes (hypertrophy) or an increase in the total number of melanocytes (hyperplasia).

A nevus (syn. freckle) is a benign focal, well-circumscribed, nonthickened region of iris hyperpigmentation resulting from an increase in melanin content of iris melanocytes. Nevi may be solitary or multiple, unilateral or bilateral, and are slowly progressive (Figs. 16 and 17). Iris melanosis is a more extensive benign change involving progressive iris pigmentation that typically begins in middle age (Figs. 18-20). Hyperpigmentation is restricted to the iridal surface but there is potential for future malignant transformation into diffuse iris melanoma and therefore careful monitoring is advised.

Chronic anterior uveitis can also result in darkening of the iris due to diffuse hyperpigmentation (Fig. 21). This arises due to stimulation of intracellular melanin production by melanocytes.

Copper-coloured iris

The iris of some cats with portosystemic shunts develops a copper or golden colour (Fig. 22). The colour change usually reverses after successful surgical occlusion of the shunt. Despite this, controversy exists as to whether there is a true disease association.

Iris atrophy

Atrophy of the iridal sphincter and dilator muscles results in thinning of the iris. This leads to mydriasis and a reduction in the pupillary light reflex (PLR). Iris atrophy may occur after prolonged inflammation (Fig. 23) or, less commonly, may be age-related.

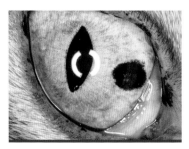

Figure 16. Iris nevus. A focal region of non-thickened dark iris pigmentation is present.

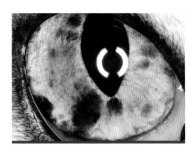

Figure 17. Iris nevi. Multifocal nonthickened darkly pigmented regions are present three years after the appearance of the initial iris nevus.

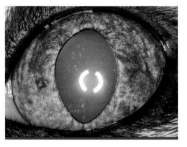

Figure 18. Iris melanosis. Diffuse iris pigmentation is present which is confined to the surface of the iris.

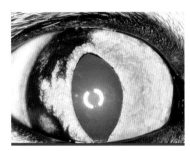

Figure 19. Iris melanosis. Dark pigmentation is present in the peripheral lateral iris, prompting careful evaluation for early diffuse iris melanoma.

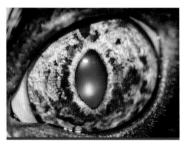

Figure 20. Iris melanosis. Extensive multifocal pigmentation of the iris surface, requiring monitoring for transformation to diffuse iris melanoma.

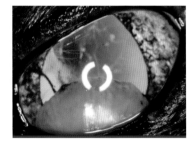

Figure 21. Chronic uveitis has resulted in anterior lens luxation, cataract and multifocal dark pigmentation of the iris surface.

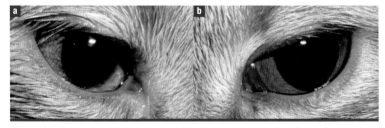

Figure 22. a) A healthy ginger cat showing a typical iris colour. b) Copper-coloured iris. A 6-month-old Domestic shorthair presented with an extra-hepatic portosystemic shunt. Both irides were copper-coloured. Courtesy of Kelly Bowlt.

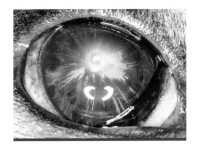

Figure 23. Iris atrophy. Ocular trauma 5 years previously had resulted in globe rupture, iris bombé and glaucoma. The inflammation and hypertension settled but regions of the iris atrophied as a result. There is a white scar in the central cornea and the tapetal reflex is bright due to retinal degeneration.

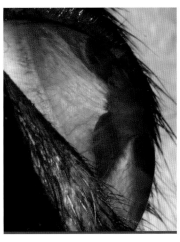

Figure 24. Anterior synechiae from a side-view perspective. The iris tissue at the border of the pupil is adhered to the cornea, both ventro-medially and ventro-laterally.

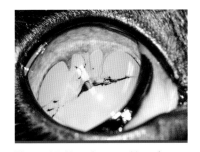

Figure 25. Posterior synechiae after recovery from uveitis. The pigment from the posterior iris surface was deposited on the anterior lens capsule when the pupil was miotic, and some adhesions of iris tissue remain. Courtesy of Filip Nachtegaele.

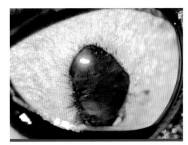

Figure 26. Posterior synechiae causing dyscoria in a cat that suffered blunt trauma that resulted in uveitis and cataract formation.

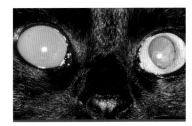

Figure 27. Lipaemic aqueous in the right eye (and very mild lipaemic aqueous in the left eye) of a young Burmese cross following a fatty meal.

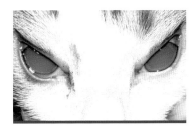

Figure 28. Bilateral lipaemic aqueous and conjunctival hyperaemia in a 12-year-old cat with diabetes mellitus secondary to chronic megestrol acetate treatment.

Synechiae

Synechiae are adhesions between the iris and other ocular structures (see Fig. 12). Anteror synechiae are most often caused by perforating ocular injury with incarceration of the iris within the wound (Fig. 24). Posterior synechiae are fibrinous adhesions of the pupillary margin of the iris or the posterior iris epithelium to the anterior lens capsule (Figs. 25 and 26). They can cause dyscoria and a reduced PLR due to mechanical restriction of movement. Adhesions forming around the entire circumference of the pupil, termed iris bombé, obstructs aqueous flow into the anterior chamber and almost invariably result in glaucoma.

Lipaemic aqueous

Lipaemic aqueous results from leakage of lipid from the systemic circulation into the anterior segment of the eye giving rise to a 'milky' appearance of the aqueous humour (Figs. 27 and 28). Lipaemic aqueous can occur as a result of primary inherited hyperliproteinaemia, such as inherited hyperchylomicronaemia in the Burmese (Kluger et al., 2009). It may occur secondary to conditions such as endocrinopathies (e.g. diabetes mellitus), obesity or iatrogenic drug therapy (e.g. glucocorticoids, megestrol acetate). The most common presentation is transient lipaemic aqueous after a fatty meal in cats with otherwise healthy eyes, which resolves spontaneously. Uveitis can be a predisposing factor, as breakdown of the blood-aqueous barrier allows lipid to enter the anterior chamber. Conversely, the presence of lipid in the anterior chamber can incite an inflammatory response, leading to uveitis. Lipid is visible if triacylglyceride levels are abnormally high (> 25mmol/l), whereas raised cholesterol levels do not cause cloudy aqueous. Where possible, the fundus should be examined to assess whether there is also lipaemia retinalis (see Chapter 11). Lipoprotein analysis tests total and esterified cholesterol, phospholipids and triacylglycerols, and lipoprotein electrophoresis differentiates the lipoproteins. After a 12-16 hour fast, 5 ml of blood should be collected in EDTA tubes and the centrifuged sample should be dispatched on the same day. If an underlying cause can be identified, successful treatment will result in resolution of the condition.

Uveitis

Uveitis is a common and very significant disorder in cats. Anterior uveitis (syn. iridocyclitis, inflammation of the iris and ciliary body) is most common as inflammation of the ciliary body (cyclitis, syn. pars planitis) rarely occurs in isolation. Posterior uveitis (syn. choroiditis, inflammation of the choroid) is almost always accompanied by inflammation of the adjacent retina, and is thus usually termed chorioretinitis. Chorioretinitis arises most often from systemic infections, especially with fungal organisms.

Clinical signs

The diverse range of the potential clinical signs of anterior uveitis is summarised in Table 1. Cats more often present with signs of chronic anterior uveitis rather than acute episodes.

Table 1. Clinical signs of uveitis.

Sign	Comments
Conjunctival/episcleral hyperaemia	Vascular engorgement of the conjunctival and episcleral vessels.
Ciliary flush	Deep peripheral corneal vascularisation with short, dark, straight vessels arising from the ciliary plexus.
Corneal oedema	Due to corneal epithelial defect (ulceration) or dysfunction of the corneal endothelium due to abnormal aqueous humour components.
Keratic precipitates (Figs. 29-31)	Scattered multifocal accumulations of inflammatory cells, pigment and fibrin attached to the corneal endothelium.
Aqueous flare (Fig. 32)	Turbidity of the aqueous from accumulation of plasma proteins.
Hypopyon (Fig. 33)	Collection of white blood cells within the anterior chamber. Typically settles ventrally.
Fibrin (Figs. 34 and 35)	A product of activation of the coagulation cascade following breakdown of the blood-aqueous barrier.
Rubeosis iridis (Fig. 36)	Neovascularisation of the iris surface.
Changes in iris colour (Fig. 37)	Usually darker and duller due to iris thickening arising from vascular dilation and stromal infiltration with inflammatory cells.
Changes in iris texture (Fig. 38)	Due to swelling, the texture of the iris can be lost and it may appear flat and featureless.
Busacca nodules (Fig. 39)	Dark multifocal inflammatory nodules of the iris due to granulomatous inflammation.
Miosis	Prostaglandin-mediated spasm of the iris constrictor muscle.
Hypotony	Reduced IOP as a result of decreased aqueous humour production and/or increased uveoscleral outflow.
Reduced vision	Due to haziness from corneal oedema, abnormal aqueous humour contents, cataract, vitreal 'snow-banking' or chorioretinitis.
Cataract	Altered aqueous humour constituents may interfere with lens metabolism and lead to cataract formation.
Lens luxation (Fig. 40)	Lens zonule breakdown may result from chronic inflammation or glaucomatous globe enlargement (buphthalmos).
Synechiae and dyscoria (Fig. 41)	Adherence of iris to either the lens (posterior synechiae) or cornea (anterior synechiae).
Iris bombé	Posterior synechiae forming around the entire circumference of the pupil obstructing aqueous flow into the anterior chamber and almost invariably resulting in glaucoma.
Glaucoma (Fig. 42)	Increased IOP can develop from iris bombé or inflammatory cells obstructing the iridocorneal angle.

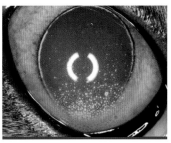

Figure 29. Diffuse multifocal keratic precipitates concentrated on the ventral aspect of the corneal endothelium in a cat with idiopathic uveitis.

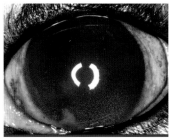

Figure 30. Multiple small keratic precipitates on the ventral corneal endothelium in a cat with uveitis associated with FIP.

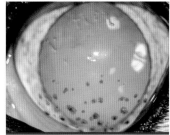

Figure 31. Multifocal darkly coloured keratic precipitates highlighted by retroillumination in a cat with lymphoplasmacytic uveitis. Courtesy of Filip Nachtegaele.

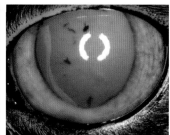

Figure 32. Aqueous flare obscuring iris detail. There is rubeosis iridis and pigment rests are present on the anterior lens capsule. A blood test was positive for FeLV antigen.

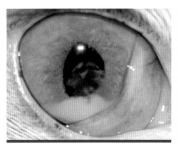

Figure 33. Hypopyon in the ventral anterior chamber along with fibrin over the pupil.

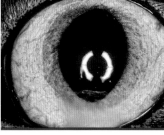

Figure 34. A fibrin clot is present in the ventral aspect of the anterior chamber, the only clear sign of uveitis in this eye with idiopathic uveitis.

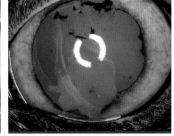

Figure 35. A fibrin clot in the anterior chamber, along with iris hyperaemia, posterior synechiae and dyscoria. The pupil has been pharmacologically dilated. FIP was later diagnosed.

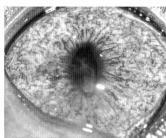

Figure 36. Rubeosis iridis is clearly visible in an inflamed eye with a blue iris. There is miosis and early cataract formation. Courtesy of Rachael Grundon.

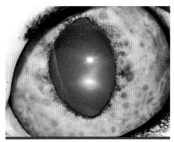

Figure 37. Iris colour change due to uveitis. The original green iris colour can be appreciated near the pupil margin. Elsewhere, there is stromal cellular infiltration with Busacca nodules and neovascularisation.

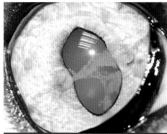

Figure 38. Iris texture change due to uveitis. There are some thickened nodules and the normal iris detail is not present. There is also fibrin in the anterior chamber and pupil dyscoria. Lymphoma was later diagnosed.

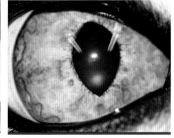

Figure 39. Busacca nodules. Multiple dark inflammatory nodules are present on the iris associated with granulomatous uveitis. Courtesy of Filip Nachtegaele.

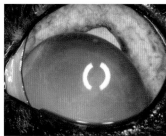

Figure 40. Chronic idiopathic anterior uveitis with poor treatment compliance resulted in sudden-onset anterior lens luxation.

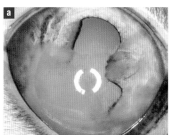

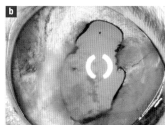

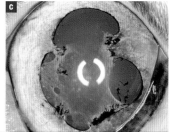

Figure 41. Unilateral idiopathic uveitis in a 7-year-old cat. a) Initial presentation. Dyscoria due to synechia, with anterior chamber fibrin and iris hyperaemia. b) Treatment with topical corticosteroids and mydriatics resulted in reduction of fibrin and a clearer view of the pink granulomatous infiltration of the iris. c) With further treatment, the inflammation resolved, but the synechiae and dyscoria remain.

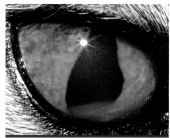

Figure 42. Secondary glaucoma due to uveitis. There was hypopyon, rubeosis iridis and dyscoria. The IOP was 67 mmHg.

Causes of uveitis

Uveitis may be infectious or noninfectious in origin. Infectious causes include feline leukaemia virus (FeLV), feline immunodeficiency virus (FIV), feline infectious peritonitis (FIP) virus, *Toxoplasma gondii*, *Bartonella henselae* and systemic fungal infections (Table 2). Noninfectious causes include trauma, immune-mediated inflammation and neoplasia. Reflex uveitis occurs in most cases of corneal ulceration, triggered by stimulation of the ophthalmic branch of the trigeminal nerve. The aetiology of uveitis can remain elusive in

as many of 70 % of cases despite diagnostic tests, in which case it may be considered idiopathic/immune-mediated (Davidson et al., 1991). Having said this, one histopathological study of 153 uveitic eyes from 139 cats identified a cause in 67 % of cases; the majority was associated with FIP, FeLV-associated lymphoma and trauma (Peiffer and Wilcock, 1991). An attempt should always be made to determine the cause because feline uveitis is often a sign of serious systemic disease.

The noneffusive or 'dry' form of FIP commonly causes uveitis along with systemic and neurological disease. It typically affects younger cats, which usually have hyperglobulinaemia, lymphocytopenia and a positive feline coronavirus titre. Common ocular signs include keratic precipitates, fibrin and hypopyon (Figs. 43 and 44). There may also be focal retinal exudates and perivascular cuffing (see Chapter 11).

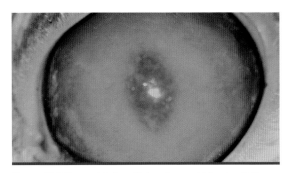

Figure 43. FIP-associated uveitis in a 1-year-old Persian. Both eyes had fibrin in the anterior chambers and miosis.

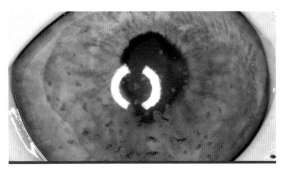

Figure 44. FIP-associated uveitis in a young cat with anorexia, weight loss and bilateral red eyes. There were multiple haemorrhagic keratic precipitates, the peripheral iris was thickened and hyperaemic, and there was miosis and ectropion uveae.

→ Preiridal fibrovascular membranes are neovascular membranes that may occur due to chronic uveitis, intraocular haemorrhage, retinal detachment, glaucoma or neoplasia.

Table 2. Infectious causes of feline uveitis.

Viruses	Bacteria	Protozoa	Fungi	Parasitic
Feline infectious peritonitis virus (FIP)	*Bartonella* spp.	*Toxoplasma gondii*	*Cryptococcus neoformans*	*Cuterebra* spp.
Feline leukaemia virus (FeLV)	*Mycobacteria* spp.	*Leishmania* spp.	*Histoplasma capsulatum*	
Feline immunodeficiency virus (FIV)			*Coccidioides immitis*	
Feline herpesvirus-1 (FHV-1)			*Blastomyces dermatitidis*	

FIV is a retrovirus that causes immunosuppression. Infection with FIV has been associated with chronic lymphoplasmacytic uveitis, which may arise due to direct viral damage or as a result of increased susceptibility to opportunistic infection (Fig. 45). The characteristic histopathological feature is of mononuclear inflammatory cell infiltrate adjacent to the base of the iris and anterior ciliary body. Pars planitis has previously been thought to occur specifically as a result of FIV infection. This appears as multifocal accumulations of inflammatory cellular infiltrates in the anterior vitreous just behind the posterior lens capsule, also termed 'snow-banking' (Fig. 46). It is no longer considered a pathognomonic sign of FIV infection, although it is still considered an important indicator of ciliary body inflammation. Potentially, leukocyte-induced lens zonular breakdown could lead to secondary lens luxation. Co-infection with *Toxoplasma gondii* further increases the likelihood of uveitis. FIV-positive cats also have a higher incidence of B-cell lymphoma which also affects the uveal tract. Diagnosis is by serum ELISA testing for circulating antibodies.

The other important feline retrovirus, FeLV, can also cause uveitis. This can arise either directly from viral-mediated uveal inflammation, or indirectly through lymphosarcoma induction by the virus. A wide variety of ocular signs can occur, including eyelid, conjunctival and orbital masses, keratitis, anterior uveal tumours, anterior uveitis, optic neuritis and retinal detachments (Fig. 47). Diagnosis is by a serum ELISA test for circulating antigen.

FHV-1 has been considered to play a role in feline uveitis, although it has been difficult to prove a causal association. In one study of 44 cats with idiopathic uveitis, FHV-1 virus was found by PCR in the aqueous humour of 12 cats, 11 of which had uveitis (Maggs et al., 1999). The conclusion was that FHV-1 can infect the intraocular tissues in cats and that this may be associated with uveitis. In another study, FHV-1 DNA could be detected in the aqueous humour but not in the blood of two cats with uveitis (Powell et al., 2010). Taken together, these data suggest that intraocular FHV-1 infection occurs and that, at least in some cats, stimulates a specific local intraocular antibody response.

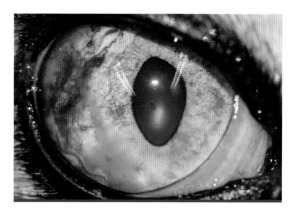

Figure 45. Unilateral uveitis with fibrin in the anterior chamber, rubeosis iridis and miosis. The cat tested positive for FIV antibody. Courtesy of Filip Nachtegaele.

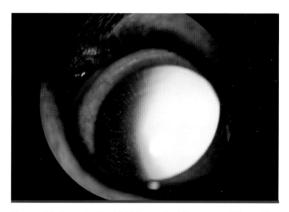

Figure 46. Pars planitis. Multiple small white accumulations of inflammatory cells are visible with an almost linear arrangement on the posterior lens capsule. The cat tested positive for FIV antibody. Courtesy of Professor Sheila Crispin.

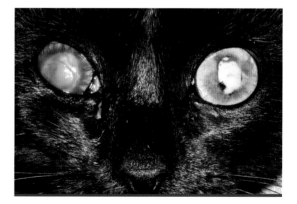

Figure 47. FeLV-associated lymphoma and uveitis in an anorexic cat with dramatic weight loss. The right eye had corneal ulceration, oedema and neovascularisation. The left eye had corneal cellular infiltrate, fibrin in the anterior chamber, miosis and posterior synechiae. Diagnosis was confirmed on post mortem.

Infection with *Toxoplasma gondii* is known to cause anterior uveitis and/or granulomatous chorioretinitis (Fig. 48). The diagnosis is achieved by an ELISA test for circulating serum IgG antibodies (suggestive of exposure; a rising titre is suggestive of active infection) and IgM antibodies (suggestive of active infection). The recommended treatment for toxoplasmosis is oral clindamycin 12.5 mg/kg twice daily for three weeks.

Bartonella henselae causes cat scratch fever in man and is transmitted by fleas. Uveitis has been observed after both experimental inoculation and naturally occurring infection. There is a very high seropositive rate (up to 93 %) among the normal cat population in areas where fleas are common, and thus it can be difficult to attribute the cause of idiopathic uveitis to bartonellosis in these circumstances. Diagnosis is by PCR or western blot analysis. The recommended treatment is oral doxycycline 10-22 mg/kg once daily for 2-6 weeks (see Chapter 3).

Systemic fungal infection is an important cause of uveitis in several geographical areas. The spores are inhaled resulting in initial infection of the respiratory tract before haematogenous dissemination to other tissues including the uveal tract. Affected cats usually present with granulomatous chorioretinitis, but granulomatous anterior uveitis may also occur. Blepharitis, optic neuritis, retinal detachment or orbital abscessation may also feature in some cases. There are usually other systemic signs such as skin or CNS disease. Diagnosis is achieved through cytology of lesions, thoracic radiography, evaluation of specific serum titres and also taking into account geographical location. Fungal organisms found to affect the feline eye include *Cryptococcus neoformans*, *Histoplasma capsulatum*, *Coccidioides immitis* and *Blastomyces dermatitidis*. Systemic antifungal treatment is required depending on the fungal organism present, such as oral fluconazole or itraconazole.

Investigation of uveitis

The diagnosis of uveitis is straight-forward, but determining the cause is more challenging. The suggested diagnostic approach is as follows:

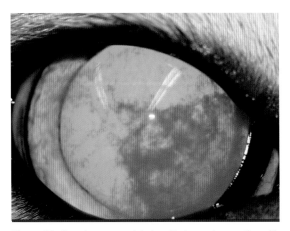

Figure 48. *Toxoplasma*-associated uveitis in a cat presenting with neurological signs. There was fibrin in the anterior chamber in both eyes. Diagnosis was confirmed by a rising IgG *Toxoplasma gondii* titre. Courtesy of Filip Nachtegaele.

Step by step guide to investigation of feline uveitis

➔ Extensive history (including concurrent diseases and medications, vaccination status, flea and worm prevention, travel, health of in-contact cats)

➔ Thorough physical and neurological examination

➔ Complete ophthalmic examination of both eyes

➔ Complete blood count, serum biochemistry panel and urinalysis

➔ Specific serological tests for the most common infectious causes, tailored according to geographical location and vaccination status:

  ➔ FIV antibody and FeLV antigen

  ➔ Feline coronavirus antibody titre

  ➔ *Toxoplasma gondii* IgG and IgM antibodies

  ➔ *Bartonella* spp. antibodies

  ➔ *Cryptococcus* spp. antigen

  ➔ Serology for other organisms endemic in the area

➔ Ocular ultrasound if the ocular media are opaque or if an intraocular mass is suspected

➔ Thoracic radiographs, abdominal ultrasound, and fine needle aspiration or biopsy of enlarged lymph nodes, masses or cutaneous nodules

➔ Aqueocentesis for cytology and potentially PCR and serological testing

Cats with serious systemic diseases may present with signs of uveitis before other clinical signs become evident. Therefore it is imperative to perform a thorough physical examination of every cat presenting with either unilateral or bilateral uveitis.

Treatment of uveitis

The goals in treating uveitis are to eliminate infectious agents, control inflammation, stabilise the blood-aqueous barrier and minimise bystander damage to intraocular structures. If the underlying cause can be identified, specific treatment is given as outlined previously. More generally, treatment with topical and systemic antiinflammatory agents is indicated. Topical corticosteroids with good corneal penetration, such as 1 % prednisolone acetate or 0.1 % dexamethasone phospate, are used initially up to six times daily. Topical corticosteroids are contraindicated if there is corneal ulceration or stromal infection. Topical mydriatics, usually 0.5-1 % tropicamide, are useful to stabilise the blood aqueous barrier, reduce pain through paralysis of the iridal sphincter and ciliary body musculature and reduce the likelihood of synechiae. However, they should be avoided if the IOP is raised. Posterior uveitis requires systemic treatment because topically applied medication does not usually achieve therapeutic concentrations in the posterior segment. Secondary glaucoma is not an uncommon sequel to uveitis, and topical glaucoma therapy may also be required (see Chapter 9).

Enucleation is required for blind, painful eyes that are not responsive to medication. This achieves elimination of pain and an opportunity for a histopathological diagnosis.

Aqueocentesis (anterior chamber paracentesis)

Samples of aqueous humour provide the opportunity for cytology, bacterial culture and susceptibility, protein measurement, antibody titres and PCR. A recent study found that in ten cats with anterior uveitis, the definitive cause was not found based on cytologic assessment of aqueous humour alone (Wiggins et al., 2014). In that study, the three cats with FIP tended to have neutrophilic aqueous compared with cats with idiopathic uveitis that tended to have a predominantly lymphoplasmacytic aqueous. Generally, aqueocentesis is most useful for the diagnosis of lymphoma (Pearl et al., 2015).

Sedation or general anaesthesia is required for restraint. The ocular surface should be cleansed with a 0.2 % povidone-iodine aqueous solution and then topical anaesthetic (e.g. 1 % proxymetacaine) is applied. A 27 or 30 G needle is used. The bulbar conjunctiva is grasped near to the site of globe entry to steady the globe. The needle is inserted (bevel up) at the limbus into the anterior chamber, keeping it parallel to the plane of the iris (Fig. 49). The tip of the needle should be watched at all times so that it does not damage the cornea, iris or lens. A small volume of aqueous (0.1 ml) can be aspirated very slowly, either via a capillary tube at the needle hub or by attaching a 1 ml syringe. A cycloplegic such as 0.5-1 % tropicamide is applied topically once, to reduce induced uveitis. The risks of the procedure include exacerbation of uveitis, inoculation of bacteria, lens damage and hyphaema due to laceration of the iris.

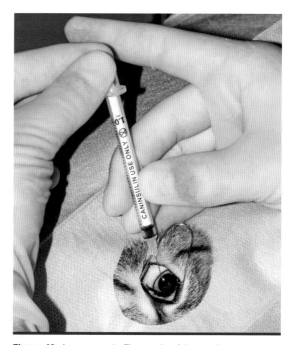

Figure 49. Aqueocentesis. The needle of the insulin syringe is inserted (bevel up) at the limbus into the anterior chamber, keeping it parallel to the plane of the iris.

Uveal neoplasia

The highly vascular uvea is a common site for primary intraocular tumours. Metastasis to the eye via haematogenous spread may occur from other sites, and direct invasion from local sites can also occur. The clinical signs of intraocular neoplasia may include the visible presence of a mass, a thickened or distorted pupil, reduced pupil mobility, hyphaema, secondary glaucoma and retinal detachment.

Diffuse iris melanoma

Diffuse iris melanoma is the most common primary intraocular neoplasm. It typically originates from the anterior surface of the iris. In the early stages there are focal or multifocal areas of hyperpigmentation with invasion of the iris stroma. Initially, it can be difficult to distinguish benign iris melanosis from melanoma formation. Diffuse iris melanoma tends to be more rapidly progressive over time (weeks to months) in both the amount and extent of pigmentation compared with benign iris melanosis. Signs such as progression of pigmentation, anterior uveitis, dyscoria, reduced pupil motility, thickening or altered texture of the iris, pigment invasion into the iridocorneal angle and free pigment in the anterior chamber are considered to be indicative of melanoma rather than melanosis (Figs. 50-52). Gonioscopy enables determination of invasion of the iridocorneal angle (Fig. 53). Secondary glaucoma may arise due to this invasion or as a result PIFM formation (see Chapter 9). In the advanced stages, the tumour may occupy the anterior and posterior chambers, and invade the sclera (Fig. 54). There is a potential for metastasis, principally to the liver and lungs, which has been reported as late as 1-3 years after enucleation (Duncan and Peiffer, 1991). The rate of metastasis has been reported to be as high as 63 %, so the clinician faces a dilemma when presented with any acquired iris pigmentation in cats (Patnaik and Mooney, 1988).

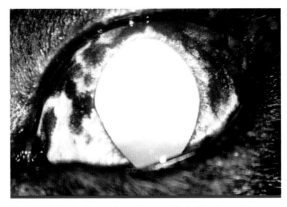

Figure 50. Early diffuse iris melanoma. Dark iris pigmentation and dyscoria. Histopathology confirmed invasion into the iris stroma but no evidence of metastasis was found on thoracic radiography and abdominal ultrasound examination.

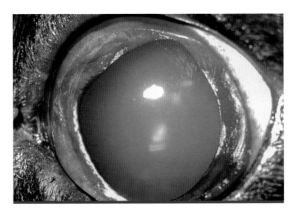

Figure 51. Diffuse iris melanoma. Note the thickened iris pigmentation with dyscoria. Posterior uveitis and glaucoma (note mydriasis) were also present. On histopathological examination, neoplastic cells were found in the scleral venous channels.

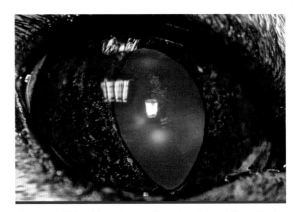

Figure 52. Diffuse iris melanoma. Extensive pigmentation of the iris surface and stroma.

→ Intraocular melanomas have a much higher tendency to metastasise in cats than in dogs. For this reason, enucleation is performed more readily and rapidly in cats.

Signs of progressive diffuse iris melanoma

→ Thickening or altered texture of the iris stroma

→ Change to pupil shape or reduced mobility of the iris

→ Pigment invasion of the iridocorneal angle

→ Free pigment in the anterior chamber

→ Secondary glaucoma

Feline intraocular sarcoma

Feline intraocular sarcomas are highly malignant intraocular neoplasms that involve the uveal tract. They are most frequently associated with a history of significant ocular trauma, and an average interval of seven years from the traumatic event to the diagnosis of the tumour has been reported (Dubielzig et al., 2010). Apart from blunt trauma, they may also arise after intraocular surgery, chronic uveitis and intravitreal gentamicin injections. There are three morphological variants; a spindle cell variant from lens epithelial cells, a round cell variant associated with B-cell lymphoma and a less common type associated with osteosarcoma/chondrosarcoma (Dubielzig et al., 2010). Clinical signs include a visible intraocular mass, uveitis, hyphaema associated with PIFMs or secondary glaucoma (Fig. 55). There is a high potential for haematogenous metastasis and local invasion through the sclera and optic nerve. The aggressive behavior of this tumour gives convincing justification for the early prophylactic enucleation of any severely damaged nonvisual feline globe.

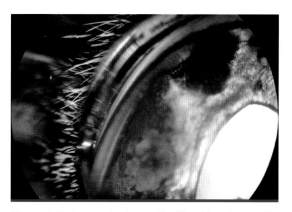

Figure 53. Drainage angle of a cat with diffuse iris melanoma. The pectinate ligament strands are heavily pigmented due to neoplastic invasion.

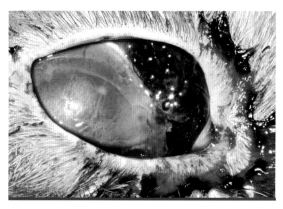

Figure 54. Extensive intraocular melanoma in the right eye of a 14-year-old Domestic shorthair invading the sclera. Ocular ultrasound revealed an extensive mass lesion almost filling the entire globe with extension across the medial globe wall. There was also total retinal detachment and the globe was enlarged. Further imaging revealed mass lesions within the liver, intestines and lungs.

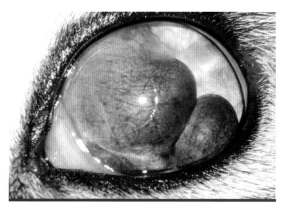

Figure 55. Intraocular sarcoma in a 7-year-old Domestic shorthair that suffered ocular trauma four years previously. The uveal tissue is grossly thickened and pigmented, and occupies the anterior chamber. There was also neoplastic extension through the posterior sclera and optic nerve.

Primary ciliary body neoplasia

Primary iridociliary epithelial tumours (both adenomas and adenocarcinomas) have been reported in cats, but are relatively uncommon (Peiffer, 1983; Dubielzig et al., 1998). They typically arise in the pars plicata of the ciliary body, and present as a pink fleshy mass visible behind the pupil (Figs. 56-58). Secondary glaucoma may occur due to mass effect or because of induction of a PIFM. They tend to be slow-growing and metastasis is not common (Dubielzig et al., 1998). Enucleation is indicated if secondary glaucoma develops.

Metastatic neoplasia

Secondary neoplasia can affect the eye as a result of metastasis from other sites, such as lymphoma and angioinvasive pulmonary carcinoma. Other rare and infrequently reported metastatic tumours to the eye include mammary and intrauterine adenocarcinoma, haemangioma and squamous cell carcinoma. Extension from neighbouring extraocular tumours such as squamous cell carcinoma (SCC) can also occur.

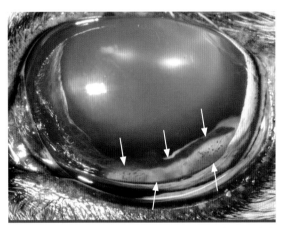

Figure 56. Ciliary body adenoma. The pupil has been pharmacologically dilated. A pink mass is visible ventrally behind the iris (arrows).

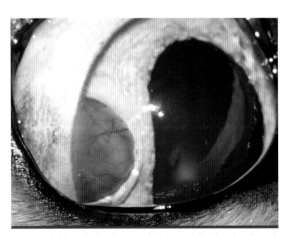

Figure 57. Ciliary body adenoma. A pink mass has invaded through the iridocorneal angle laterally.

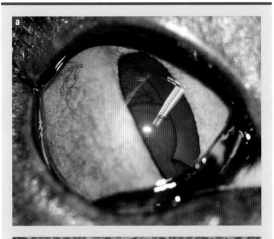

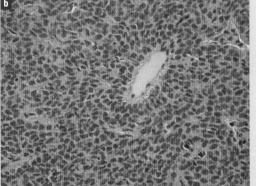

Figure 58. Ciliary body adenoma in a 12-year-old Domestic shorthair. a) A clinical photograph shows a large pink mass laterally, visible behind the pupil. Courtesy of Filip Nachtegaele. b) Perivascular palisading of iridociliary epithelial cells at 200× magnification (haematoxylin and eosin). Courtesy of Karen Dunn, FOCUS-EyePathLab.

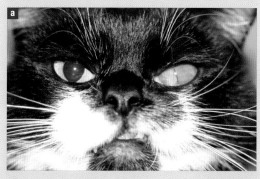

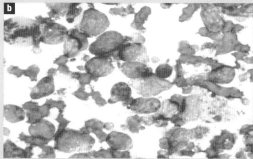

Figure 59. a) Lymphoma in the left eye causing gross thickening and hyperaemia of the iris, due to neoplastic invasion. b) Cytology of a fine needle biopsy from a renal mass in the same cat. The predominant cells are lymphoblasts.

→ It is recommended that all enucleated globes are submitted for histopathological examination. Adnexal tissue including the eyelids and extraocular muscles are dissected from the globe before fixation in 10 % formalin.

Lymphoma

Lymphoma is the most common secondary intraocular tumour (Fig. 59) and may be associated with FIV or FeLV infection. FeLV can directly induce neoplasia whereas FIV indirectly results in neoplasia due to its immunosuppressive effects. Clinically, lymphoma usually presents with signs of inflammation/uveitis but fleshy pink intraocular masses may be present. Secondary glaucoma may develop due to obstruction of the aqueous humour outflow pathways. Cytology of the aqueous humour is considered to be valuable diagnostically as there is a high yield of affected cells as the tumour readily exfoliates (Pearl et al., 2015). It is considered worthwhile to achieve an early and accurate diagnosis as a recent study has shown that many of these tumours are B-cell lymphomas, which are generally more amenable to chemotherapy than T-cell lymphomas (Ota-Kuroki et al., 2013).

Angioinvasive pulmonary carcinoma

Sometimes referred to as 'feline lung-digit syndrome', primary angioinvasive pulmonary adenocarcinoma has an unusual pattern of metastasis to atypical sites, including the skin, eyes, skeletal muscle and bone (Goldfinch and Argyle, 2012). Extensive invasion of the choroid by neoplastic cells can occur, with subsequent ischaemic necrosis and retinal degeneration. Posterior segment metastasis has been reported (Davidson, 1999) (see Chapter 11).

References

Colitz CM (2005). Feline uveitis: diagnosis and treatment. *Clinical Techniques in Small Animal Practice*; 20:117-120.

Davidson M (1999). Angioinvasive pulmonary carcinoma with posterior segment metastasis in four cats. *Veterinary Ophthalmology*; 2:125-131.

Davidson MG, Nasisse MP, English RV et al. (1991). Feline anterior uveitis: a study of 53 cases. *Journal of the American Animal Hospital Association*; 27(1):77-83.

Dubielzig RR, Ketring K, McLellan GJ et al. (2010) Non-surgical trauma. In: *Veterinary Ocular Pathology. A Comparative Review*. Saunders Elsevier, chapter 5:97-103.

Dubielzig RR, Steinberg H, Garvin H et al. (1998). Iridociliary epithelial tumors in 100 dogs and 17 cats: a morphological study. *Veterinary Ophthalmology*; 1:223-231.

Duncan DE, Peiffer RL (1991). Morphology and prognostic indicators of anterior uveal melanomas in cats. *Progress in Veterinary and Comparative Ophthalmology*; 1:25-32.

Gemensky-Metzler AJ, Wilkie DA, Cook CS (2004). The use of semiconductor diode laser for deflation and coagulation of anterior uveal cysts in dogs, cats and horses: a report of 20 cases. *Veterinary Ophthalmology*; 7:360-368.

Goldfinch N, Argyle D (2012). Feline lung-digit syndrome: unusual metastatic patterns of primary lung tumours in cats. *Journal of Feline Medicine and Surgery*; 14:202-208.

Kalishman JB, Chappell R, Flood LA et al. (1998). A matched observational study of survival in cats with enucleation due to diffuse iris melanoma. *Veterinary Ophthalmology*; 1:25-29.

Kluger EK, Hardman C, Govendir M et al. (2009). Triglyceride response following an oral fat tolerance test in Burmese cats, other pedigree cats and domestic crossbred cats. *Journal of Feline Medicine and Surgery*; 11:82-90.

Linn-Pearl RN, Powell, RM, Newman HA et al. (2015). Validity of aqueocentesis as a component of anterior uveitis investigation in dogs and cats. *Veterinary Ophthalmology*; DOI: 10.1111/vop. 12245.

Maggs D (2009). Feline uveitis. An 'intraocular lymphadenopathy'. *Journal of Feline Medicine and Surgery*; 11:167-182.

Maggs DJ, Lappin MR, Nasisse MP (1999). Detection of feline herpesvirus-specific antibodies and DNA in aqueous humor from cats with or without uveitis. *American Journal of Veterinary Research*; 60:932-936.

Ota-Kuroki J, Ragsdale JM, Bawa B et al. (2014). Intraocular and periocular lymphoma in dogs and cats: a retrospective review of 21 cases (2001-2012). *Veterinary Ophthalmology*; 17(6):389-96.

Patnaik AK, Mooney S (1988). Feline melanoma: a comparative study of ocular, oral, and dermal neoplasms. *Veterinary Pathology Online*; 25:105-112.

Peiffer RL (1983). Ciliary body epithelial tumours in the dog and cat; a report of thirteen cases. *Journal of Small Animal Practice*; 24:347-370.

Peiffer Jr RL, Wilcock BP (1991). Histopathologic study of uveitis in cats: 139 cases (1978-1988). *Journal of the American Veterinary Medical Association*; 198:135.

Powell CC, McInnis CL, Fontenelle JP et al. (2010). *Bartonella* species, feline herpesvirus-1, and *Toxoplasma gondii* PCR assay results from blood and aqueous humor samples from 104 cats with naturally occurring endogenous uveitis. *Journal of Feline Medicine and Surgery*; 12:923-928.

Wiggans KT, Vernau W, Lappin MR et al. (2014). Diagnostic utility of aqueocentesis and aqueous humor analysis in dogs and cats with anterior uveitis. *Veterinary Ophthalmology*; 17:212-220.

9

Glaucoma

Introduction

Feline glaucoma is an under-diagnosed condition due to the insidious onset of clinical signs, very gradual progression of disease and limited availability of suitable tonometers in general practice. A comprehensive review of the condition has been published (McLellan and Miller, 2011). Glaucoma in cats most commonly occurs as a sequel to chronic intraocular inflammation and treatment can be challenging.

What is glaucoma?

The 'glaucomas' constitute a large, diverse group of disorders that share the common feature of pathologically high intraocular pressure (IOP) which interferes with retinal and optic nerve function. Glaucoma is, thus, a neurodegenerative disease and is associated with disruption of axoplasmic flow and microcirculation of the optic nerve head, loss of retinal ganglion cells and their axons, cupping of the optic disc, optic nerve atrophy and visual impairment or blindness.

Aqueous humour dynamics

Normally there is an equilibrium between the production and drainage of aqueous humour resulting in a relatively constant IOP. Impairment of aqueous drainage interrupts this balance, leading to increased IOP which is potentially damaging to the eye.

Aqueous humour is produced by the nonpigmented epithelium of the ciliary body and secreted into the posterior chamber. Aqueous may then leave the eye via one of two main pathways (Figs. 1 and 2). In the cat, the majority (> 97 %) of aqueous leaves the eye via the 'conventional' drainage route. Aqueous humour circulates from the posterior chamber via the pupil into the anterior chamber and then crosses the iridocorneal angle into the sieve-like trabecular meshwork before being drained from the eye by the venous angular aqueous plexus which feeds into the scleral venous plexus and then into the systemic circulation.

An alternative route of drainage, the uveoscleral or 'unconventional' route, accounts for about 3 % of aqueous outflow in the cat. In this situation, aqueous

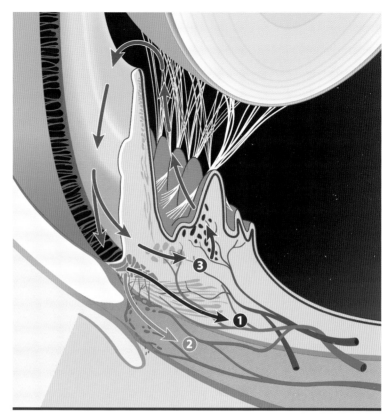

Figure 1. Aqueous humour formation and drainage pathways. Aqueous is formed by the ciliary body and flows from the posterior chamber through the pupil and into the anterior chamber (red arrows). Aqueous is drained from the eye by one of three ways. 1. Drainage of aqueous occurs mainly though the pectinate ligament and trabecular meshwork into the aqueous plexus and scleral venous circulation ('conventional' pathway). 2. Aqueous may pass into the ciliary cleft and then the choroidal and suprachoroidal spaces, and enter the scleral venous circulation ('unconventional' pathway). 3. A small volume of aqueous may drain through the anterior iris face and the interstitial spaces of the ciliary body musculature.

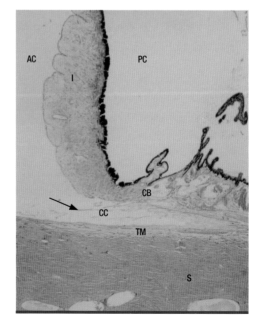

Figure 2. Photomicrograph of the normal feline iridocorneal angle.
AC = anterior chamber.
I = iris.
PC = posterior chamber.
CC = ciliary cleft.
CB = ciliary body.
TM = corneoscleral trabecular meshwork.
S = sclera.
The arrow represents the entrance to the drainage angle, the site of the pectinate ligament. Courtesy of Karen Dunn, FOCUS-EyePathLab.

passes through the ciliary body and choroid via the supraciliary and suprachoroidal spaces, and from there it passes through the sclera and episcleral tissues into the orbit for drainage into the systemic circulation.

Investigation of glaucoma

Tonometry

Instruments used to measure IOP include the indentation Schiotz, the applanation Tono-Pen® and the rebound TonoVet® tonometers (Fig. 3). Measurements vary between the instruments so it is important to consistently use the same tonometer when monitoring the IOP of an individual patient. The Schiotz tonometer is difficult to use in the conscious cat. The Tono-Pen® requires topical anaesthesia but is suitable for use in the cat. Rebound tonometry is becoming increasingly popular because of the ease of use and excellent patient compliance. Topical anaesthesia is not required as there is such light impact on the cornea, which is of benefit if the eye is fragile or painful. A recent study found that the TonoVet® provides readings much closer to the true IOP than the Tono-Pen®, and that the former is superior in accurately detecting elevations of IOP in cats in a clinical setting (McLellan et al., 2013).

Ophthalmoscopy

Ophthalmoscopy is also essential for diagnosis of the type of glaucoma and for on-going monitoring. It is used for detection of signs of globe enlargement (buphthalmos), investigation of an underlying cause (e.g. uveitis), to assess for secondary effects such as lens luxation and to estimate IOP-related damage to the retina and optic disc.

Gonioscopy

Gonioscopy is the examination technique used to view the iridocorneal drainage angle or, more specifically, the opening to the ciliary cleft. The cat has a relatively deep anterior chamber and a wide iridocorneal angle compared to other species. The pectinate ligament fibres which span the iridocorneal angle are normally slender, sparse and slightly branching.

The ciliary cleft, which contains the trabecular meshwork, is normally long and wide (Fig. 4). Because of the deep anterior chamber, it is possible to examine much of the feline angle without a goniolens by direct observation using focal illumination. However, the use of a goniolens magnifies the view, and is advised in order to reliably examine the structures. In glaucomatous cats the iridocorneal angle may not be fully closed but usually appears recessed posteriorly, especially if the globe is enlarged.

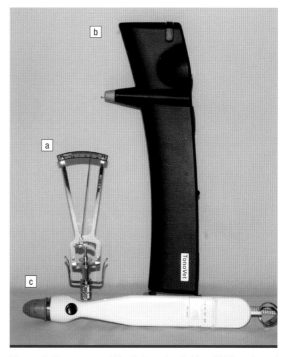

Figure 3. Tonometers. a) The indentation Schiotz. b) The rebound TonoVet®. c) The applanation Tono-Pen®.

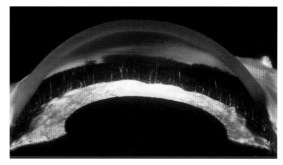

Figure 4. Macrohistology photograph of the drainage angle of a normal cat displaying fine pectinate ligament fibres and a deep anterior chamber. Courtesy of John Mould.

Normal intraocular pressure

Normal feline IOP is generally 10-25 mmHg. However, the range is somewhat variable as there are many factors that can influence it, and these are summarised in Tables 1 and 2. Apart from a raised IOP, asymmetry of readings between the eyes is also considered a risk factor for glaucoma, with a difference of 5 mmHg or more considered significant. Such a discrepancy should prompt a thorough ocular examination for clinical signs of glaucoma or uveitis.

Table 1. Normal IOP according to the type of tonometer used.

Tonometer	Normal IOP in cats (mmHg ± SD)	Reference
Schiotz	21.6 ± 5	Miller and Pickett, 1992
Tono-Pen®	19.7 ± 5.6	Miller et al., 1991
TonoVet®	20.74 ± 7.07	Rusanen et al., 2010

Table 2. Factors known to influence IOP in normal cats.

Factor	Effect on IOP	Reference
Time of day	Lowest mid-afternoon, highest at night	Del Sole et al., 2007
Age	Normal IOP for young cats: 20.2 ± 5.5 mmHg. Normal IOP for cats ≥ 7 years: 12.3 ± 4.0 mmHg	Kroll et al., 2001
Reproductive status	Oestrus increases IOP	Ofri et al., 2002
Topical tropicamide	Increases IOP in treated eyes, and also in contralateral, nontreated eyes	Stadtbaumer et al., 2002
Topical atropine	Increases IOP in treated eyes	Stadtbaumer et al., 2006
Sedative and anaesthetic drugs (except ketamine)	Reduces IOP	
Systemic ketamine	Increases IOP	Hahnenberger, 1976
Restraint around the neck	Increases IOP	

Clinical signs of glaucoma

Feline glaucoma is typically insidious in onset and owners may be unaware of a problem until it has been present for some time. The eye may appear larger in size (buphthalmos, Fig. 5). Conjunctival and episcleral congestion are usually present but tend to be less obvious than in dogs with glaucoma (Figs. 6 and 7). There may be corneal oedema, especially peripherally, mydriasis and vision impairment. Secondary lens subluxation or luxation may arise due to stretching and breaking of the lens zonules as globe enlargement ensues (Fig. 8). Optic nerve cupping is present in chronic glaucoma (Fig. 9), but is much more difficult to appreciate in the cat compared to the dog because the feline optic disc is small and dark owing to the lack of myelin.

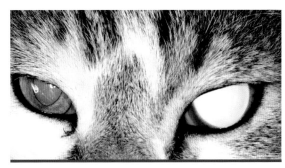

Figure 5. Buphthalmos of the left eye of a Domestic shorthair with glaucoma due to untreated chronic uveitis. Note the mydriasis and widened palpebral aperture.

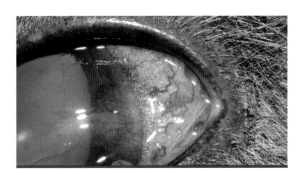

Figure 6. Glaucoma due to aqueous humour misdirection syndrome in a 9-year-old Burmese. Note pronounced conjunctival hyperaemia, peripheral keratitis and mydriasis.

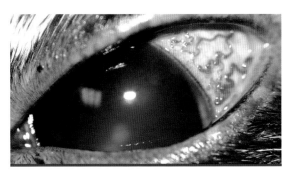

Figure 7. Pronounced episcleral congestion and mydriasis in a 4-year-old Domestic shorthair with primary glaucoma.

→   Buphthalmos is difficult to appreciate in the cat because the sclera is not normally visible. Increased size of the palpebral aperture may be the most obvious sign.

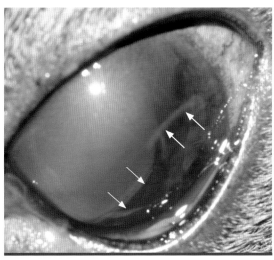

Figure 8. Glaucoma due to aqueous humour misdirection syndrome in a 9-year-old Burmese. Note buphthalmos, conjunctival hyperaemia, corneal oedema, break in Descemet's membrane (white arrows), mydriasis and lens subluxation (yellow arrows).

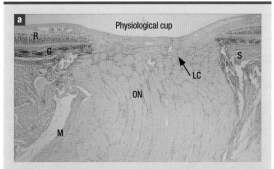

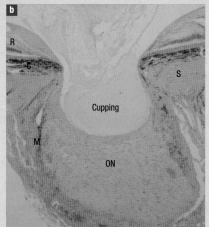

Figure 9. a) Photomicrograph of the normal feline optic nerve head region. R = retina. C = choroid. S = sclera. ON = optic nerve. LC = lamina cribosa. M = meninges. b) Photomicrograph of the optic nerve head region in a cat with secondary glaucoma showing a deeply cupped optic nerve head. Note condensed basophilic vitreous material collected within the cup. Courtesy of Karen Dunn, FOCUS-EyePathLab.

Types of feline glaucoma

Primary glaucoma

In contrast to the dog, primary (i.e. inherited) glaucoma in cats is very uncommon. In one study (Blocker and van der Woerdt, 2001) glaucoma was secondary in 87 % of 93 glaucomatous feline eyes. A histological study found primary glaucoma in three of 131 enucleated feline eyes (Wilcock et al., 1990). Primary glaucoma is diagnosed when no other cause can be attributed to the pathological elevation of IOP. Breed predispositions have been described which is suggestive of an inherited aetiology. Congenital glaucoma may be unilateral or bilateral, and arises as a result in maldevelopment of the aqueous drainage outflow pathways (Fig. 10). Primary open angle glaucoma has been reported in Domestic short- and long-haired and Burmese cats (Jacobi and Dubielzig, 2008; Wilcock et al., 1990). The histopathology of open angle glaucoma was described in a study of eight enucleated eyes from eight cats (Jacobi and Dubielzig, 2008). All had an open iridocorneal angle with an open ciliary cleft.

Pectinate ligament dysplasia (syn. goniodysgenesis), which is significantly associated with canine primary closed angle glaucoma, has been described in a group of closely related Siamese cats with congenital glaucoma (McLellan et al., 2004). A colony of Siamese cats affected with congenital glaucoma was created as an animal model to research the condition. They display

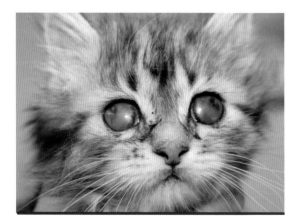

Figure 10. Bilateral congenital glaucoma in a 5-week-old European longhair. Buphthalmos, corneal oedema and pigmentation are present. Courtesy of Filip Nachtegaele.

> → The majority of cases of feline glaucoma are secondary, with chronic uveitis being the most common underlying cause.
>
> → Most cats with glaucoma are presented late in the course of disease because the initial signs can be subtle and go unnoticed.

slowly progressive clinical progression with elongated ciliary processes, globe enlargement and spherophakia. Histologically, they have arrested development of the uveal trabecular meshwork and angular aqueous plexus along with uveal hypoplasia (McLellan et al., 2006). Pectinate ligament dysplasia can also be one feature of eyes with multiple ocular malformations. Primary closed angle glaucoma associated with pectinate ligament dysplasia has been described in six Burmese cats in Australia (Hampson et al., 2002), but is rare.

Secondary glaucoma

Secondary glaucoma is far more common. It arises as a result of an antecedent intraocular disease process that results in impairment of drainage of aqueous humour and a subsequent increase in IOP.

Chronic anterior uveitis

Feline glaucoma occurs most frequently as a result of chronic uveitis. Causes of uveitis in cats include infectious diseases, trauma and neoplasia, but chronic idiopathic lymphoplasmacytic uveitis is the most common (see Chapter 8). Uveitis leads to raised IOP through obstruction of the iridocorneal angle by inflammatory cells and debris such as fibrin and red blood cells (Fig. 11). Synechiae can also form, with adhesions between the iris at the margin of the pupil and the anterior lens capsule (posterior synechiae) or, less commonly, the corneal endothelium (anterior synechiae, see Fig. 12 Chapter 8). Iris bombé results when posterior synechiae form around the entire pupil margin, obstructing the flow of aqueous humour into the anterior chamber (Fig. 12). Chronic inflammation can also lead to lens luxation and secondary glaucoma.

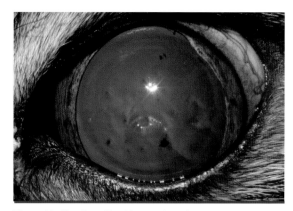

Figure 11. Chronic uveitis with secondary glaucoma. Note prominent scleral vessels, mydriasis, darkened iris, posterior synechiae and multifocal iris rests (black spots of pigment on the anterior lens capsule).

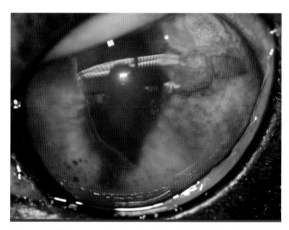

Figure 12. Glaucoma due to chronic lymphoplasmacytic uveitis in a 5-year-old European shorthair. There is chemosis, keratic precipitates on the ventral corneal endothelium, iris hyperaemia and iris bombé. The IOP was 49 mmHg. Courtesy of Filip Nachtegaele.

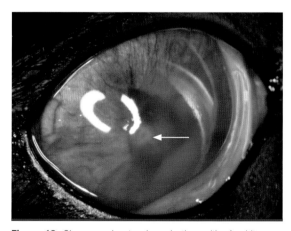

Figure 13. Glaucoma due to phacoclastic uveitis. A white scar indicates the site of a previous corneal penetration injury (arrow). Rupture of the lens capsule resulted in uveitis with miosis, and both fibrin and hypopyon in the anterior chamber. The IOP was 44 mmHg.

Intraocular neoplasia

The second most common cause of glaucoma in cats is intraocular neoplasia. The most common primary feline intraocular neoplasm is diffuse iris melanoma but feline intraocular sarcoma and iridociliary epithelial tumours are also encountered with some frequency. Lymphoma is the most common secondary intraocular neoplasm of the eye although, rarely, it can affect the eye primarily. Raised IOP develops through infiltration of the drainage pathway by neoplastic cells, formation of peripheral anterior synechiae or preiridal fibrovascular membranes and secondary inflammation.

Lens disorders

Anterior lens luxation can cause glaucoma through obstruction of aqueous flow. There is a very low incidence of primary lens luxation in cats and, instead, it usually arises as a result of chronic uveitis or buphthalmos and subsequent lens zonule damage.

Lens perforations can lead to severe phacoclastic uveitis or septic implantation syndrome, both of which can result in glaucoma (Fig. 13).

Intraocular haemorrhage

The most common causes of intraocular haemorrhage are systemic hypertension, trauma and bleeding disorders. Raised IOP may occur as a result of the acute accumulation of blood cells within the iridocorneal angle and ciliary cleft or the chronic formation of anterior and posterior synechiae. Persistent rebleeding, for example with preiridal fibrovascular membrane development, is more likely to result in glaucoma than a single bleed.

Aqueous humour misdirection syndrome

Aqueous humour misdirection syndrome (syn. ciliovitreolenticular glaucoma or 'malignant' glaucoma) is apparently unique to the cat. In this syndrome, aqueous is misdirected posteriorly into the vitreous humour and displaces the iris-lens diaphragm anteriorly. This results in a uniformly shallow anterior chamber, compromise of the iridocorneal angle and ciliary cleft and a progressively raised IOP (Czederpiltz et al., 2005) (Figs. 14-16). It typically develops

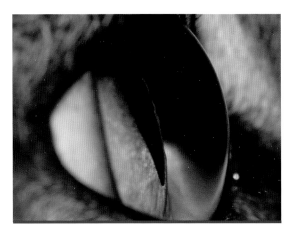

Figure 14. A normal eye of an adult Domestic shorthair. The anterior chamber is the area between the cornea and the iris, and is deep. Courtesy of John Mould.

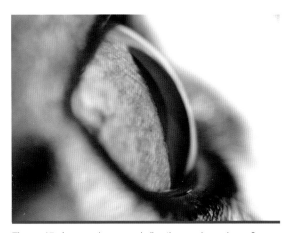

Figure 15. Aqueous humour misdirection syndrome in an 8-year-old Domestic shorthair. The iris and lens are displaced anteriorly resulting in a very shallow anterior chamber. The IOP was 33 mmHg.

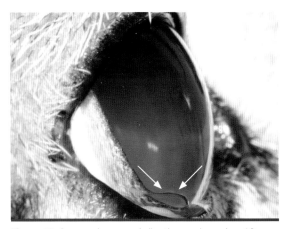

Figure 16. Aqueous humour misdirection syndrome in a 12-year-old Domestic shorthair. There is mydriasis and a very shallow anterior chamber as a result of anterior displacement of the lens. The IOP was 42 mmHg. There was also a small persistent pupillary membrane (PPM, arrows).

slowly and many affected cats appear to tolerate the increase in IOP well, not showing overt signs of discomfort and retaining vision for some time. Medical management with topical carbonic anhydrase inhibitors is recommended in an attempt to reduce the IOP, but the condition inevitably progresses very slowly over time. Surgical treatment in the form of phacoemulsification and anterior vitrectomy may be attempted in cases that respond poorly to medical treatment.

Uveal cysts

Uveal cysts are not common in cats (see Chapter 8) and, when they do arise, tend to remain attached to the posterior iris. Occasionally they displace the iris forwards resulting in shallowing of the anterior chamber and subsequent increase in IOP (Fig. 17). In this situation, removal of the cysts is recommended to normalise IOP. This can be achieved by using laser treatment to coagulate and deflate the cysts, or by an irrigation and aspiration procedure.

Treatment of glaucoma

Medical treatment of glaucoma in cats has limited reported success. A retrospective study of 82 glaucomatous cats reported successful medical management in 58 % of cases (Blocker and van der Woerdt, 2001). The apparent poor response to medical therapy is most likely explained by a combination of factors including delayed presentation of cases, the secondary nature of the condition and the limited efficacy of human glaucoma drugs in the cat. There is often a poor tolerance to topical medication due to adverse local and systemic side effects which can lead to poor patient and owner compliance, further confounding treatment.

Medical treatment

Medical treatment of glaucoma is outlined in Chapter 3. As chronic uveitis is the most common cause, in some cases, management of uveitis with topical and systemic antiinflammatories control the disease process enough to reduce the IOP and specific antihypertensive therapy may not be required. However, a study of normal cats found an increase of 5-10 mmHg

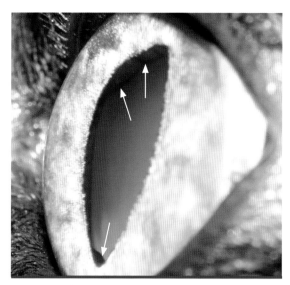

Figure 17. Multiple uveal cysts of the posterior iris, some of which are visible and shown with arrows. The anterior chamber is shallow as a result, and the IOP was 27 mmHg.

in IOP after 2-3 weeks of treatment 2-3 times daily with topical corticosteroids, and steroid-induced ocular hypertension should be considered in cats with raised IOPs receiving topical or systemic corticosteroid treatment (Bhattacherjee et al., 1999).

Topical carbonic anhydrase inhibitors remain the first line treatment in the management of feline ocular hypertension and work by reducing aqueous humour production. Carbonic anyhydrase inhibitors do not exacerbate uveitis and do not cause miosis, reducing the chance of pupil block (obstruction of aqueous flow from the posterior to the anterior chamber). Examples include 2 % dorzolamide and 1 % brinzolamide which are applied every 8-12 hours. In normal cats and those with primary congenital glaucoma, dorzolamide significantly reduces IOP (Sigle et al., 2011). Brinzolamide has no effect on IOP in normal cats (Gray et al., 2003) but, when administered three times daily, it did significantly lower IOP and blunt circadian fluctuation in IOP in glaucomatous cats although to a lesser degree than dorzolamide (McLellan et al., 2009).

Topical beta-blockers, such as betaxalol and timolol, are also widely used. They reduce IOP through blockade of beta-adrenergic receptors in the nonpigmented ciliary epithelium should be applied every 8-12 hours. There are no reports on the efficacy of betaxalol in cats, but 0.5 % timolol maleate reduced IOP by 22 %

in normal cats (Wilkie and Latimer, 1991), and recommended frequency of application is every 8-12 hours. Ocular side effects include local irritation, conjunctival hyperaemia and miosis. Adverse systemic side effects include bradycardia and vomiting and thus it has been suggested that the lower 0.25 % solution may be more appropriate in cats.

The use of topical prostaglandin analogues is ill-advised in cats due to their apparent lack of efficacy and because of their potential to exacerbate uveitis, which is often present.

Surgical treatment

When the general health of the cat permits surgical intervention, there are some additional options for glaucoma treatment. These involve either providing an alternative route of drainage for aqueous humour (gonioimplantation) or reducing its production (cyclodestructive procedures). Gonioimplantation involves the placement of a valved drainage tube to shunt aqueous humour from the anterior chamber of the eye usually to the subconjunctival space. However, obstruction of the drainage tube with inflammatory material is a real problem, particularly as uveitis is the main underlying cause of feline glaucoma. Cyclodestructive procedures involve either laser cyclophotocoagulation or cyclocryotherapy. However, both cyclophotocoagulation and cyclocryotherapy result in intraocular inflammation which is counterintuitive in cats with secondary glaucoma as a result of lymphoplasmacytic uveitis.

Owing to the late presentation and high incidence of secondary glaucoma, the most common surgical procedure performed for treatment of glaucoma is enucleation of the globe (see Chapter 4). Enucleation is indicated for irreversibly blind or painful eyes and when neoplasia is present. An alternative to enucleation, globe evisceration with placement of an intraocular prosthesis, achieves the goal of pain elimination. However, the risk of on-going neoplasia (most commonly diffuse iris melanoma), future intraocular sarcoma development, extrusion of the implant through wound failure, corneal disease, epithelial downgrowth and a suboptimal cosmetic appearance make this procedure much less attractive than the practical approach of enucleation.

References

Bhattacherjee P, Paterson CA, Spellman JM et al. (1999). Pharmacological validation of a feline model of steroid-induced ocular hypertension. *Archives of Ophthalmology*; 117:361-364.

Blocker T, van der Woerdt A (2001). The feline glaucomas: 82 cases (1995-1999). *Veterinary Ophthalmology*; 4:81-85.

Czederpiltz JM, La Croix NC, van der Woerdt A et al. (2005). Putative aqueous humor misdirection syndrome as a cause of glaucoma in cats: 32 cases (1997-2003). *Journal of the American Veterinary Medical Association*; 227:1434-1441.

Del Sole MJ, Sande PH, Bernades JM et al. (2007). Circadian rhythm of intraocular pressure in cats. *Veterinary Ophthalmology*; 10:155-161.

Gray HE, Willis AM, Morgan RV (2003). Effects of topical administration of 1 % brinzolamide on normal cat eyes. *Veterinary Ophthalmology*; 6:285-90.

Hahnenberger RW (1976). Influence of various anesthetic drugs on the intraocular pressure of cats. *Albrecht von Graefes Archiv für klinische und experimentelle Ophthalmologie*; 199:179-186.

Hampson EC, Smith RI, Bernays ME (2002). Primary glaucoma in Burmese cats. *Australian Veterinary Journal*; 80:672-680.

Jacobi S, Dubielzig RR (2008). Feline primary open angle glaucoma. *Veterinary Ophthalmology*; 11:162-165.

Kroll MM, Miller PE, Rodan I (2001). IOP measurements obtained as part of a comprehensive geriatric health examination from cats seven years of age or older. McLellan GJ, Miller PE (2011). Feline glaucoma – a comprehensive review. *Veterinary Ophthalmology*; 14:15-29.

McLellan GJ, Kemmerling JP, Kiland JA (2013). Validation of the TonoVet® rebound tonometer in normal and glaucomatous cats. *Veterinary Ophthalmology*; 16:111-118.

McLellan GJ, Betts D, Sigle K, Grozdanic S (2004). Congenital glaucoma in the Siamese cat – a new spontaneously occurring animal model for glaucoma research (Abstract). *35th Annual Meeting of the American College of Veterinary Ophthalmologists*; Washington, DC.

McLellan GJ, Kuehn MH, Ellinwood NM et al. (2006). A feline model of primary congenital glaucoma – histopathological and genetic characterization (Abstract). *Association for Research in Vision and Ophthalmology Annual Meeting*; Fort Lauderdale, FL.

McLellan GJ, Lin T-L, Hildreth S et al. (2009). Diurnal IOP and response to topically administered 1 % brinzolamide in a spontaneous feline model of primary congenital glaucoma (Abstract). *Annual Meeting of the Association for Research in Vision and Ophthalmology*; Fort Lauderdale, FL.

Miller PE, Pickett JP (1992). Comparison of the human and canine Schiotz tonometry conversion tables in clinically normal cats. *Journal of the American Veterinary Medical Association*; 201:1017-1020.

Miller PE, Pickett JP, Majors LJ et al. (1991). Evaluation of two applanation tonometers in cats. *American Journal of Veterinary Research*; 52:1917-1921.

Rusanen E, Florin M, Hassig M et al. (2010). Evaluation of a rebound tonometer (Tonovet) in clinically normal cat eyes. *Veterinary Ophthalmology*; 13:31-36.

Ofri R, Shub N, Galin Z et al. (2002). Effect of reproductive status on intraocular pressure in cats. *American Journal of Veterinary Research*; 63:159-162.

Sigle KJ, Camaño-Garcia G, Carriquiry AL et al. (2001). The effect of dorzolamide 2 % on circadian IOP in cats with primary congenital glaucoma. *Veterinary Ophthalmology*; 4:48-53.

Stadtbaumer K, Frommlet F, Nell B (2006). Effects of mydriatics on intraocular pressure and pupil size in the normal feline eye. *Veterinary Ophthalmology*; 9:233-237.

Stadtbaumer K, Kostlin RG, Zahn KJ (2002). Effects of topical 0.5 % tropicamide on intraocular pressure in normal cats. *Veterinary Ophthalmology*; 5:107-112.

Wilcock BP, Peiffer RL, Jr, Davidson MG (1990). The causes of glaucoma in cats. *Veterinary Pathology*; 27:35-40.

Wilkie DA, Latimer CA (1991). Effects of topical administration of timolol maleate on IOP and pupil size in cats. *American Journal of Veterinary Research*; 52:436-440.

10

The lens

Embryology, anatomy and function

Development of the lens begins early on in embryogenesis. The lens is derived from a region of surface ectoderm which thickens to form the lens placode. The placode then invaginates and detaches to form a hollow sphere – the lens vesicle. Primary lens fibres fill this vesicle and will go on to form the embryonic nucleus (Fig. 1). Secondary lens fibres originate from anterior cuboidal epithelial cells and differentiate at the lens equator. They surround the primary lens fibres extending both anteriorly and posteriorly, their ends meeting to form the lens sutures. In cats, the union of the sutures forms an upright 'Y' pattern anteriorly, and an inverted 'Y' pattern posteriorly (Fig. 2). These suture lines can be difficult to discern but become more obvious with advancing age. Successive lens fibres grow throughout life surrounding the inner, earlier fibres, similar to the layers of an onion. The developing lens derives its nutrition from the hyaloid artery, tunica vasculosa lentis and pupillary membrane (Fig. 3). These structures usually completely atrophy in early kittenhood before eyelid opening. Thereafter, the lens becomes dependent on the surrounding aqueous and vitreous humours for nutrition and waste removal. The lens metabolises glucose as its main energy source predominantly via anaerobic glycolysis.

Once lens development is complete, it is a transparent avascular biconvex disc (Fig. 4). It has a central nucleus, which is surrounded by the cortex, and is contained within an acellular capsule. The anterior lens capsule is considerably thicker than the posterior. The lens is held in position by the support of zonules, which extend from the equator of the lens and, in the cat, insert in the valleys between the ciliary processes of the ciliary body (Fig. 5). It is positioned in the patellar fossa, on the anterior face of the vitreous.

Lens transparency is dependent on several factors:

- Lack of blood supply, pigment and a relative state of dehydration.
- Low cellularity.
- Lack of organelles and nuclei within the lens fibres.
- Lens proteins are predominantly soluble and are arranged in a highly organised lattice pattern.

a) **The lens placode.**
Day 17 of gestation.

b) **The thickened lens placode in the surface ectoderm starts to invaginate into the neuroectoderm.**
Day 18 of gestation.

c) **The lens vesicle develops as the invagination proceeds.**
Day 21 of gestation.

d) **The lens vesicle is lined with epithelium.**
Day 25 of gestation.

e) **The posterior cells elongate to become primary lens fibres.**
Days 25-30 of gestation.

f) **The embryonic lens nucleus forms as the primary lens fibres fill the lumen.**
Day 30 of gestation.

Figure 1. Embryological development of the lens.

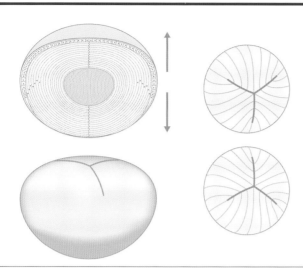

Figure 2. Illustration of lens development and Y sutures. The nuclei of the epithelial cells are at the equator, the site of transformation of epithelial cells into lens fibres. These fibres do not quite reach the poles but instead meet fibres from the opposite equator, forming the Y-shaped suture pattern.

Loss of transparency results in cataract formation. This can arise through several processes including oxidative damage, altered proteinase activity and abnormalities of metabolism.

The main function of the lens is to refract light, focusing images onto the retina for sharp vision. Removal of the lens, for example by phacomemulsification cataract surgery, therefore results in extreme long-sightedness (hypermetropia). To return the feline eye to emmetropia after phacoemulsification, insertion of a 53 D artificial lens into the remaining capsular bag is required. The lens is also involved in accommodation, the process by which the eye can change its optical power to bring objects at different distances into focus on the retina. In many species, such as man, lens accommodation is achieved by altering lens curvature. The feline lens capsule, however, has very low elasticity making significant alterations in lens curvature impossible. Instead, the feline lens accommodates by being moved anteriorly and posteriorly in a process called translation. The feline lens can be translated up to 0.6 mm, achieving up to 8 D of accommodation.

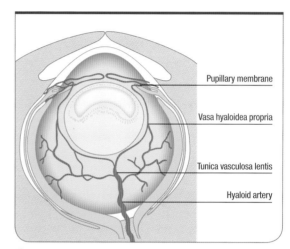

Pupillary membrane

Vasa hyaloidea propria

Tunica vasculosa lentis

Hyaloid artery

Figure 3. Illustration of developing lens vascular supply.

→ The refractive power of the feline lens is 53 D, being higher than that of the dog and human.

→ The feline lens is approximately 7.5 mm thick, 9-10 mm in equatorial diameter and has a volume of 0.5 ml.

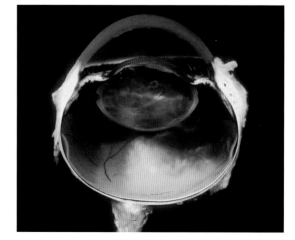

Figure 4. Gross pathology photograph of a section through a normal cat's eye, demonstrating the normal position and shape of the lens. Courtesy of John Mould.

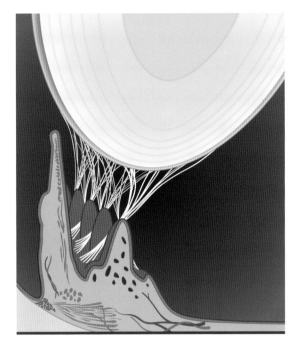

Figure 5. Illustration of ciliary zonules inserting on the lens. In the cat, the ciliary zonules insert in the valleys between the ciliary processes of the ciliary body.

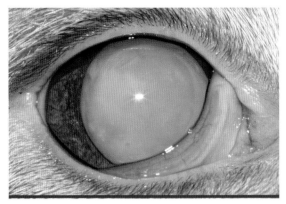

Figure 6. Microphthalmos with mature cataract. The nictitans is prominent owing to the abnormally small globe.

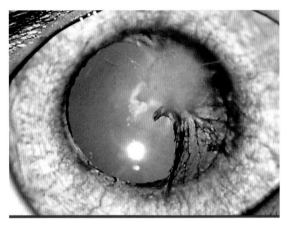

Figure 7. Anterior segment dysgenesis (ASD) causing adherent leukoma (white corneal opacity caused by adherence of anterior uveal tissue to the corneal endothelium). Pigmented persistent pupillary membrane remnants extend from the iris collarette to the corneal endothelium and a focal posterior polar cataract is present.

Congenital anomalies

Congenital lens anomalies are not very common in cats. Because of the timing of lens development at an important stage of embryogenesis of the eye, it is not uncommon for congenital lens anomalies to coexist with other ocular abnormalities, such as microphthalmia (Fig. 6), eyelid agenesis, persistent pupillary membranes (Fig. 7) and posterior segment colobomas. Anterior segment dysgenesis is the term used to describe a spectrum of developmental conditions affecting the cornea, iris and lens (Fig. 7). Congenital cataracts are occasionally encountered affecting either the nucleus or the lens capsules. Persistent hyperplastic tunica vasculosa lentis and persistent hyperplastic primary vitreous (PHTVL/PHPV) have also been reported in cats causing opacification of the posterior lens capsule and cortex (Allgoewer and Pfefferkorn, 2001). Other possible congenital lens abnormalities include an abnormally large lens (macrophakia), an abnormally small lens (microphakia) or complete lens absence (aphakia) (Benz et al., 2011; Molleda et al., 1995).

Acquired anomalies of the lens

Nuclear sclerosis

Nuclear sclerosis is a normal aging process of the lens that occurs in all cats aged 10 years and older (Figs. 8-10). Over time, as successive new lens fibres are formed, the older ones in the nucleus become compressed. The optical properties of the nucleus are altered and light is scattered causing the nucleus to develop a milky appearance. Nuclear sclerosis is occasionally misdiagnosed as cataract although the two conditions can be easily distinguished by distant direct ophthalmoscopy (see Chapter 1, Fig. 10). Nuclear sclerosis is not thought to impair vision in cats, and therefore no treatment is necessary.

ADVANCING STAGES OF NUCLEAR SCLEROSIS

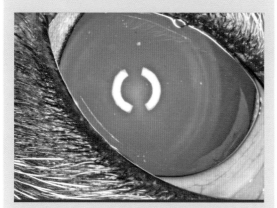

Figure 8. Nuclear sclerosis. Within the pupil, a faint ring is visible around the nucleus in this 10-year-old cat.

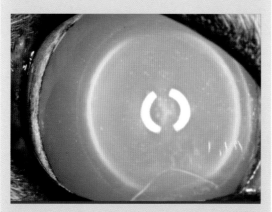

Figure 9. Nuclear sclerosis. A more obvious ring of nuclear sclerosis is seen within the pupil in a 13-year-old cat.

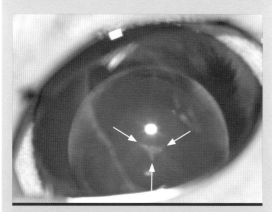

Figure 10. Pronounced nuclear sclerosis with a ring surrounding the nucleus in a 17-year-old cat. A central circular halo is visible within the dilated pupil, representing advanced nuclear sclerosis of the lens. There is also a small triradiate posterior polar cataract (arrows).

Cataracts

A cataract is defined as an opacity of the lens or its capsule. Cataracts are most commonly classified by their extent of lens involvement as illustrated in Table 1. In cats, primary (presumed inherited) cataracts are particularly rare and may either be congenital or developmental (Figs. 11-13). Secondary cataracts are far more common and may occur as a result of traumatic injury (Figs. 14-17), chronic uveitis (Figs. 17-20), lens luxation (Figs. 21 and 22), glaucoma (Fig. 23) and senility (Figs. 24 and 25). Occasionally, the cause of cataracts is unknown (Figs. 26 and 27). The most common cause of cataract in cats is chronic anterior uveitis (Olivero et al., 1991). Cataracts caused by intraocular inflammation usually begin in the peripheral cortex and may gradually progress to maturity. Penetrating corneal injuries (e.g. caused by cat scratches) causing lens capsular rupture can lead to progressive cataract formation or be associated with septic implantation which can be disastrous to the eye unless treated immediately and appropriately (Dalesandro et al., 2011; Paulsen and Kass, 2012 and Bell et al., 2013). Primary infectious causes of cataracts are rare but have been reported in association with infection with *Encephalitozoon cuniculi* (Benz et al., 2011). Metabolic cataracts have been reported in kittens fed commercial milk replacer deficient in arginine (an essential amino acid for the cat). A cross-sectional study of 2000 normal cats showed that 50 % had evidence of cataract by 12 years of age and all cats over 17 years of age had some form of lens opacity (Williams and Heath, 2006). Diabetic cataracts are much less common in cats than in dogs and, when they do occur, are usually very slowly progressive. The low incidence of cataracts in diabetic cats relates to the low activity of aldose reductase in the feline lens (Richter et al., 2002).

→ Nuclear sclerosis is easily distinguished from cataracts by distant direct ophthalmoscopy. It has little effect on vision.

Table 1. Types of cataracts according to lens involvement.

Stage	Illustration	Features	Ability to examine fundus	Vision status
Incipient		< 15 % of lens volume affected Large tapetal reflex present	Detailed examination possible	Usually good although impairment possible if visual axis involved
Immature (incomplete)		15 % up to almost entire lens volume may be affected Tapetal reflex reduced but still present	Examination usually possible but may be limited	Varies according to extent
Mature (complete)		Entire lens is affected Loss of tapetal reflex	Examination not possible	Blind
Hypermature		Cataract liquefaction and resorption with loss of lens volume and capsule wrinkling and plaques Partial tapetal reflex may be restored	Examination may be possible again	Usually blind Retinal detachment and/or secondary glaucoma common

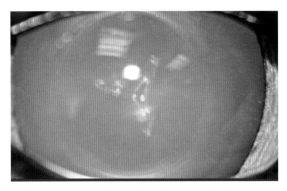

Figure 11. Y-shaped cataract involving the anterior suture lines of the lens, along with a perinuclear halo due to early nuclear sclerosis in an 11-year-old cat.

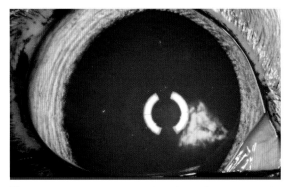

Figure 12. Triangular posterior polar subcapsular cataract to the right of the flash artefact.

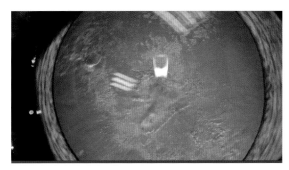

Figure 13. Extensive anterior subcapsular/cortical progressive cataract.

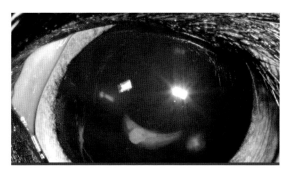

Figure 14. Penetrating cat-claw injury. There is a small dorsal corneal scar and a crescent-shaped rupture of the anterior lens capsule. A small amount of lens cortex has herniated through the lens capsular tear.

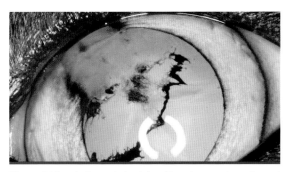

Figure 15. Penetrating cat-claw injury. There is corneal scarring and anterior cortical cataract formation. The pigmented opacities on the anterior lens capsule represent 'iris rests' resulting from previous contact of the posterior iris with the anterior lens capsule during a period of anterior uveitis and accompanying miosis.

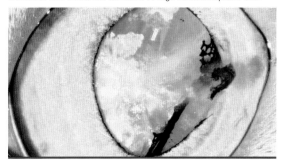

Figure 16. A previous cat-claw injury penetrated the cornea and lens causing lens capsule rupture and resulting in a hypermature cataract.

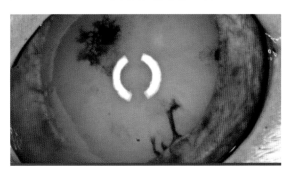

Figure 17. Chronic uveitis of two years' duration with rubeosis iridis, posterior synechiae, 'iris rests' on the anterior lens capsule and a mature cataract.

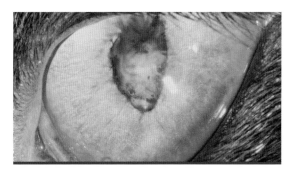

Figure 18. Chronic uveitis has resulted in miosis, posterior synechiae and a hypermature cataract.

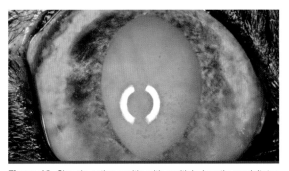

Figure 19. Chronic active uveitis with multiple keratic precipitates on the corneal endothelium, rubeosis iridis and a mature cataract.

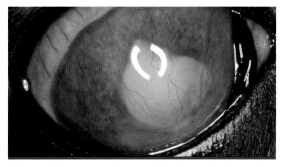

Figure 20. Chronic active keratouveitis with episcleral congestion, corneal vascularisation, pronounced rubeosis iridis, dyscoria and a mature cataract.

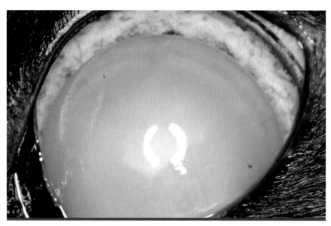

Figure 21. Anterior lens luxation. A spherical lens with a mature cataract lies anterior to the iris.

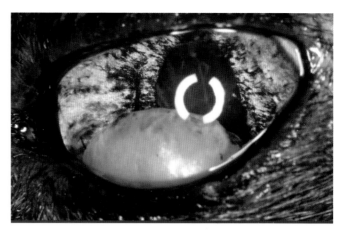

Figure 22. Chronic anterior lens luxation. The lens exhibits a hypermature cataract and is visible within the ventral anterior chamber. The iris is hyperpigmented as a result of chronic uveitis.

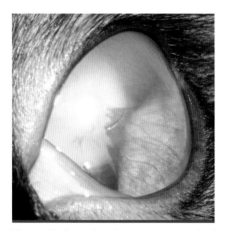

Figure 23. Secondary glaucoma as a result of chronic anterior uveitis. The globe is enlarged (buphthalmic) and there is corneal oedema, iris swelling, posterior synechiae and a subluxated cataractous lens.

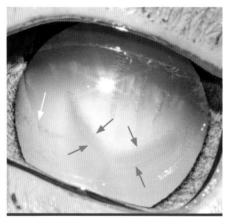

Figure 24. Mature cataract in an older cat with no evidence of uveitis. The Y-suture clefts (red arrows) and cortical vacuolation (white arrow) are visible.

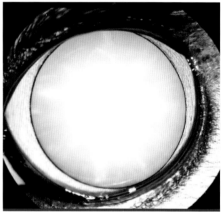

Figure 25. Mature cataract in a geriatric cat with no evidence of uveitis.

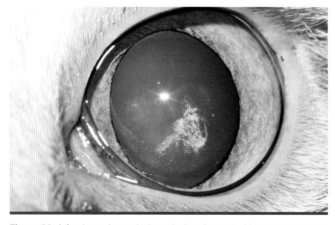

Figure 26. A focal anterior cortical opacity in a 6-month-old cat, with an otherwise normal lens.

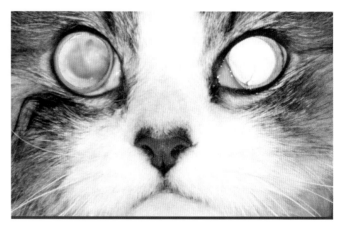

Figure 27. A nuclear cataract in the right eye of a 14-month-old Domestic longhair. The left lens was normal.

Cataracts are assessed for position, extent and density. A full examination of both the affected and contralateral eye may yield clues as to the cause. Sight-impairing cataracts can be removed by phacoemulsification surgery. This highly specialised procedure involves cataract extraction through a small (3 mm) peripheral corneal incision. A small window is made in the anterior lens capsule – the capsulorhexis. The phacoemulsification hand-piece is introduced through the corneal incision and the cataract is emulsified using high-frequency ultrasonic vibrations before being aspirated from the eye. A synthetic intraocular lens is usually then inserted in the remaining capsular bag in order to return the eye to emmetropia. These artificial lenses are species specific and, in the cat, a refractive power of 53 D is required to achieve emmetropia. Careful aftercare is imperative and involves the frequent use of topical medications and reexaminations. The most common immediate postoperative complications in cats include postoperative ocular hypertension and corneal ulceration which can usually be treated very

successfully. More long-term potential complications include posterior capsular opacification, glaucoma and retinal detachment (Cobo et al., 1984). The prognosis after cataract surgery is very good and success rates appear to be higher in cats than dogs, as they seem to suffer from less postoperative intraocular inflammation and secondary glaucoma (Figs. 28 and 29).

Lens luxation

Lens luxation is the displacement of the lens from its normal position either anteriorly into the anterior chamber or posteriorly into the vitreous chamber (posterior segment) (Figs. 30-35). It occurs most commonly as a secondary condition usually as a result of chronic anterior uveitis or glaucoma. Primary (presumed inherited) lens luxation is rare in cats but has been reported occurring either as a congenital or as a developmental abnormality (Payen et al., 2011; Molleda et al., 1995). Other ocular defects such as microphakia and goniodysgenesis or systemic abnormalities such as cardiac malformations may also be present.

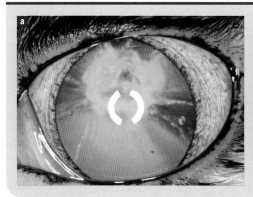
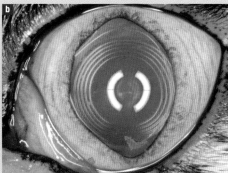

Figure 28. a) A progressive posterior subcapsular cataract with radiating cortical extensions beginning to cause visual impairment in an one-eyed cat. b) The same eye one day after phacoemulsification surgery and implantation of a synthetic intraocular lens.

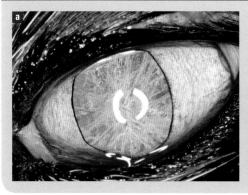
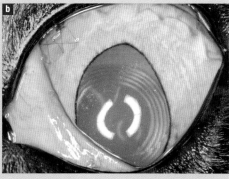

Figure 29. a) A progressive maturing cataract with cortical vacuolation. b) The same eye one day after phacoemulsification surgery and implantation of a synthetic intraocular lens. The sutured 3 mm corneal incision is present at the 10 o'clock position.

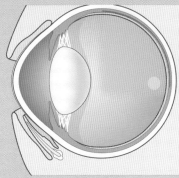

a. Normal lens position.

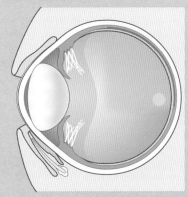

b. Anterior lens luxation into the anterior chamber.

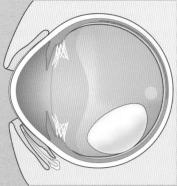

c. Posterior lens luxation into the vitreous chamber.

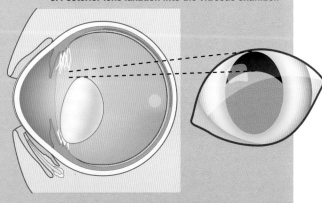

d. Aphakic crescent with lens subluxation.

Figure 30. Normal and abnormal lens positions in the feline eye.

→ Lens luxation is often a bilateral condition so both eyes should be thoroughly examined for signs of lens luxation, uveitis and glaucoma.

Clinical signs of lens luxation include mild to moderate signs of ocular discomfort and episcleral congestion. Anterior lens luxation can cause focal corneal oedema resulting from direct contact of the luxated lens with the corneal endothelium. The anteriorly luxated lens may also interrupt aqueous humour dynamics and outflow leading to raised intraocular pressure which, in turn, can cause more generalised corneal oedema. Anterior lens luxation is much less commonly associated with acute glaucoma in cats than in dogs. This can be explained by the relatively deep feline anterior chamber. Chronic glaucoma, however, is more common and usually results in blindness owing to irreversible damage to the retinal ganglion cells and their axons (see Chapter 9). If the intraocular pressure remains elevated this can also lead to globe enlargement (buphthalmos). Examination of the contralateral eye is important as uveitis, the most common cause of lens luxation, is often a bilateral condition. Investigation for proper causes of feline uveitis is required if this is present (see Chapter 8). The intraocular pressure of the contralateral eye should be measured also, as glaucoma is a painful and blinding condition that can either be the cause or the result of lens luxation.

Treatment of lens luxation involves surgical removal of the lens via intracapsular lens extraction (Figs. 36 and 37) and treatment of any attendant intraocular inflammation and/or raised intraocular pressure. The prognosis depends on many factors including chronicity and whether or not glaucoma is present, but is usually favourable with success rates of up to 90 % being reported (Olivero et al., 1991).

For blind and painful eyes with no hope of restoration of vision (Fig. 38), enucleation is usually advised on welfare grounds. Long-term monitoring of the remaining eye is usually necessary as the initial cause of luxation usually affects both eyes.

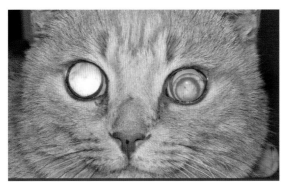

Figure 31. Anterior lens luxation in the left eye. The border of the luxated lens is visible and there is an aphakic crescent. The displaced lens is becoming cataractous.

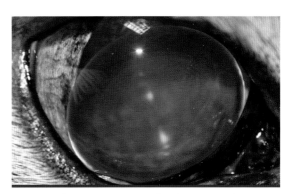

Figure 32. The large disc-shaped lens is occupying the anterior chamber due to acute anterior lens luxation.

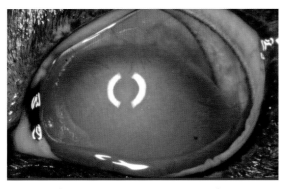

Figure 33. Chronic uveitis with anterior luxation of a cataractous lens. There is also chemosis and corneal vascularisation.

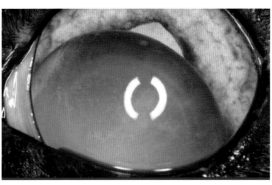

Figure 34. Chronic uveitis with rubeosis iridis has resulted in anterior lens luxation, and the lens is starting to become opaque.

→ Clinical signs of lens luxation are often more insidious, and acute glaucoma is less common in the cat than in the dog.

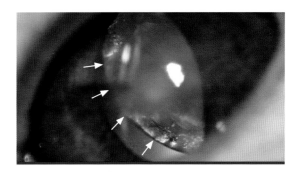

Figure 35. The edge of the lens is visible within the pupil behind the iris (arrows). There is progressive cortical opacification in this posteriorly luxated lens.

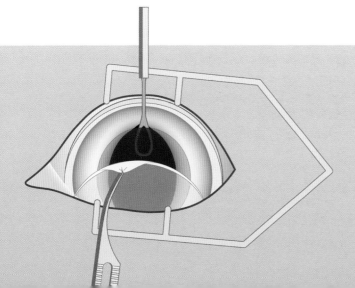

Figure 36. Illustration of intracapsular lens extraction surgery for anterior lens luxation. After creating a large limbal incision and injecting viscoelastic, the cornea is gently retracted with a forceps such as Colibri forceps. A lens loop is gently inserted posterior to the lens and the lens is gradually extracted from the eye.

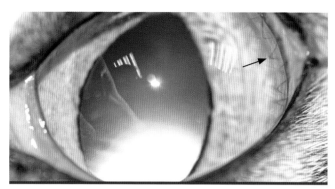

Figure 37. Appearance of an eye three days after intracapsular lens extraction surgery for an anteriorly luxated lens. Part of the large peripheral corneal incision is visible (arrow), sutured with absorbable suture in a continuous pattern.

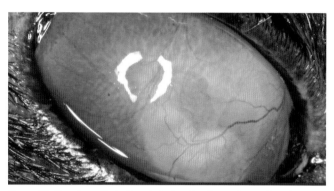

Figure 38. Chronic uveitis led to anterior lens luxation and secondary glaucoma. Progressive corneal oedema and vascularisation occurred and the glaucoma did not respond to topical treatment.

Examination tip

B-mode ultrasonography is a very useful method to examine the position and density of the lens when direct examination is precluded by disease and/or opacities of the ocular adnexa or anterior segment (Fig. 39).

Figure 39. a) B-mode ultrasound of a normal feline lens. The normal lens cortex and ▶ nucleus are hypoechoic whereas the capsule is hyperechoic. The equatorial diameter of the lens is 116 mm and the anterior-posterior thickness is 77 mm. b) Intumescent cataract. The entire lens demonstrates increased echogenicity. c) Anterior lens luxation. The lens is recognised as a smooth spherical structure within the anterior chamber. The relative increased echogenicity reflects cataractous changes within the lens. d) Posterior lens luxation. The cataractous lens is recognised as a spherical structure of high echogenicity within the posterior (vitreal) segment. e) Linear foreign body penetrating the lens (yellow arrow). The retina was inflamed and is seen to be thickened in this image (white arrow).

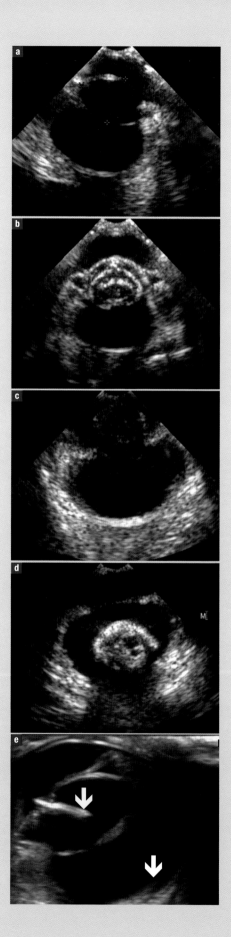

References

Allgoewer I, Pfefferkorn B (2001). Persistent hyperplastic tunica vasculosa lentis and persistent hyperplastic primary vitreous (PHTVL/PHPV) in two cats. *Veterinary Ophthalmology*; 4:161-164.

Bell CM, Pot SA, Dubielzig RR (2013). Septic implantation syndrome in dogs and cats: a distinct pattern of endophthalmitis with lenticular abscess. *Veterinary Ophthalmology*; 16:180-185.

Benz P, Maass G, Csokai J et al. (2011). Detection of *Encephalitozoon cuniculi* in the feline cataractous lens. *Veterinary Ophthalmology*; 14(Suppl 1):37-47.

Benz P, Walde I, Gumpenberger M et al. (2011). Macrophakia in three cats. *Veterinary Ophthalmology*; 14(Suppl 1):99-104.

Cobo LM, Ohsawa E, Chandler D et al. (1984). Pathogenesis of capsular opacification after extracapsular cataract extraction. An animal model. *Ophthalmology*; 91:857-863.

Dalesandro N, Stiles J, Miller M (2011). Septic lens implantation syndrome in a cat. *Veterinary Ophthalmology*; 14(Suppl 1):84-87.

Molleda JM, Martín E, Ginel PJ et al. (1995). Microphakia associated with lens luxation in the cat. *Journal of the American Animal Hospital Association*; 31:209-212.

Olivero DK, Riis RC, Dutton AG et al. (1991) Feline lens displacement: a retrospective analysis of 345 cases. *Progress in Veterinary and Comparative Ophthalmology*; 1:239-244.

Paulsen ME, Kass PH (2012). Traumatic corneal laceration with associated lens capsule disruption: a retrospective study of 77 clinical cases from 1999 to 2009. *Veterinary Ophthalmology*; 15:355-368.

Payen G, Hänninen RL, Mazzucchelli S et al. (2011). Primary lens instability in ten related cats: clinical and genetic considerations. *Journal of Small Animal Practice*; 52:402-410.

Richter M, Guscetti F, Spiess B (2002). Aldose reductase activity and glucose-related opacities in incubated lenses from dogs and cats. *American Journal of Veterinary Research*; 63:1591-1597.

Williams DL, Heath MF (2006). Prevalence of feline cataract: results of a cross-sectional study of 2000 normal animals, 50 cats with diabetes and one hundred cats following dehydrational crises. *Veterinary Ophthalmology*; 9:341-349.

11

The vitreous and fundus

Anatomy and function

The vitreous is an elastic hydrogel that occupies the posterior segment of the globe (Fig. 1). It is composed of 99 % water with the remaining 1 % largely made up of collagen fibres, hyalocytes (resident vitreal cells) and hyaluronic acid. Embryologically, the vitreous plays an important role in the nourishment of the lens as it harbours the hyaloid artery and tunica vasculosa lentis. The developed vitreous is transparent to enable transmission of light and it provides support to the globe and intraocular tissues. The anterior vitreous supports the lens within its patellar fossa and the posterior vitreous helps maintain close contact of the neurosensory retina with the retinal pigment epithelium (RPE). The vitreous base is attached in the region of the ciliary body.

The fundus can be defined as the posterior region of the eye that is viewed via the pupil during ophthalmoscopy. The fundus thus always includes the retina, optic nerve and choroid but also may include, in those animals where it can be visualised, the sclera. The retina is composed of ten layers and is divided into the inner, sensory retina and the outer, nonsensory retina (Fig. 2). The inner retina is composed of nine layers with the photoreceptors (rods and cones) located outermost (Fig. 3). The photoreceptors are stimulated by light photons to convert chemical energy into electrical energy in a process called phototransduction. The electrical impulses created are then transmitted, via bipolar cells within the inner nuclear layer, to the inner ganglion cells and optic nerve to the brain for visual processing. Other than bipolar cells, the inner nuclear layer also contains the cell bodies of amacrine and horizontal cells which modulate the electrical signals, and Müller cells which have a supportive role and contribute to the formation of the outer and inner limiting membranes of the retina. The RPE is the outermost layer of the retina, is nonsensory and is immediately adjacent to the choroid. From inside out, the choroid is composed of the choriocapillaris, tapetum and stroma which contains medium to large-sized blood vessels. Adjacent to the choroid is the sclera which, together with the cornea, forms the globe's fibrous tunic.

The tapetum is located within the choroid between the choriocapillaris and choroidal stroma. It tends to be more uniform in cats than in dogs and is a roughly triangular, reflective structure in the dorsal fundus (Fig. 4). The adult tapetum usually takes on a yellow-green appearance although, in some

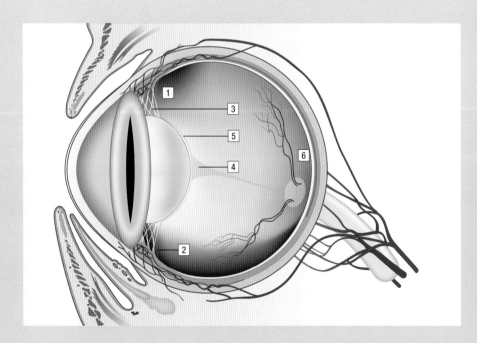

Figure 1. Location and anatomy of vitreous.
1. Vitreous base
2. Anterior vitreous face
3. Lens zonular fibres
4. Cloquet's canal
5. Hyaloideocapsular ligament
6. Posterior vitreous

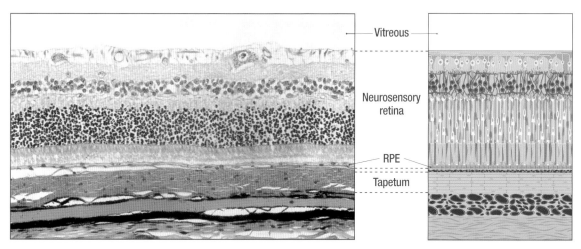

Figure 2. Photomicrograph (haematoxylin and eosin) showing histological section of normal feline tapetal fundus.

Figure 3. Illustration of normal retinal architecture.

individuals, it may appear blue or even be absent (Figs. 5-9). The tapetum is visible during ophthalmoscopy owing to the absence of melanin within the overlying RPE of the tapetal fundus. The nontapetal fundus is usually dark brown as a result of a high concentration of melanin granules within the RPE in this region. In blue-eyed cats there may be no tapetum and no pigment within the RPE. In this situation the normal radial striping of the choroidal vessels may be seen against the white sclera (Figs. 9 and 10). The developing tapetum initially takes on a lilac appearance in the first few weeks after eyelid opening. At eight weeks it appears blue (Fig. 11) and then gradually assumes a more yellow-green colouration. The feline tapetum is particularly well developed and is, on average, 15-20 cell layers deep and may be even thicker centrally. The tapetum owes its reflectivity to the presence of specialised cells called iridocytes which, in the cat, are full of riboflavin rodlets. The tapetum functions to reflect light that has passed through the retina back to the photoreceptors for a second chance of stimulation.

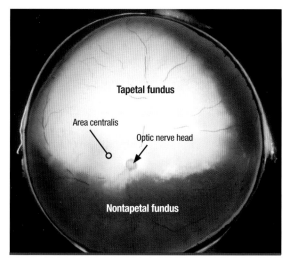

Figure 4. Gross photograph of feline fundus taken from a transected formalin-fixed globe. Courtesy of John Mould.

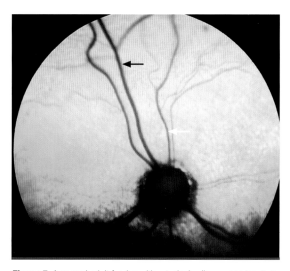

Figure 5. A normal adult fundus with a typical yellow-green tapetum. Note the retinal arterioles (white arrow) and veins (black arrow).

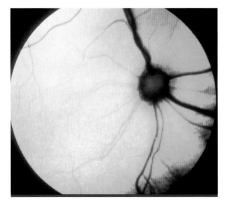

Figure 6. A normal adult fundus with a yellow-green tapetum.

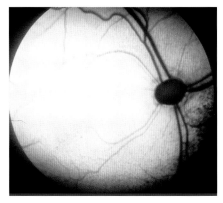

Figure 7. A normal adult fundus with a yellow tapetum.

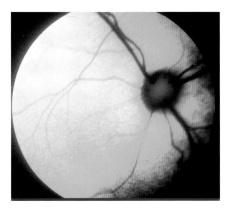

Figure 8. A normal adult fundus with a blue-green tapetum.

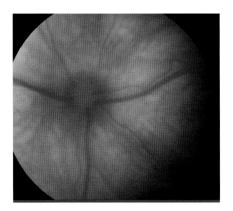

Figure 9. A normal adult fundus in a 6-year-old Siamese with blue irides. There is no tapetum or choroidal pigmentation. Courtesy of Professor Sheila Crispin.

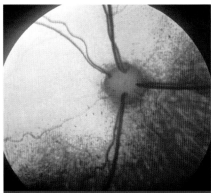

Figure 10. A normal fundus of a 10-year-old Siamese. The RPE and choroid are nonpigmented in the nontapetal fundus allowing visualisation of the choroidal vessels and underlying white sclera.

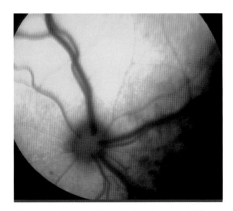

Figure 11. A normal fundus of an 8-week-old kitten. Note the typical blue appearance of the developing tapetum.

The optic disc is located in the ventral tapetal fundus and in a corresponding location in atapetal eyes. It is usually grey owing to the absence of myelin and usually appears 'cupped' with blood vessels dipping into it over its edge (Fig. 10). The optic nerve head can occasionally be myelinated in which case it appears white and large (macropapilla) and peripapillary myelinated nerve fibres may be present and are considered normal variation (Figs. 12-14). Typically, three major pairs of cilioretinal arterioles and veins originate from the periphery of the optic disc. These vessels arc around the area centralis which is devoid of arterioles and veins (although a capillary network is present). The area centralis is located 3-4 mm dorsolateral to the optic disc and is a region of relatively high cone density (Fig. 4). Cones are responsible for visual acuity and colour detection. Visual acuity in the cat, however, is relatively poor being 5-9 times less than that of man. Cats, on the other hand, have excellent night vision owing to the presence of a rod-dominated retina. Furthermore, there are species-specific alterations in the composition of the inner nuclear layer tied to the large fraction of rod photoreceptors which likely represents the cat's evolutionary adaptation to nocturnal behaviour (Macneil et al., 2009). The visual streak is closely related to the area centralis and is defined as the region of the fundus with highest ganglion cell density. The visual streak takes the form of

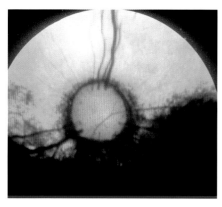

Figure 12. Macropapilla. The optic nerve head is myelinated and large. This is normal variation and vision is unaffected.

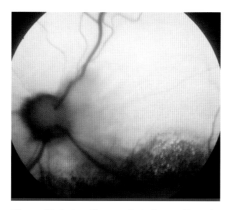

Figure 13. Peripapillary myelinated nerve fibres. An example of normal variation.

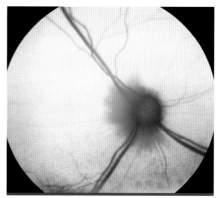

Figure 14. Peripapillary myelinated nerve fibres. An example of normal variation.

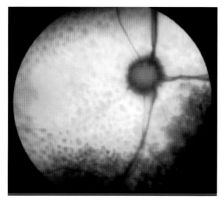

Figure 15. Retinal dysplasia of unknown cause in a 6-month-old Domestic shorthair. The cat was otherwise healthy and the lesions were nonprogressive.

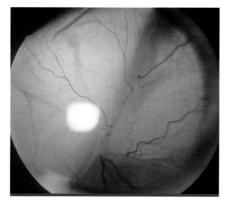

Figure 16. Total retinal dysplasia with total retinal detachment in a 3-month-old Domestic shorthair.

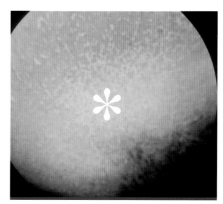

Figure 17. Aplasia of the retina and optic nerve head in an 8-week-old Domestic shorthair. The expected location of the optic nerve head is indicated (asterisk).

a near horizontal band approximately 3 mm dorsal to the optic disc and is thought to make a significant contribution to the pupillary light reflex in the cat (Thompson et al., 2010).

Congenital abnormalities of the vitreous and fundus

The vitreous

Persistent hyperplastic tunica vasculosa lentis/persistent hyperplastic primary vitreous (PHTVL/PHPV) is rare but has been reported in cats causing opacification of the posterior lens capsule and cortex (Allgoewer and Pfefferkorn, 2001). Persistent hyaloid artery is even rarer.

The fundus

Retinal dysplasia is uncommon but can have a number of causes. The most commonly cited cause in cats is intrauterine infection with feline leukaemia (FeLV) or feline panleucopaenia (FPV) viruses. Inherited retinal dysplasia, as seen in certain dog breeds, is not well characterised in cats but is seen occasionally and may be multifocal or total in manifestation (Figs. 15 and 16). A rod-cone photoreceptor dysplasia leading to retinal degeneration has been documented in the Abyssinian (see later). Optic disc hypoplasia is uncommon and optic disc aplasia is extremely rare but both have been reported in cats (Fig. 17).

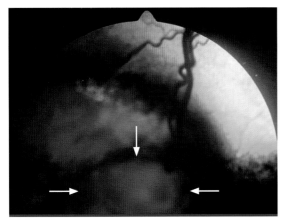

Figure 18. Posterior segment coloboma affecting the optic nerve head, peripapillary retina and choroid allowing visualisation of the white sclera dorsal to the optic nerve head (arrows).

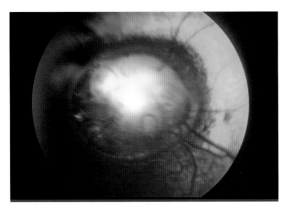

Figure 19. Posterior segment coloboma affecting the optic nerve head and peripapillary retina. The image is focused on the retina and, hence, the optic nerve tissue appears out of focus owing to the colobomatous defect.

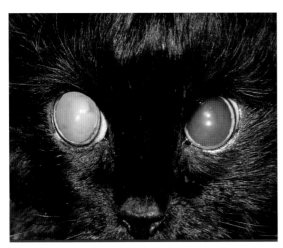

Figure 20. Haemorrhage within the anterior vitreous in a 14-year-old Domestic shorthair with systemic hypertension. This blind cat has bilateral mydriasis and the right eye has a bullous retinal detachment.

Fundus colobomas are rare in cats but when they do occur they usually affect the optic nerve head and peripapillary retina, choroid and sclera (Figs. 18 and 19). They are termed 'typical' when they occur ventrally at the 6 o'clock position and 'atypical' at other locations. Colobomas of the posterior segment may occur in isolation or in conjunction with other congenital ocular abnormalities such as retinal dysplasia, persistent pupillary membrane and eyelid agenesis (eyelid coloboma). Posterior segment colobomas may be an incidental finding but, if extensive, can cause visual deficits and blindness.

Acquired diseases of the vitreous and fundus

Acquired diseases of the vitreous

The vitreous may be affected by cellular infiltrates from contiguous inflammation of the posterior uveal tract and retina. Large collections of inflammatory cells within the anterior vitreous are often described as 'pars planitis' although the retina, rather than the choroid, may be the primary site of inflammation. Potential causes of such inflammation include feline immunodeficiency virus (FIV), feline infectious peritonitis (FIP) and toxoplasmosis. Although avascular itself, rupture of vessels within the ciliary body, choroid or retina may result in haemorrhage within the vitreous (Fig. 20). Possible causes include trauma, systemic hypertension, inflammation and neoplasia. Although primary vitreal neoplasia has not been reported, the vitreous may become involved by extension of neoplasia affecting neighbouring ocular tissues.

Acquired diseases of the fundus
Retina and choroid
Lysosomal storage diseases

These are rare, progressive, inherited diseases caused by a deficiency of a specific lysosomal enzyme. There is a resultant accumulation of enzyme substrate within cellular lysosomes which leads to cell death and resultant disease. Multiple organs are usually involved but this depends on the specific disease. Examples of lysosomal storage diseases which can affect the retina in cats include GM1-gangliosidosis, α-mannosidosis, mucolipidosis II and mucopolysaccharidosis VI.

Vascular disease

Haemorrhage

Haemorrhage within the posterior segment is not uncommon in the cat and there are many possible causes. Haemorrhage occurs when there is rupture of blood vessels and thus, in the posterior segment, this may originate from the ciliary body, retina or choroid.

Hypertensive retinopathy

Hypertensive retinopathy occurring secondary to systemic hypertension is fairly common in geriatric cats and is usually secondary to chronic renal insufficiency or, less frequently, hyperthyroidism. Hypertrophic cardiomyopathy is a common finding in cats with systemic hypertension but is usually thought to occur as a result of the hypertension rather than cause it. Hypertensive retinopathy is particularly prevalent in cats with systolic blood pressures above around 170 mmHg and female neutered cats appear to be at increased risk (Sansom et al., 2004). The eye is a particularly sensitive target organ of systemic hypertension as its precise function depends on vascular integrity. The accessibility of the fundus for direct examination yields itself to the detection of very early signs of systemic hypertension. It is recommended that all cats over the age of 10 years and those with previously diagnosed chronic renal disease and hyperthyroidism should receive funduscopy and blood pressure measurement on an annual basis. Any cat diagnosed with hypertension should receive thorough investigation into the underlying cause and all hypertensive cats should be evaluated for cardiac disease. Early diagnosis and prompt treatment are important to prevent the development of severe, devastating and irreversible damage to the eye. Prolonged systemic hypertension causes damage to retinal and choroidal capillaries and arterioles which leads to leakage of plasma into the surrounding tissues (retinal and choroidal oedema). More severe vascular damage leads to rupture of vessel walls and haemorrhage, and total retinal detachment is thought to result from choroidal effusion and ischaemic damage to the RPE.

Clinically, the earliest detectable signs of hypertension on funduscopy are tortuosity of the retinal arterioles (Fig. 21) and retinal oedema with focal bullae (Figs. 22 and 23). More severe disease is associated with haemorrhage and, depending on which vessels are involved, focal haemorrhages may be subretinal, intraretinal or preretinal with haemorrhage in each location having a typical appearance (Figs. 24-26). Massive retinal and choroidal haemorrhages are usually associated with retinal detachment and blood within the vitreous which may also migrate through the pupil manifesting as hyphaema (Figs. 27-29). When haemorrhage within the anterior segment is severe, secondary glaucoma may develop. The typical presentation of a cat with hypertensive retinopathy, however, is of acute blindness associated with total retinal detachment with varying extents of anterior and posterior segment haemorrhage (Figs. 27 and 30-32).

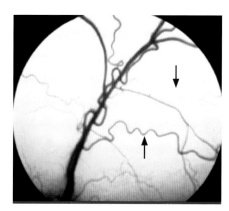

Figure 21. Hypertensive retinopathy. Tortuosity of the retinal arterioles (arrows) in a 10-year-old cat with a systolic blood pressure of 190 mmHg.

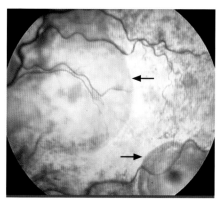

Figure 22. Hypertensive retinopathy. Large retinal bullae (detachments) are present within the tapetal fundus (arrows).

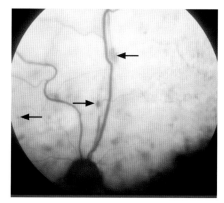

Figure 23. Hypertensive retinopathy. The retinal arterioles are attenuated, there is retinal oedema and some small intraretinal haemorrhages (arrows).

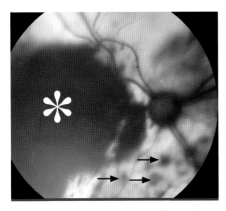

Figure 24. Hypertensive retinopathy. Subretinal (asterisk) and intraretinal (arrows) haemorrhages along with widespread retinal oedema.

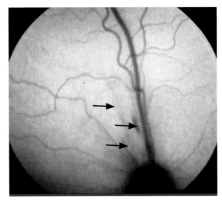

Figure 25. Hypertensive retinopathy. Three streaks of haemorrhage are present within the nerve fibre layer of the retina adjacent to the optic nerve head between the 11 and 12 o'clock positions (arrows).

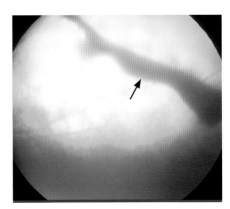

Figure 26. Hypertensive retinopathy. A preretinal, 'keel-shaped' haemorrhage is present (arrow).

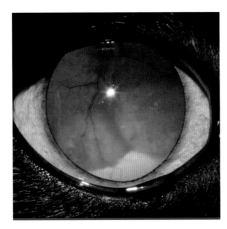

Figure 27. Hypertensive retinopathy. There is total retinal detachment with the retina visible because it has been displaced anteriorly.

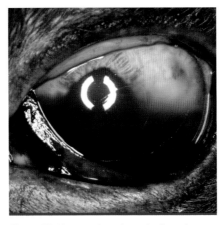

Figure 28. Hypertensive retinopathy. Posterior segment haemorrhage has migrated anteriorly and is present as diffuse hyphaema.

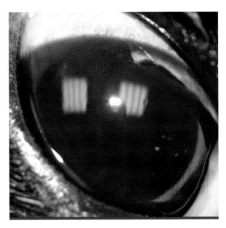

Figure 29. Hypertensive retinopathy. Haemorrhage arising within the posterior segment has migrated anteriorly (hyphaema) and there is a formed blood clot within the anterior chamber.

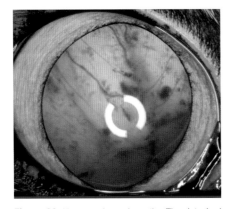

Figure 30. Hypertensive retinopathy. The detached and haemorrhagic retina is adjacent to the posterior lens capsule.

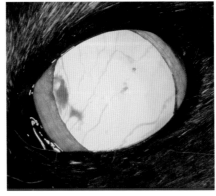

Figure 31. Hypertensive retinopathy. The detached and haemorrhagic retina is adjacent to the posterior lens capsule.

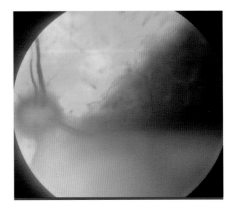

Figure 32. Hypertensive retinopathy. The retina ventral to the optic nerve head has detached. Evidence of previous intraretinal haemorrhages can be seen within the tapetal fundus.

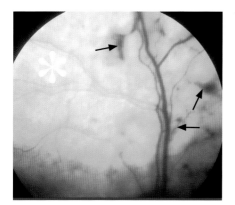

Figure 33. Hypertensive retinopathy. Antihypertensive medication has resulted in retinal reattachment. There is moderate tapetal hyperreflectivity indicating retinal degeneration (asterisk) and several blood clots from previous retinal haemorrhages (arrows).

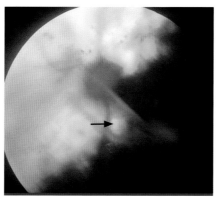

Figure 34. Hypertensive retinopathy two months after initial diagnosis and treatment. Antihypertensive medication has resulted in retinal reattachment. A fibrous traction band is present resulting from previous haemorrhage (arrow).

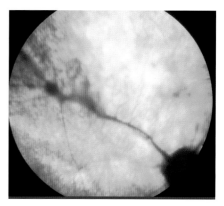

Figure 35. Hypertensive retinopathy six months after initial diagnosis and treatment. Antihypertensive medication resulted in early retinal reattachment but there is evidence of retinal degeneration with tapetal hyperreflectivity and vascular attenuation present and the cat remained blind.

Treatment of systemic hypertension involves treatment of the primary cause (usually chronic kidney disease) as well as antihypertensive medications. If treatment is instigated early, then even very large retinal detachments can resolve and vision be restored, but this does depend on the extent of the initial damage to the retina (Figs. 33-35). The antihypertensive medication of choice in the cat is amlodipine, a calcium channel blocker. Initially a dose of 0.625-1.25 mg amlodipine orally once daily is administered and funduscopy and blood pressure measurement are repeated after seven days. The amlodipine dose can be increased to 1.25 mg once daily if response is unsatisfactory and the later addition of an ACE inhibitor, such as benazepril, can help improve control in recalcitrant cases. Once normotension is achieved, reevaluation is required at least every six months.

Diabetic and megoestrol acetate retinopathy

Diabetic retinopathy is not well characterised in the cat but has been acknowledged especially when diabetes mellitus has resulted from prolonged administration of megoestrol acetate. The ophthalmoscopic signs are identical to those of hypertensive retinopathy (Figs. 36 and 37) and thus are more likely explained by systemic hypertension rather than glycaemic status *per se*.

Anaemic retinopathy

In its mildest form, anaemic retinopathy appears as a relative pallor of the retinal vessels. Profound anaemia, with haematocrit less than 10 % and haemoglobin concentrations less than 5 g/dL, is associated with retinal haemorrhages (Fig. 43). It is thought that anaemia leads to hypoxic damage of the vascular endothelium with resultant fragility of the vascular walls.

Lipaemia retinalis

Lipaemia retinalis describes the ophthalmoscopically visible presence of lipoproteins (specifically chylomicrons or very low density lipoproteins (VLDL)) within retinal vessels and is most obvious over the dark nontapetal fundus. The retinal vessels become white to cream in colour and appear wider than normal but do not seem to exhibit other overt pathology (Figs. 38 and 39). The finding of lipaemia retinalis, however, is useful in the diagnosis of systemic hyperlipoproteinaemia for which there are several causes. In cats, hyperlipoproteinaemia is most commonly associated with diabetes mellitus, hypothyroidism and prolonged treatment with corticosteroids and/or megoestrol acetate. It may, however, occur as a result of a primary familial abnormality of lipid metabolism. Successful treatment of any identifiable underlying cause is associated with resolution of the condition.

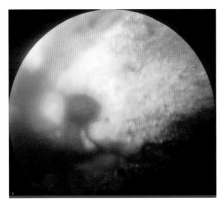

Figure 36. Areas of retinal detachment and degeneration in a cat which became diabetic and hypertensive after prolonged oral administration of megoestrol acetate. Systolic blood pressure was 210 mmHg.

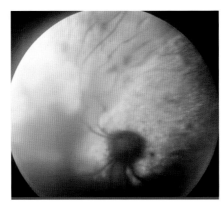

Figure 37. Areas of retinal detachment and degeneration in a cat which became diabetic after prolonged oral administration of megoestrol acetate. Systolic blood pressure was recorded as 220 mmHg.

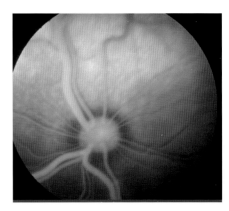

Figure 38. The lipaemia retinalis in this 4-week-old cat was created experimentally and resolved once the diet was changed. Courtesy of Professor Sheila Crispin.

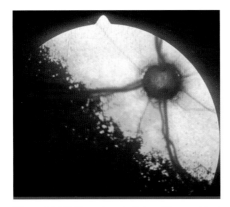

Figure 39. Mild lipaemia retinalis in a 12-year-old cat after a fatty meal. Note the 'strawberry milkshake' appearance of the blood within the retinal vessels.

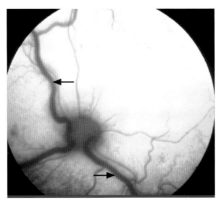

Figure 40. Hyperviscosity retinopathy in a 6-month-old Birman with FIP. The retinal veins are engorged with blood (arrows). Courtesy of Professor Sheila Crispin.

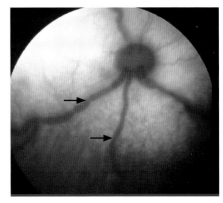

Figure 41. Hyperviscosity retinopathy in a 6-month-old Birman with FIP. The retinal veins are engorged with blood (arrows). Courtesy of Professor Sheila Crispin.

Hyperviscosity retinopathy

Hyperviscosity syndrome usually arises as a result of an increase in the concentration of blood plasma proteins (hyperproteinaemia) but may alternatively be a consequence of an abnormally elevated concentration of red blood cells (polycythaemia). In cats, hyperproteinaemia is most commonly associated with multiple myeloma and elevated IgG levels (monoclonal gammopathy) but may also occur with chronic systemic inflammatory conditions such as systemic lupus erythematosus and FIP (polyclonal gammopathies). Polycythaemia can either be primary (i.e. polycythaemia vera) or secondary as a consequence of

cardiorespiratory disease. Systemic signs of hyperviscosity syndrome vary but include lethargy, anorexia, weight loss, neurological disturbance and heart murmur. The most common funduscopic findings are engorged and tortuous retinal vessels, retinal haemorrhages and papilloedema although retinal detachment can also occur (Figs. 40 and 41).

Chorioretinitis

Owing to the intimate relationship between the retina and the choroid, they are rarely affected by inflammatory disease in isolation. Funduscopic signs of active chorioretinitis include oedema, exudates, cellular infiltrate

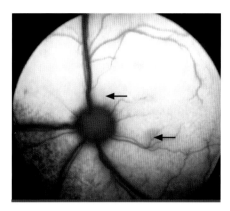

Figure 42. Hyperviscosity retinopathy, vasculitis and papillitis in an 8-month-old Domestic shorthair with FIP. The retinal veins are engorged. Note the oedema surrounding the optic nerve head and terminations of the finer vessels (arrows). Courtesy of Professor Sheila Crispin.

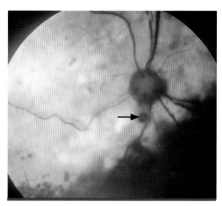

Figure 43. Active chorioretinitis of unknown cause. There is generalised retinal oedema with early detachment and a small intraretinal haemorrhage near the optic nerve head (arrow).

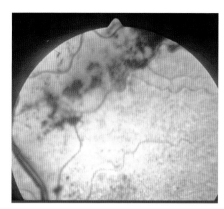

Figure 44. Active chorioretinitis of unknown cause. There is intraretinal haemorrhage accompanied by cellular infiltrate. Courtesy of Professor Sheila Crispin.

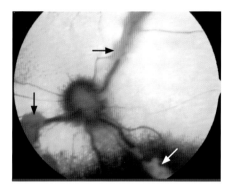

Figure 45. Dense and extensive accumulation of inflammatory cells around the retinal vessels (perivascular 'cuffing') in a 14-month-old Chinchilla with bilateral posterior uveitis associated with FIP (arrows). Courtesy of Professor Sheila Crispin.

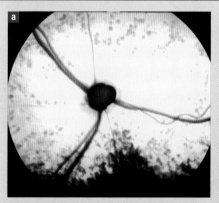 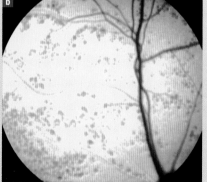

Figure 46. a) and b). Active chorioretinitis. The multiple focal areas of hyporeflectivity within the tapetal fundus represent cellular infiltration in this FIV-positive cat.

and haemorrhages (Figs. 42-46). When inflammation is severe, retinal detachment often ensues (Fig. 47). Evidence of previous episodes of chorioretinitis is often discovered as an incidental finding when the eye is examined for other reasons. These inactive, postinflammatory retinopathies usually appear as well demarcated areas of retinal degeneration with pigmentary changes. In the tapetal fundus, areas of hyperreflectivity are usually evident with or without pigment deposition (Figs. 48 and 49). In the nontapetal fundus, there is often pigment loss (Fig. 50). The most common cause of feline chorioretinitis is infection with viral, bacterial, fungal or parasitic agents although the aetiology may remain elusive.

Viral chorioretinitis

FIP is the most common viral cause of chorioretinitis. Fundus involvement is more commonly reported with the 'dry' form of the disease, with areas of pyogranulomatous inflammation present and sometimes appearing as cuffing around retinal vessels (Fig. 45). Haemorrhages are also common and the optic nerve may also be involved in the inflammatory process. FeLV has also been associated with chorioretinitis but the inflammation usually relates to infiltration with neoplastic cells in metastatic lymphoma rather than as a result of any direct cytopathic viral effect (Fig. 51). The role of FIV in chorioretinitis is even less clear (Figs. 46 and 52).

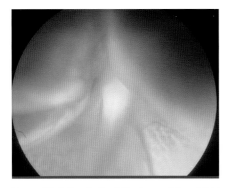

Figure 47. Active chorioretinitis. Accumulation of fluid between the RPE and neurosensory retina in this case of chorioretinitis has led to exudative retinal detachment.

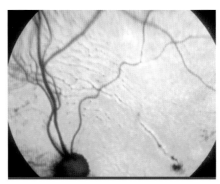

Figure 48. Postinflammatory chorioretinopathy. There is an unusual linear pattern of pigment deposition in the tapetal fundus associated with areas of hyperreflectivity.

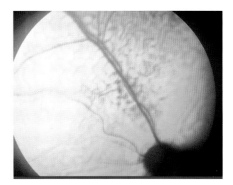

Figure 49. Postinflammatory chorioretinopathy. There is an unusual reticulated pattern of pigment deposition and associated tapetal hyperreflectivity. The retina surrounding the optic nerve head remains detached.

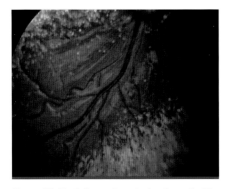

Figure 50. Postinflammatory chorioretinopathy. The RPE and choroid have become depigmented in a focal area of the nontapetal fundus.

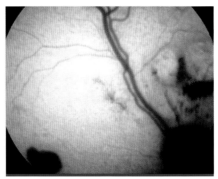

Figure 51. Feline leukaemia. There are areas of subretinal and intraretinal haemorrhages in this FeLV-positive cat.

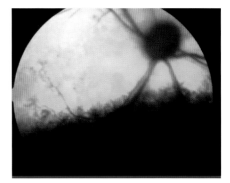

Figure 52. Active chorioretinitis and papillitis. This cat was FIV-positive and had an elevated *Toxoplasma gondii* IgM titre.

Bacterial chorioretinitis

Any systemic bacterial infection can potentially lead to chorioretinitis although the inflammation is rarely confined to the fundus, with panuveitis or endophthalmitis being more common scenarios. Chorioretinitis has been reported in association with mycobacterial disease with *Mycobacterium bovis* and *Mycobacterium simiae* reported as potential aetiological agents. Funduscopic findings are of granulomatous-appearing lesions, haemorrhages and retinal detachment (Fig. 53).

Fungal chorioretinitis

Chorioretinitis is a frequent finding in cats with systemic mycotic infections. Cryptococcosis is the most common feline systemic mycosis but histoplasmosis, blastomycosis and coccidioidomycosis are also reasonably common depending on geographic location.

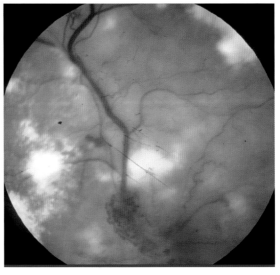

Figure 53. A 4-year-old Domestic shorthair with mycobacterial chorioretinitis. The retina is detached and demonstrates multiple areas of haemorrhage. The choroid is affected by cream-pink granulomatous inflammation. Courtesy of Dr Keith Barnett.

Typically, granulomatous inflammation is present and the anterior uvea may also be involved (Fig. 54).

Parasitic chorioretinitis

Toxoplasma gondii is the most commonly implicated parasitic cause of feline chorioretinitis. Toxoplasmosis, however, is rarely confirmed in cats without systemic signs of disease or which have not been experimentally infected with this protozoal agent. Fundus changes include focal areas of retinal oedema and cellular infiltration, bullous retinal detachments and retinal haemorrhages (Figs. 55 and 56). More advanced and chronic cases often exhibit signs of granulomatous anterior uveitis. Coinfections with FeLV and/or FIV are reasonably common (Fig. 52). Ophthalmomyiasis interna posterior describes parasitic larval migration within the posterior segment of the eye. Signs of previous parasitic larval migration are usually an incidental finding in otherwise normal cats with multiple curvilinear tracks present within the retina. *Cuterebra* sp. larva has been identified as the cause in one case which had signs of panuveitis and systemic disease (Wyman et al., 2005).

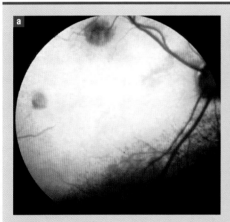
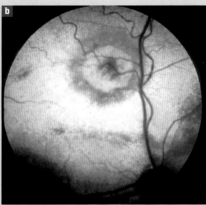
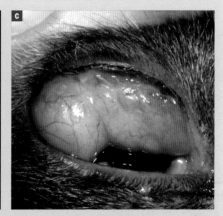

Figure 54. Systemic cryptococcosis in a 12-year-old Siamese. a) Note the active, focal granulomatous chorioretinitis lesions. b) After treatment with systemic antifungal medications, a chorioretinal scar remains. c) *Cryptococcus neoformans* was identified on culture of a biopsy sample from the upper eyelid.

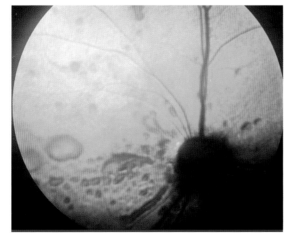

Figure 55. Multiple retinal bullae in the tapetal fundus in a 3-month-old cat. Severe respiratory disease was also present and a diagnosis of toxoplasmosis was made based on clinical signs and serological testing.

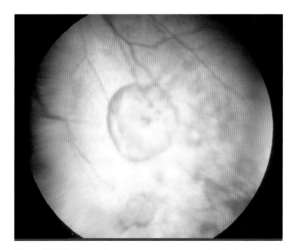

Figure 56. Multiple retinal bullae and generalised retinal oedema in a 12-month-old Domestic shorthair with weight loss and respiratory disease. A diagnosis of toxoplasmosis was reached.

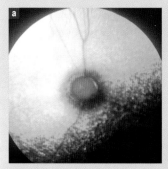 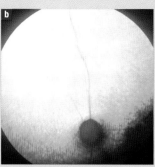 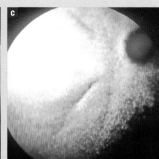 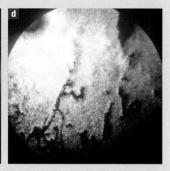

Figure 57. Advancing stages of retinal degeneration in Abyssinians with cone-rod dysplasia. a) 11-week-old kitten with moderate retinal degeneration. b) 24-week-old kitten with severe retinal degeneration. c) 8-month-old kitten with total retinal degeneration. The degenerate retina exhibits marked tapetal hyperreflectivity. d) 2-year-old cat with total retinal degeneration. The degenerated retina exhibits marked hyperreflectivity and there is pigment deposition. Courtesy of Dr Keith Barnett.

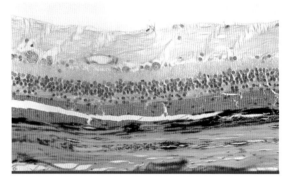

Figure 58. Photomicrograph of the retina of a 6-month-old Abyssinian with cone-rod dysplasia. The photoreceptors are no longer present. Courtesy of Dr Keith Barnett.

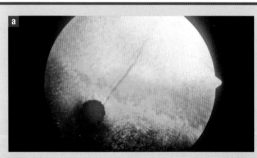

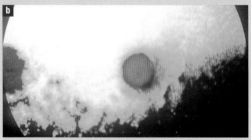

Figure 59. a) and b) Advanced retinal degeneration in two 5-year-old Abyssinians with photoreceptor degeneration. Courtesy of Dr Keith Barnett.

Retinal degeneration

Documented causes of feline retinal degeneration include inherited dysplasias and dystrophies, nutritional imbalances, drug toxicities and, as described above, inflammation.

Inherited retinal degenerations

Photoreceptor dysplasia

An inherited abnormality of rod and cone development which leads to their degeneration prior to maturation has been reported in the Abyssinian. The disease is very early in onset and the cones appear to be affected before the rods. The tapetum appears dull with lack of detail from approximately eight weeks of age and more advanced signs of retinal degeneration progress rapidly (tapetal hyperreflectivity, nontapetal depigmentation and vascular attenuation) (Fig. 57). Histologically, the photoreceptor layer is completely absent by six months of age (Fig. 58). This cone-rod dysplasia is inherited in an autosomal dominant fashion and caused by a single base pair deletion in the CRX gene (Menotti-Raymond et al., 2010).

Photoreceptor degeneration

The Abyssinian is also affected by a later onset photoreceptor degeneration which is inherited in an autosomal recessive fashion. Disease onset occurs from around 18 months of age and, although progression and funduscopic signs can vary between individuals, typical signs of advanced degeneration are usually present by 4-6 years of age (Fig. 59). The disease is

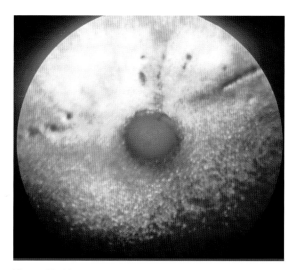

Figure 60. Advanced suspected inherited retinal degeneration in a 10-year-old Siamese.

caused by a mutation in the CEP290 gene and the same mutation has been found in Somalis with suspected inherited retinal degeneration (Menotti-Raymond et al., 2007; Narfström et al., 2009). The Persian also exhibits a similar autosomal recessive retinal degeneration although the mutation has not yet been identified (Rah et al., 2005). In some countries, a suspected inherited retinal degeneration of late onset is also seen with reasonable frequency in the Siamese, although the disease has not been studied in any detail in this breed (Fig. 60).

Taurine deficiency retinopathy/Feline central retinal degeneration

Taurine deficiency retinopathy and feline central retinal degeneration are synonymous. Taurine is an essential amino acid in the cat and a dietary content of at least 500 ppm is required to prevent retinal and cardiac disease – where taurine levels and requirements are highest. The first ophthalmoscopic sign of taurine deficiency is a dull, granular appearance in the region of the area centralis, just dorsolateral to the optic nerve head (Fig. 61a). This area of the tapetal fundus then appears hyperreflective and a similar lesion develops just dorsomedial to the optic nerve head (Figs. 61b-d). These lesions later coalesce before more widespread signs of retinal degeneration become apparent. Although the early ophthalmoscopic signs of taurine deficiency are generally considered pathognomonic

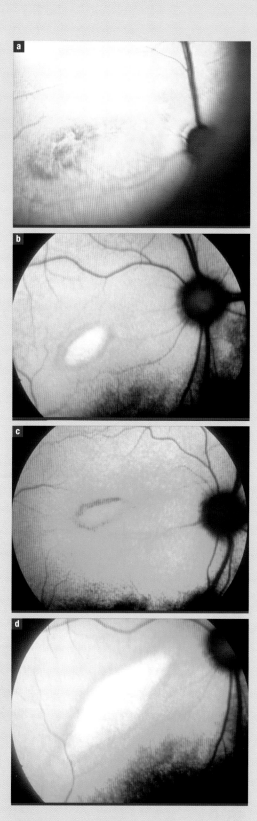

Figure 61. Taurine deficiency retinopathy. a) The earliest sign is a granular appearance of the area centralis which is dorsolateral to the optic nerve head. Courtesy of Claudia Hartley. b), c) and d) A well demarcated area of tapetal hyperreflectivity then develops in the region of the area centralis.

for the disease, plasma taurine concentrations should always be measured with values less than 40 nmol/ml considered as diagnostic of deficiency. If diagnosis is achieved and dietary deficiency corrected before complete retinal degeneration has occurred, then disease progression can be arrested, although any pre-existing retinal degeneration cannot be reversed. All cats with taurine deficiency retinopathy should receive a thorough cardiac evaluation.

Fluoroquinolone-induced retinal degeneration

Enrofloxacin has been associated with acute retinal degeneration in cats when used systemically above the manufacturer's current dose rate recommendation (2.5 mg/kg every 12 hours). The drug may potentially even be retinotoxic when used at the recommended dose rate in particularly susceptible cats such as geriatrics and those with renal or hepatic impairment. Visual deficits and funduscopic and electroretinographic evidence of profound retinal degeneration can be present within 24-72 hours of drug administration. Histological studies have revealed the outer retina to show evidence of pathology first with rod degeneration preceding that of cones (Ford et al., 2007) (Fig. 62). The retinal degeneration appears to be permanent although some cats may appear to retain some vision. A molecular basis for susceptibility to the drug's effects has been documented in cats (Ramirez et al., 2011). The ABCG2 transporter protein functions to restrict distribution of fluoroquinolones across the blood-retinal barrier. Feline ABCG2 has been shown to be defective in its function compared to other species which is thought to allow for the potential build-up of photoactive and potentially retinotoxic fluoroquinolones within the retina. Although the evidence for retinotoxicity is most clear for enrofloxacin, other fluoroquinolones may have similar effects. Orbifloxacin, when administered at doses much higher than the manufacturer's recommendations, resulted in funduscopic and histological evidence of retinal degeneration in one study (Turnidge, 1999). Pradofloxacin and marbofloxacin, even when used at very high doses, however, have not been shown to be retinotoxic (Wiebe and Hamilton, 2002; Messias et al., 2008).

Neoplasia of the retina and choroid

Primary neoplasia is rare but choroidal melanocytoma has been reported (Semin et al., 2011). Secondary neoplasia appears to be much more common with

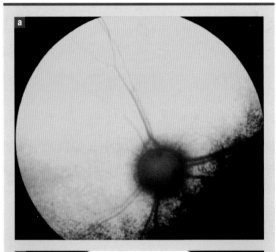

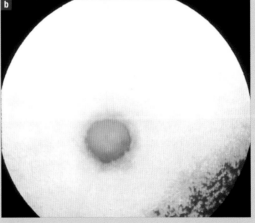

Figure 62. Fluoroquinolone-induced retinal degeneration. a) This cat received 20 mg/kg enrofloxacin orally for five days and became acutely blind. One week after blindness, the tapetum is mildly hyperreflective and mild retinal vascular attenuation is present. b) The same cat five weeks later. The tapetum is markedly hyperreflective, severe retinal vascular attenuation is present and the optic nerve head is atrophic. Courtesy of Dr David Gould.

→ Enrofloxacin has been associated with acute retinal degeneration.

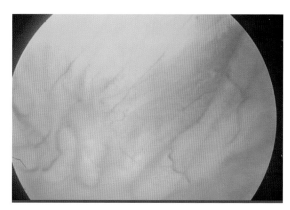

Figure 63. Total retinal detachment as a result of subretinal metastatic lymphoma.

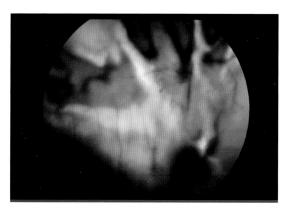

Figure 64. Angioinvasive pulmonary carcinoma. Retinal necrosis is present with typical tan-coloured wedge-shaped lesions appearing to fan out from the optic nerve head.

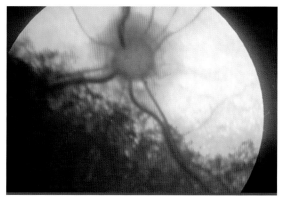

Figure 65. Papilloedema. The optic nerve head is hazy and the vessels no longer appear to dip into it. There is accompanying oedema of the peripapillary region.

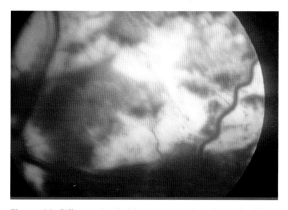

Figure 66. Diffuse subretinal haemorrhage in a 4-month-old cat with hydrocephalus.

metastatic lymphoma being most frequently encountered (Fig. 63). Angioinvasive pulmonary carcinoma has also been shown to have the potential for metastasis to the choroid (Cassotis et al., 1999). The neoplastic emboli within the choroidal vessels lead to ischaemic necrosis of the choroid and retina which, on funduscopy, appear as wedge-shaped tan lesions within the tapetal fundus (Fig. 64).

Optic nerve head
Papilloedema
Papilloedema, that is noninflammatory swelling of the optic nerve head, is infrequently recognised in the cat, perhaps owing to the normal dark and 'cupped' optic nerve head in this species (Fig. 65). Papilloedema is caused by elevated intracranial pressure which in turn is usually due to an inflammatory or neoplastic

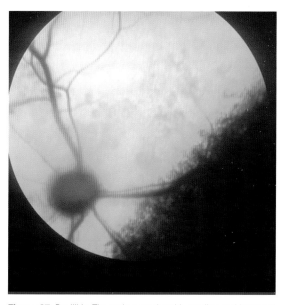

Figure 67. Papillitis. The optic nerve head is swollen and hazy and the lack of fundus detail is consistent with chorioretinitis.

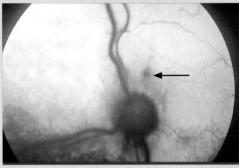

Figure 68. Papillitis. The optic nerve head is swollen and hazy and there is a small haemorrhage adjacent to it (arrow).

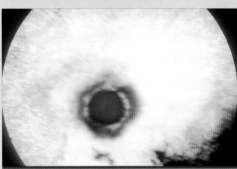

Figure 69. Optic nerve head atrophy as a result of end-stage retinal degeneration.

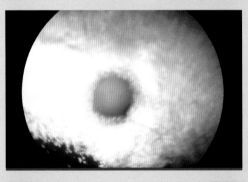

Figure 70. Optic nerve head atrophy as a result of end-stage retinal degeneration.

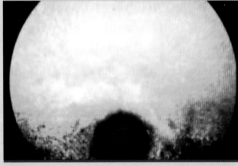

Figure 71. Optic nerve head atrophy as a result of end-stage retinal degeneration.

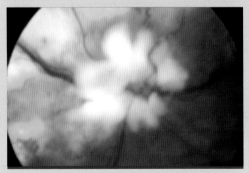

Figure 72. Neoplastic infiltration of the optic nerve head in a cat with metastatic lymphoma. Courtesy of Professor Sheila Crispin.

process within the brain but may also result from systemic hypertension or hydrocephalus (Fig. 66). In cats, FIP is probably the most common cause of intracranial inflammation. Meningioma is the most common primary intracranial neoplasm, and lymphoma is the most common secondary one.

Papillitis

Papillitis refers to inflammation of the optic nerve head and is thus readily diagnosed on ophthalmoscopy. The optic nerve head may be inflamed as part of a contiguous inflammatory process within the retina and choroid or, more commonly, as part of more widespread optic neuritis. Signs of papillitis include swelling and haemorrhages and adjacent retinal detachments or other signs of chorioretinitis (Figs. 66-68). Potential causes include FIP, toxoplasmosis and cryptococcosis.

Optic atrophy

Optic atrophy is an end-stage process resulting from the death of retinal ganglion cells and their axons. Potential causes include retinal degeneration, glaucoma, proptosis and previous optic neuritis (Figs. 69-71). Another important possible cause of blindness and subsequent optic nerve atrophy is iatrogenic trauma at the level of the optic chiasm, caused by enucleation of the contralateral globe (Chapter 12).

Optic nerve neoplasia

Optic nerve neoplasia is very uncommon in the cat but possible causes include meningioma (primary) and lymphoma (secondary) (Fig. 72). The optic nerve may also be involved by extension of post-traumatic intraocular sarcoma.

References

CASSOTIS NJ, DUBIELZIG RR, GILGER BC et al. (1999). Angioinvasive pulmonary carcinoma with posterior segment metastasis in four cats. *Veterinary Ophthalmology*; 2:125-131.

FORD MM, DUBIELZIG RR, GIULIANO EA et al. (2007). Ocular and systemic manifestations after oral administration of a high dose of enrofloxacin in cats. *American Journal of Veterinary Research*; 68:190-202.

MACNEIL MA, PURRIER S, RUSHMORE RJ (2009). The composition of the inner nuclear layer of the cat retina. *Visual Neuroscience*; 26:365-374.

MAGGIO F, DEFRANCESCO TC, ATKINS CE et al. (2000). Ocular lesions associated with systemic hypertension in cats: 69 cases (1985-1998). *Journal of the American Veterinary Medical Association*; 217:695-702.

MESSIAS A, GEKELER F, WEGENER A et al. (2008). Retinal safety of a new fluoroquinolone, pradofloxacin, in cats: assessment with electroretinography. *Documenta Ophthalmologica*; 116:177-191.

MENOTTI-RAYMOND M, DECKMAN KH, DAVID V et al. (2010). Mutation discovered in a feline model of human congenital retinal blinding disease. *Investigative Ophthalmology and Visual Science*; 51:2852-2859.

MENOTTI-RAYMOND M, DAVID VA, SCHÄFFER AA et al. (2007). Mutation in CEP290 discovered for cat model of human retinal degeneration. *Journal of Heredity*; 98:211-220.

NARFSTRÖM K, DAVID V, JARRET O et al. (2009). Retinal degeneration in the Abyssinian and Somali cat (rdAc): correlation between genotype and phenotype and rdAc allele frequency in two continents. *Veterinary Ophthalmology*; 12:285-291.

RAH H, MAGGS DJ, BLANKENSHIP TN et al. (2005). Early-onset, autosomal recessive, progressive retinal atrophy in Persian cats. *Investigative Ophthalmology and Visual Science*; 46:1742-1747.

RAMIREZ CJ, MINCH JD, GAY JM et al. (2011). Molecular genetic basis for fluoroquinolone-induced retinal degeneration in cats. *Pharmacogenetics and Genomics*; 21:66-75.

SANSOM J, ROGERS K, WOOD JL (2004). Blood pressure assessment in healthy cats and cats with hypertensive retinopathy. *American Journal of Veterinary Research*; 65:245-252.

SEMIN MO, SERRA F, MAHE V et al. (2011). Choroidal melanocytoma in a cat. *Veterinary Ophthalmology*; 14:205-208.

THOMPSON S, WHITING RE, KARDON RH et al. (2010). Effects of hereditary retinal degeneration due to a CEP290 mutation on the feline pupillary light reflex. *Veterinary Ophthalmology*; 13:151-157.

TURNIDGE J (1999). Pharmacokinetics and pharmacodynamics of fluoroquinolones. *Drugs*; 58 (Suppl 2):29-36.

WIEBE V, HAMILTON P (2002). Fluoroquinolone-induced retinal degeneration in cats. *Journal of the American Veterinary Medical Association*; 221:1568-1571.

WYMAN M, STARKEY R, WEISBRODE S et al. (2005). Ophthalmomyiasis (interna posterior) of the posterior segment and central nervous system myiasis: *Cuterebra* spp. in a cat. *Veterinary Ophthalmology*; 8:77-80.

Neuro-ophthalmology

The neuro-ophthalmic examination

Systematic assessment of the neuro-ophthalmic responses and reflexes is an essential part of the ophthalmic examination. If the anatomical bases of the various tests are understood, the results of the neuro-ophthalmic examination often afford expedient results in the neuro-anatomical localisation of pathological lesions.

Vision testing

Cats can be extremely uncooperative during vision testing and, sometimes, more than one test is required to fully establish a cat's vision status, particularly in the consulting room environment.

The menace response

The menace response is the most commonly employed test of vision (Fig. 1). It is a learned response and may be absent in kittens less than 12 weeks of age. The response is elicited by a menacing gesture to the eye of interest whilst the other eye is covered. Furthermore, the gesture can be performed medially and laterally to the eye to assess the two different visual fields. The first afferent component of the menace response is the retina and thus clear ocular media are required for initial stimulation of the pathway. From the retina, the response is relayed via the optic nerve (CN II), optic chiasm, optic tract, lateral geniculate nucleus and optic radiation to the visual cortex located in the caudal parietal and occipital lobes of the forebrain. From the visual cortex, there are anterior projections to the motor cortex and then to the facial nucleus and then facial nerve (CN VII). The facial nerve supplies motor fibres to the orbicularis oculi muscle which effects blinking – the normal response of this test. Any lesion along this pathway can cause a reduced or absent menace response. In addition, there are also undefined interactions of the facial nucleus with the cerebellum and so cerebellar disease can also result in absence of the menace response.

In the cat, around two thirds (~67 %) of optic nerve axons cross over to the contralateral side of the brain at the level of the optic chiasm. This means that the left visual cortex receives the lateral third of the total axons of the left eye (~33 %) and the central and medial two thirds of the total axons of the right eye (~67 %). If the menace response is negative, the examiner should next assess whether the palpebral reflex is present and complete to rule out facial paralysis or paresis. If the cat cannot blink, then presence of vision may still be indicated by globe retraction (mediated by the abducent nerve, CN VI) with accompanying nictitans protrusion or turning of the head (mediated by the accessory nerve, CN XI). If the menace response is absent then vision testing by other means should be performed.

The tracking response

The tracking response involves dropping a light object (to avoid air movement and noise), such as a cotton wool ball, within the visual field being assessed. Alternatively, a moving light source such as a laser pointer

> → An absent menace response may be due to blindness, inability to blink, cerebellar disease or an uncooperative patient.

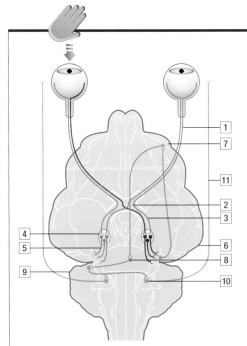

1. Optic nerve
2. Optic chiasm
3. Optic tract
4. Lateral geniculate nucleus
5. Optic radiation
6. Occipital cortex
7. Primary motor cortex
8. Pontine nucleus
9. Cerebellar cortex
10. Facial nucleus
11. Facial nerve

Figure 1. The menace response.

can be used to the same effect. The tracking response is useful in kittens and inquisitive cats although some stoic yet visual individuals may not respond consistently.

The visual placing response

The visual placing response involves carrying the cat towards a table edge. One eye can be covered at a time to assess the vision of each eye separately. A cat with vision should extend its forelimbs towards the table surface before its limbs make contact with it.

Maze tests and obstacle courses

Maze tests and obstacle courses performed in different lighting conditions can be very useful in assessing vision in dogs. Cats, however, often do not cooperate and so they are of limited use in this species.

Light reflexes

The pupillary light and dazzle reflexes are true reflexes and therefore do not need to be learned. These pathways do not involve the visual cortex, and thus they do not assess vision. Both of these reflexes, used in conjunction with the menace response, are particularly useful in the neuro-anatomical localisation of visual deficits.

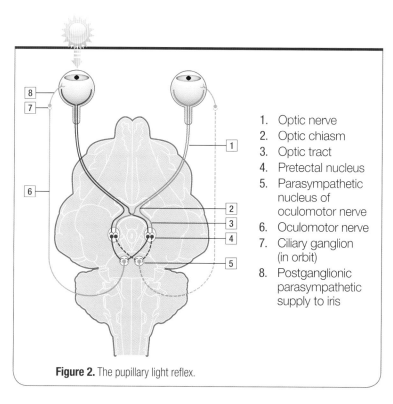

1. Optic nerve
2. Optic chiasm
3. Optic tract
4. Pretectal nucleus
5. Parasympathetic nucleus of oculomotor nerve
6. Oculomotor nerve
7. Ciliary ganglion (in orbit)
8. Postganglionic parasympathetic supply to iris

Figure 2. The pupillary light reflex.

The pupillary light reflex and swinging flashlight test

The pupillary light reflex

The pathways involved in the pupillary light reflex are illustrated in Figure 2. Following retinal stimulation with light, the reflex is relayed by the optic nerve (CN II) to the optic chiasm, where crossing to the contralateral side occurs, and then to the pretectal nucleus. Further crossing occurs between the pretectal nuclei. From the pretectal nucleus the pathway continues to the parasympathetic nucleus of the oculomotor nerve (CN III) which is located within the midbrain. Preganglionic parasympathetic fibres then travel ipsilaterally within the oculomotor nerve across the middle cranial fossa beside the pituitary gland. The fibres then travel to the orbit where they synapse in the ciliary ganglion. Postganglionic fibres then pass via short ciliary nerves to enter the globe adjacent to the optic nerve and course anteriorly to innervate the ciliary body and pupillary sphincter muscle. The cat has two short ciliary nerves, the malar nerve providing lateral and the nasal nerve providing medial innervation. It is this pattern of innervation that is responsible for the potential phenomenon of hemidilation of the feline pupil (so called 'D' or 'reversed D' pupil) (Fig. 3). Each eye has two types of pupillary light reflex: the direct and the consensual (or indirect). The direct refers to the response of the pupil of the illuminated eye. The consensual reflex refers to the simultaneous response of the pupil of the contralateral eye. In a normal situation, both pupils should constrict although the extent of constriction of the pupil of the contralateral eye will not be as great because of the decussation of ~67 % of optic nerve axons at the optic chiasm.

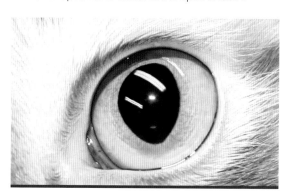

Figure 3. Reverse D-shaped pupil in a 9-year-old Domestic shorthair indicating abnormal function of the nasal ciliary nerve of the left eye. Courtesy of Filip Nachtegaele.

The swinging flashlight test

The swinging flashlight test is a useful additional variation of the pupillary light reflex (Fig. 4). To perform it, the examiner shines a light into the first eye. The normal response is for the pupil of both the illuminated and nonilluminated eye to constrict. The examiner then swings the light to the other eye. The normal response is for the second pupil to remain constricted or to constrict even further. The abnormal response is for the pupil to dilate upon direct light stimulation and this result constitutes a positive swinging flashlight test, or so-called Marcus-Gunn sign. This finding is highly suggestive of a prechiasmal lesion i.e. a lesion in the retina or proximal optic nerve, or both.

The dazzle reflex

The dazzle reflex tests the function of most of the same neurological components as the menace response but with a major key difference (Fig. 5). The dazzle reflex is subcortical and, as such, cannot be used to fully assess vision. An intensely bright light source is shone into the eye of interest and the appropriate response is a partial or complete blink. A negative response implies subcortical blindness or a facial nerve (CN VII) lesion.

The palpebral and corneal reflexes

The afferent component of the palpebral and corneal reflexes is the trigeminal nerve (CN V). The eyelids are predominantly innervated by the ophthalmic branch of the trigeminal nerve medially and the maxillary branch laterally although there is some overlap. Thus the palpebral reflex should be performed at both the medial and lateral canthi to assess both branches. The normal response is a blink elicited by innervation of the orbicularis oculi muscle by the facial nerve (CN VII). An absent palpebral reflex therefore may result from a defect of either the trigeminal or facial nerves (Figs. 6 and 7). The corneal reflex is not performed as part of a routine ophthalmic examination but only when there is suspicion of trigeminal nerve dysfunction. A fine wisp of cotton wool is applied to the central cornea. The normal response is globe retraction mediated by the abducent nerve (CN VI) which innervates the retractor bulbi muscle and a blink in cats with normal facial

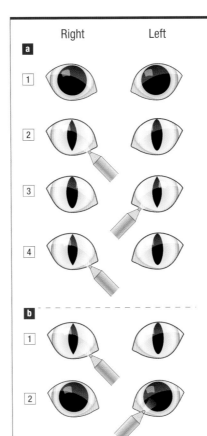

Figure 4. The swinging flashlight test.

a) The normal (negative) swinging flashlight test. 1. In a darkened room both pupils are dilated. 2. A bright light source is directed into the right eye and both pupils constrict. The left pupil constricts to a slightly lesser degree than the right. 3. The bright light source is then immediately directed into the left eye. The left pupil constricts further and the right pupil dilates very slightly. 4. The light source is redirected into the right eye and slight reconstriction of the pupil occurs.

b) The abnormal (positive) swinging flashlight test (Marcus-Gunn pupil). 1. When the light source is directed into the normal right eye, both pupils constrict. 2. When the light source is immediately directed into the abnormal left eye, both pupils dilate. The left eye demonstrates a Marcus-Gunn pupil and the finding is suggestive of a left prechiasmal lesion.

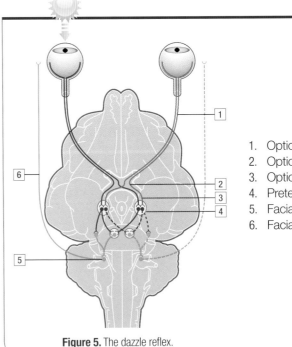

1. Optic nerve
2. Optic chiasm
3. Optic tract
4. Pretectal nucleus
5. Facial nucleus
6. Facial nerve

Figure 5. The dazzle reflex.

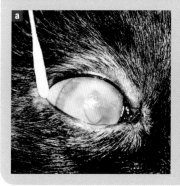
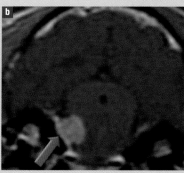

Figure 6. Defect of the maxillary branch of the trigeminal nerve in a 4-year-old Domestic shorthair. a) The cat does not blink when the lateral palpebral reflex is assessed. Ability to blink was confirmed with a dazzle reflex, ruling out facial nerve paralysis. This cat also has neurotrophic keratitis. b) Transverse T1W postcontrast MR image of the brain at level of the mesencephalon showing enlargement of the right trigeminal nerve (arrow) and secondary compression of the tegmentum of the mesencephalon. Differential diagnoses included peripheral nerve sheath tumour, meningioma and lymphoma.

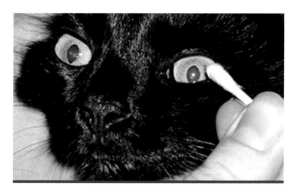

Figure 7. Idiopathic left facial nerve paralysis in a 5-year-old Domestic shorthair. The cat does not blink on assessment of the corneal or palpebral reflexes. Globe retraction and nictitans protrusion indicated normal function of the trigeminal and abducent nerves.

Examination tip

When interpreting dorsal and transverse MR (magnetic resonance) images, the left side of the image represents the right side of the patient.

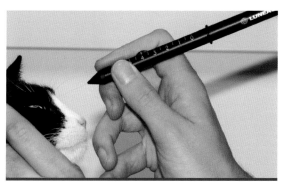

Figure 8. Use of the Cochet-Bonnet aesthesiometer.

nerve function. Globe retraction results in passive protrusion of the nictitans. Corneal sensation may be measured by aesthesiometry, for example with a Cochet-Bonnet aesthesiometer (Fig. 8).

The vestibulo-ocular reflex and physiological nystagmus

The pattern of innervation and actions of the extraocular muscles are illustrated in Figure 9. These muscles are responsible for movement of the globe and maintaining it in a central resting position. The extraocular muscles of each eye function synergistically to enable coordinated and simultaneous movements of both eyes. Normal eye position and movement require input to the nuclei of the nerves which supply the extraocular muscles (the oculomotor (CN III), trochlear (CN IV) and abducent (CN VI) nerves) from the vestibular apparatus. The function of the extraocular muscles and their respective nerves is assessed in the routine ophthalmic examination by the vestibulo-ocular reflex. To perform this, the head is moved in both directions along the horizontal and vertical planes. The normal response is for the eyes to jerk in the direction of head movement and then to slowly return to their original position. This involuntary slow-quick pattern of eye movement is also known as physiological nystagmus. Spontaneous pathological nystagmus results from asymmetrical input from the two vestibular systems to the nuclei of the cranial nerves which supply the extraocular muscles. Nystagmus usually has a fast and a slow phase although it may be pendular in which case no such distinctive phases are present.

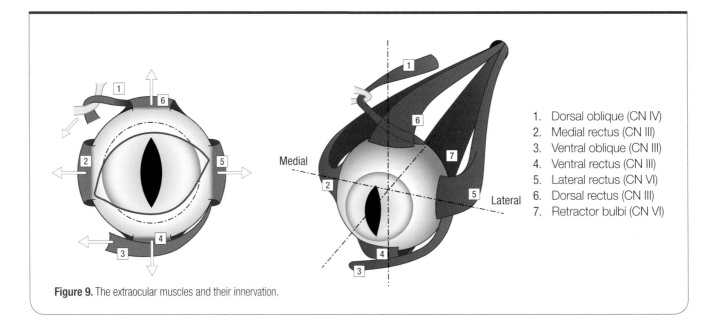

Figure 9. The extraocular muscles and their innervation.

1. Dorsal oblique (CN IV)
2. Medial rectus (CN III)
3. Ventral oblique (CN III)
4. Ventral rectus (CN III)
5. Lateral rectus (CN VI)
6. Dorsal rectus (CN III)
7. Retractor bulbi (CN VI)

Autonomic innervation of the eye and adnexa

Parasympathetic innervation

Oculomotor-parasympathetic innervation to the pupillary sphincter muscle has already been discussed. Parasympathetic supply of ocular structures, however, also originates within the nucleus of the facial nerve (CN VII). These parasympathetic fibres travel with the facial nerve before synapsing in the pterygopalatine ganglion. Postganglionic parasympathetic fibres are formed here and then go on to supply the lacrimal, palatine and nasal glands.

Sympathetic innervation

First-order sympathetic neurons (upper motor neurons) originate within the hypothalamus and rostral midbrain and pass caudally within the tectotegmental spinal pathway to synapse in the T1-T3 spinal cord segments. Second-order neurons (preganglionic sympathetic fibres) leave the ventral horn of the spinal cord here and travel cranially within the vagosympathetic trunk and synapse in the cranial cervical ganglion. Third-order neurons (postganglionic sympathetic fibres) then course ventromedially to the tympanic bulla and are distributed to supply structures of the head including the smooth muscle of the orbit and eyelids and the pupillary dilator muscle. Sympathetic

innervation of the eye is illustrated in Figure 10. Any lesion along this pathway can result in the signs of Horner's syndrome (see below).

Ophthalmic manifestations of neurological disease

Disorders of the autonomic nervous system

Horner's syndrome

Horner's syndrome refers to the spectrum of abnormal signs resulting from disruption of the sympathetic nerve supply to the eye and adnexa. The main clinical features in the cat are miosis, eyelid ptosis, protrusion of the nictitans and enophthalmos. Horner's syndrome can result from a lesion at any level of the sympathetic pathway and thus the syndrome can be further categorised as first-, second- or third-order. Potential causes include cranial spinal lesions, brachial plexus avulsion, otitis media, orbital disease, iatrogenic surgical manipulation and idiopathic. Idiopathic Horner's syndrome is less common in the cat than in the dog, is usually postganglionic in nature and tends to spontaneously resolve within 6-8 weeks. Localisation of the lesion responsible for Horner's syndrome requires diagnostic imaging in the form of radiography/CT of the cranial thorax and CT/MRI of the head. Pharmacological testing with a direct-acting sympathomimetic drug

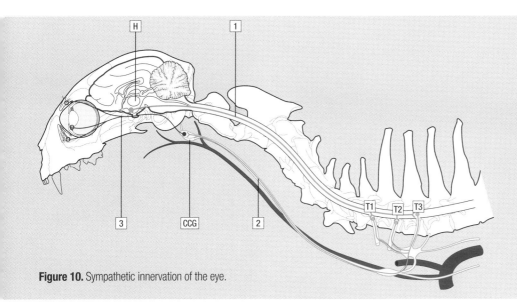

Figure 10. Sympathetic innervation of the eye.

1. First order neuron (tectotegmental spinal tract)
2. Second order neuron (vagosympathetic trunk)
3. Third order neuron
H. Hypothalamus
CCG. Cranial cervical ganglion
T1. First thoracic spinal cord segment
T2. Second thoracic spinal cord segment
T3. Third thoracic spinal cord segment

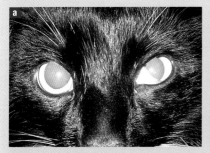
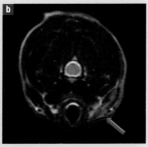

Figure 11. Second-order Horner's syndrome in a 3-year-old Domestic shorthair. a) There is left-sided upper eyelid ptosis, nictitans protrusion and miosis. b) Transverse T2W MR image at the level of the C2 vertebra. There is increased signal intensity of the tissue surrounding the left external and internal jugular veins, the common carotid artery, and the vagosympathetic trunk (arrow).

Causes of anisocoria

Mydriasis (unilateral)
→ Retinal or optic nerve (CNII) disease
→ Oculomotor nerve (CNIII) lesion (ophthalmoplegia)
→ Congenital iris anomaly or age-related iris atrophy
→ Glaucoma
→ Pharmacological dilation
→ Cerebellar lesions

Miosis (unilateral)
→ Anterior and reflex uveitis
→ Horner's syndrome

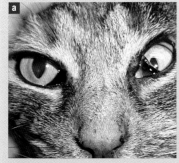
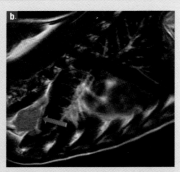

Figure 12. Second-order Horner's syndrome in a 9-year-old Domestic shorthair. a) There is left-sided nictitans protrusion and miosis. b) Left parasagittal T2W MR image of the thorax. A mass is present in the cranial mediastinum (arrow) underlying the T1 and T2 vertebrae.

can also help differentiate between second- and third-order Horner's syndrome. When one drop of 0.25-1 % phenylephrine is applied to an eye where there is a third-order (postganglionic) lesion, mydriasis will occur within 20 minutes owing to denervation hypersensitivity of the pupillary dilator muscle. If the lesion involves the first-order (upper motor neuron) or second-order (preganglionic) neurons, pupil dilation is much slower because the dilator muscle is not hypersensitised. Clinical examples of different orders of Horner's syndrome are represented in Figures 11-13.

Pourfour du Petit syndrome

In humans, Pourfour du Petit syndrome is used to describe a host of clinical signs attributed to hyperactivity of the sympathetic nervous system. These signs are opposite to, and may precede, those of Horner's syndrome and include mydriasis, a widened palpebral fissure and exophthalmos. A similar condition has been reported in cats following iatrogenic trauma to the middle ear (Boydell, 2000).

Dysautonomia (Key-Gaskell syndrome)

Feline dysautonomia involves widespread autonomic (parasympathetic and sympathetic) dysfunction including supply to the eye and adnexa. Ophthalmic signs are bilateral and include unresponsive mydriasis, reduced tear production and nictitans protrusion (Fig. 14). Systemic signs include dehydration, xerostomia, dysphagia, regurgitation, constipation and urinary retention. The cause of feline dysautonomia is unknown and definitive ante mortem diagnosis is rarely achieved as it requires histological examination of autonomic ganglia. That said, the results of pharmacological testing may support a diagnosis of dysautonomia. In this instance, a drop of a direct-acting parasympathetic agent such as 0.1 % pilocarpine is applied to the eye. A dilated pupil with parasympathetic denervation will be hypersensitive to the drug and rapidly constrict whereas a normal pupil will show little, if any, response. Treatment of feline dysautonomia involves supportive therapy but the prognosis is usually poor.

Disorders of globe position and movement

Strabismus

Strabismus refers to abnormal globe position and results from lesions to the cranial nerves that supply the extraocular muscles (the oculomotor (CN III), trochlear (CN IV) and abducent nerve (CN VI)) or their nuclei (see Fig. 9). It can also occur as a direct result of disease of the extraocular muscles themselves or elsewhere within the orbit. If strabismus is restricted to only certain head positions then a lesion within the ipsilateral vestibular system should be suspected.

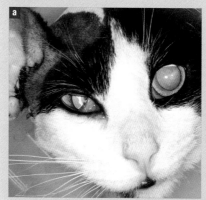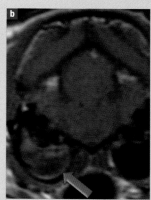

Figure 13. Third-order Horner's syndrome in an 8-year-old Domestic shorthair. a) Right-sided Horner's syndrome developed following total ear canal ablation and bulla osteotomy. b) Presurgical transverse T1W postcontrast MR image at the level of the middle ear. The changes in the right bulla (arrow) are consistent with a diagnosis of otitis media.

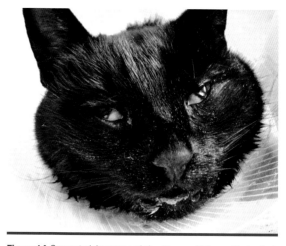

Figure 14. Suspected dysautonomia in a 5-year-old Domestic shorthair. There was mydriasis, nictitans protrusion, xerostomia and dysphagia.

Strabismus and nystagmus associated with ocular albinism

The Siamese has been extensively studied as a model of visual system anomalies associated with reduced ocular pigmentation although other hypopigmented breeds may also be affected. Retinal hypopigmentation in the Siamese results in misrouting of optic nerve (CN II) axons so that a greater percentage cross over at the optic chiasm. The most common sign is convergent strabismus although nystagmus may also be present (Fig. 15).

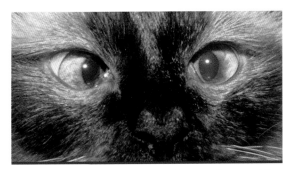

Figure 15. Convergent strabismus in a Siamese. Courtesy of Professor Sheila Crispin.

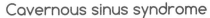

→ Internal ophthalmoplegia = paralysis of iris and ciliary body musculature

→ External ophthalmoplegia = paralysis of extraocular muscles

Cavernous sinus syndrome

The paired cavernous sinuses reside within the middle cranial fossa of the skull. The cavernous sinus, as well as housing a collection of veins, also acts as a conduit for the oculomotor (CN III), trochlear (CN IV) and facial (CN VII) nerves and the ophthalmic and maxillary branches of the trigeminal nerve (CN V). Cavernous sinus syndrome refers to the array of clinical signs associated with a lesion within the region of one or both of the cavernous sinuses of the brain. Ophthalmic signs usually result from lesions to the oculomotor nerve (which is the most dorsally located of the nerves within the sinus) and include a fixed dilated pupil (internal ophthalmoplegia), ventrolateral strabismus (external ophthalmoplegia) and upper eyelid ptosis. In cats, internal ophthalmoplegia is often the only presenting sign (Figs. 16 and 17). This is because the parasympathetic fibres which supply the pupillary sphincter muscle are located superficial and medial to the motor fibres making them more susceptible to compression as a result of disease of the pituitary gland. Neoplasia is the most common disease process causing cavernous sinus syndrome with lymphoma and meningioma being the most frequent diagnoses (Guevar et al., 2013).

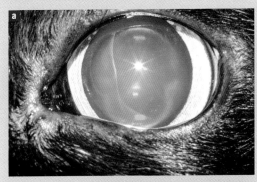

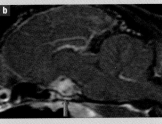

Figure 16. a) Internal ophthalmoplegia of the left eye in a 12-year-old Domestic shorthair. Note mydriasis. b) Midline sagittal T1W postcontrast MR image of the brain revealed the presence of an extra-axial lesion in the region of the middle cranial fossa (arrow). The lesion was causing ventral displacement of the pituitary gland and the hypothalamus.

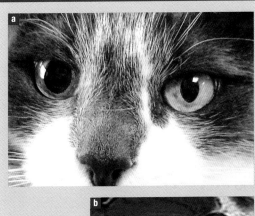

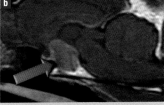

Figure 17. a) Internal ophthalmoplegia of the right eye in a 9-year-old Domestic shorthair. b) Midline sagittal T1W postcontrast MR images of the brain. There is a well-defined spherical/ovoid extra-axial mass arising from the pituitary fossa and indenting the overlying hypothalamus (arrow). The suspected diagnosis was a pituitary adenoma.

Causes of neuro-ophthalmic disease

Congenital

Hydrocephalus

Congenital internal hydrocephalus is rarer in the cat than in the dog. Any breed may be affected but a recessive mode of inheritance has been presumed in the Siamese. The accumulation of cerebrospinal fluid within the ventricular system leads to ventricular dilation and elevated intracranial pressure with subsequent brain atrophy. The most common clinical signs associated with congenital internal hydrocephalus are blindness and visual deficits, gait abnormalities, seizures and obtunded mentation (Biel et al., 2013). Medical and surgical treatment options are available but prognosis is usually guarded to poor. One study investigated the use of a ventriculoperitoneal shunt in six cats, with five of these showing an improvement in clinical signs after shunt placement (Biel et al., 2013).

Acquired

Infectious causes of neuro-ophthalmic disease

Viral

Feline infectious peritonitis (FIP), as well as being an important cause of uveitis, may also cause neurological disease. The ocular and nervous systems are more likely to be involved in the noneffusive ('dry') form of the disease. The neuro-ophthalmic signs vary according to the regions of the central nervous system (CNS) affected by disease but may include visual deficits, reduced vestibulo-ocular reflexes and nystagmus (Fig. 18).

Feline leukaemia virus (FeLV), like FIP, may be associated with signs of both uveitis and neuro-ophthalmic disease. Pupil abnormalities are often cited as one manifestation of FeLV-related disease and may be caused by direct invasion of the ciliary ganglia or short ciliary nerves by the virus itself or by lymphocytic infiltration of the uveal tract in cases of lymphoma in FeLV-positive cats (Nell et al., 1998). Reported pupil anomalies include anisocoria, dyscoria (including hemidilation, see Fig. 3) and spastic pupil syndrome. Spastic pupil syndrome, or static anisocoria, occurs when a miotic pupil fails to dilate upon dark adaptation.

Parasitic

Cerebral coenurosis has been reported in a number of species including the cat (Huss et al., 1994). The cyst is usually identified to be that of *Taenia serialis* which has a canid-lagomorph life cycle and the cat may become infected as an accidental intermediate host. Neurological signs vary according to location and size of the cyst but include obtunded mentation and blindness (Fig. 19). Surgical excision may be possible but the prognosis is generally guarded to poor.

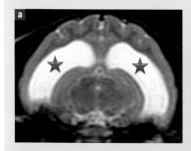
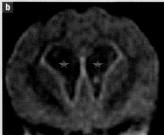

Figure 18. a) Transverse T2W (at the level of the mesencephalon) and b) T2W FLAIR MR images (at the level of the basal nuclei) of the brain of a 10-month-old Birman with suspected FIP. The cat had positional nystagmus and reduced vestibulo-ocular reflexes. There is marked distension of the lateral ventricles (stars) and obstructive hydrocephalus.

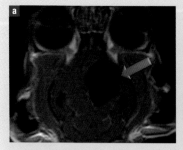
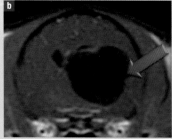

Figure 19. a) Dorsal and b) transverse (at the level of the thalamus) T1W postcontrast MR images of the brain of a 2-year-old Birman with cerebral coenurosis (confirmed at post mortem). There is a well-demarcated, intra-axial cystic structure within the frontal and parietal lobes of the left cerebral hemisphere (arrows). The cat was blind and had absent vestibulo-ocular reflexes.

Bacterial

Bacteria may gain access to the CNS via a variety of routes including haematogenous, extension of contiguous infection and direct implantation. Treatment includes prolonged administration of systemic antibiotic and antiinflammatory medications, and surgical drainage of abscesses may also be indicated in some cases (Figs. 20-24).

Fungal

Cryptococcosis is the most common fungal disease of the feline CNS with infections with *Cryptococcus neoformans* and *Cryptococcus gattii* being responsible for the vast majority of cases. The nasal cavity is the initial site of infection and the CNS may then become infected via direct extension or haematogenous spread. Neuro-ophthalmic manifestations include nystagmus, mydriasis and visual deficits (Sykes et al., 2010).

Inner and middle ear disease

Otitis media/interna usually results from extension of otitis externa caused by infections with bacteria, yeasts, fungi or parasites (Fig. 24). Inner and middle ear disease can also be caused by neoplasia (Figs. 25 and 26), polyps, trauma (Fig. 27) and iatrogenically (see Fig. 12). Possible neuro-ophthalmic signs associated with middle ear disease include facial nerve (CN VII) paralysis, Horner's syndrome and neurogenic keratoconjunctivitis sicca. If inner ear disease is present, signs of peripheral vestibular syndrome will also be evident (Negrin et al., 2010).

Idiopathic meningoencephalitis

Nonsuppurative meningoencephalitis of unknown origin is a relatively frequent finding in cats. In one study of 33 cats, diagnostic testing for 18 different known infectious agents, including viruses, bacteria and prion protein, was performed. In 20 cats (61 %), no evidence of any infectious agent was identified (Schwab et al., 2007).

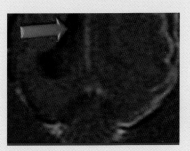

Figure 20. Dorsal T1W postcontrast MR image of the brain of an 8-year-old Domestic shorthair which presented with depressed mental status, right-sided blindness and absent vestibulo ocular reflexes. There is thickening and contrast-enhancement of the meninges associated with fluid accumulation in the subarachnoid space of the left frontal, parietal and temporal lobes with mass effect to the right (arrow). A small puncture wound was also identified in the parietal bone. The diagnosis was intracranial abscessation secondary to a cat bite.

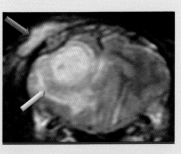

Figure 22. Transverse T2W MR image through the frontal lobes of the brain of an 8-year-old Domestic shorthair which presented with obtundation and left-sided proprioceptive deficits and blindness. There are right-sided subcutaneous (red arrow) and intracranial (green arrow) mass lesions communicating via a defect of the frontal/parietal bone consistent with abscessation.

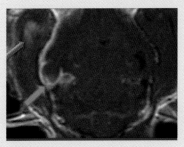

Figure 21. Dorsal T1W postcontrast MR image of the brain of a 14-year-old Domestic shorthair with bacterial meningoencephalitis secondary to a cat bite. There is marked thickening and enhancement of the meninges over the right side of the brain (blue arrow). There is also contrast enhancement of the overlying right temporal muscle (red arrow).

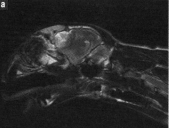
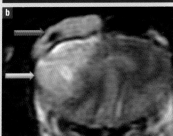

Figure 23. a) Right parasagittal and b) transverse T2W MR images of the head of a 7-year-old Domestic shorthair which presented with obtundation and visual deficits. There is increased signal intensity in the right frontal sinus (red arrow) and underlying frontal lobe of the brain (green arrow) consistent with infectious sinusitis and intracranial abscessation.

Figure 24. Transverse T2W MR image of the brain at the level of the middle ear of a 5-year-old Burmese. The cat presented with vestibular ataxia, reduced vestibulo-ocular reflexes and absent right menace response. There is right-sided middle ear disease with para-aural abscessation (red arrow) extending intracranially with secondary meningitis, obstructive hydrocephalus and brainstem compression/oedema (green arrow). ▶

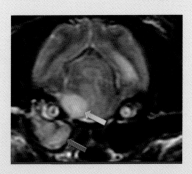

Metabolic

Neuronal ceroid-lipofuscinosis

The neuronal ceroid-lipofuscinoses (NCLs) are recessively inherited neurodegenerative lysosomal storage diseases, characterised by the accumulation of auto-fluorescent lipopigments within the CNS and peripheral tissues including the retina. A form of NCL has recently been characterised in three cats which exhibited generalised signs of neurological disease including visual deficits (Chalkley et al., 2013). Histopathological examination of post mortem tissues revealed widespread abnormal accumulation of storage product within the CNS and visual pathways including the lateral geniculate nucleus and retina.

Thiamine deficiency

Thiamine deficiency is most common in anorexic cats or those fed exclusively on raw fish-based diets. Thiamine concentrations may also be below the recommended levels in some commercially available canned diets which are either nutritionally imbalanced or contain certain food preservatives (Markovich et al., 2013 and 2014). Thiamine deficiency results in polioencephalomalacia of the oculomotor and vestibular nuclei, the caudal colliculus and lateral geniculate body, and so neuro-ophthalmic abnormalities are a common presentation. Common presenting signs include anorexia, salivation, mydriasis, ataxia, cervical ventroflexion, seizures, twitching and loss of righting reflexes. Serum thiamine concentration can be measured, and supplementation of deficient cats with vitamin B complex containing thiamine can improve clinical signs. Left untreated, signs progress to coma and death.

Trauma

Head trauma is a common cause of brain injury. If the neurological abnormalities are identified and treated early enough then many cats can recover (Figs. 27 and 28).

Neoplasia of the CNS

Intracranial neoplasia can cause an array of neuro-ophthalmic signs depending on lesion location, extent and behaviour. Potential and reported signs include blindness, strabismus, nystagmus and pupil abnormalities. Investigation usually requires MRI of the brain

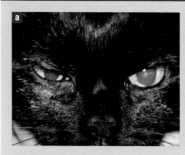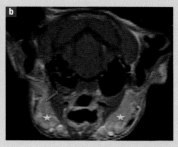

Figure 25. a) Right-sided Horner's syndrome in a 7-year-old Domestic shorthair. b) Transverse T1W postcontrast MR image of the head revealed enlarged retropharyngeal lymph nodes (green stars) and increased signal intensity within the right middle ear (red arrow). A diagnosis of metastatic lymphoma was made.

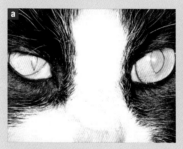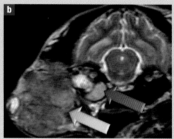

Figure 26. a) Right-sided Horner's syndrome in a 12-year-old Domestic shorthair which had an adenocarcinoma removed from the right ear canal six years previously. b) Transverse T2W MR image of the head (at the level of the caudal mesencephalon) revealed regrowth of the mass (green arrow) with extension into the middle ear cavity (red arrow).

with or without accompanying analysis of cerebrospinal fluid. Potential primary neoplasms include meningioma, ependymoma, oligodendroglioma, pituitary adenoma and choroid plexus tumours (see Fig. 17, Figs. 29-34). Meningioma is the most common tumour of the brain in cats and, dependent on location, may be amenable to treatment by surgical resection (Fig. 35). The most common secondary tumour is lymphoma which usually results from metastatic spread of primary abdominal lymphoma. Rarely, however, it can occur as a presumed solitary ocular lesion with potential spread to the CNS or *vice versa* (Giordano et al., 2013, Wiggans et al., 2013) (Fig. 36). Reported neuro-ophthalmic abnormalities associated with lymphoma include ophthalmoplegia, hemidilated pupil and blindness (Nell et al., 1998; Guevar et al., 2013). The brain may also be affected by extension of local neoplasms which breach the calvarium, such as sarcomas (Fig. 37).

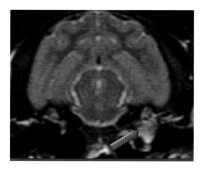

Figure 27. Transverse T2W MR image of the head (at the level of the mesencephalon) of a 6-month-old Domestic shorthair that developed peripheral vestibular syndrome after being attacked by a dog. There is fluid (presumably blood) accumulation within the left bulla (arrow).

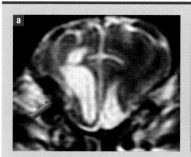
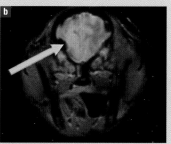

Figure 28. MR images of the head of a 2-year-old Domestic shorthair which presented with episodic circling and absent left menace response six months after a road traffic accident. a) The T2W image shows an old fracture of the right frontal bone (red arrow) with underlying compensatory hydrocephalus due to atrophy of the frontal lobe. b) The gradient echo image reveals a blood clot (green arrow).

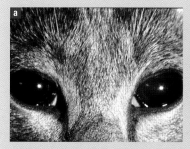
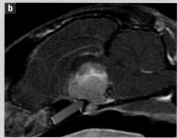
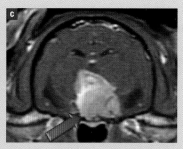

Figure 29. a) Bilateral internal ophthalmoplegia in a 14-year-old Domestic shorthair which also lacked menace responses. b) Midline sagittal postcontrast and c) transverse T1W postcontrast MR image, at the level of the pituitary gland, revealed an irregularly oval mass of marked heterogeneous contrast enhancement, thought to be a pituitary neoplasm, within the middle cranial fossa (arrows) displacing the thalamus caudally, the interthalamic adhesion dorsally, and the rostral midbrain caudally.

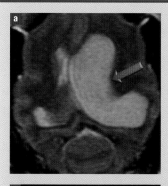
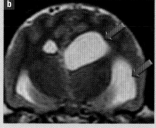

Figure 30. a) Dorsal and b) transverse T2W MR images, at the level of the thalamus, of the brain of an 8-year-old Domestic shorthair with ataxia and right-sided blindness. There is a mass lesion within the left lateral ventricle (arrows) resulting in secondary obstructive hydrocephalus, midline shift, caudal transtentorial herniation and herniation of the cerebellum through the foramen magnum.

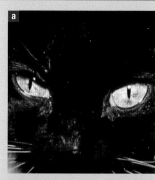
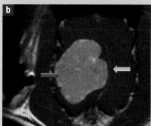

Figure 31. a) Bilateral miosis in a 9-year-old Domestic shorthair which presented with obtundation. b) Dorsal T1W postcontrast MR image of the brain revealed a large extra-axial mass, thought to be a meningioma, in the right temporal and parietal lobes (red arrow). There is severe mass effect with midline shift to the left (green arrow).

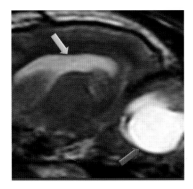

Figure 32. Right parasagittal T2W MR image of the brain of an 8-year-old Domestic shorthair with ataxia with a tendency to fall to the left and absent left menace response. There is a right-sided extra-axial cystic lesion at the level of the cerebellum and fourth ventricle (red arrow) with secondary obstructive hydrocephalus mostly of the lateral ventricles (green arrow). The main differential diagnoses are cystic meningioma, nerve sheath tumour and lymphoma.

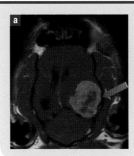
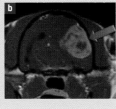

Figure 33. a) Dorsal and b) transverse T1W postcontrast MR images of the brain (at the level of the caudal thalamus) of a 9-year-old Domestic shorthair which presented with ataxia and absent right menace response. There is a large left-sided extra-axial parietal mass, thought to be a meningioma, characterised by marked heterogeneous contrast enhancement (arrows).

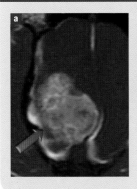
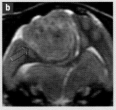

Figure 34. a) Dorsal T1W postcontrast and b) transverse T2W MR images of the brain, at the level of the caudal third ventricle, of an 8-year-old Domestic shorthair with ataxia and positional vertical nystagmus. There is a large mass (arrows) characterised by heterogeneous signal on T2W images and which is moderately and heterogeneously contrast enhancing dorsolateral to the right parietal and occipital lobes causing severe mass effect with compression of both cerebral hemispheres and the brainstem.

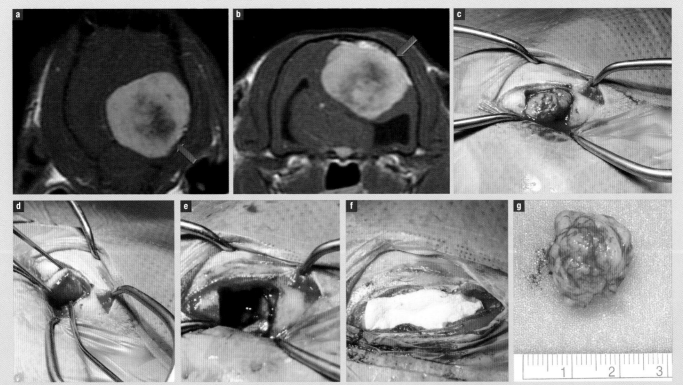

Figure 35. a) Dorsal and b) transverse T1W postcontrast images of the brain, at the level of the pituitary gland, of a 9-year-old Domestic shorthair with absent menace responses, ataxia, and falling to the right. There is a mass dorsolateral to the left parietal lobe causing severe mass effect with compression of both cerebral hemispheres and the brainstem (arrows). c) A left-sided rostrotentorial craniectomy is performed to reveal the mass. d) The mass is dissected free and removed leaving a defect. e) The defect is covered with collagen, as shown in f). The excised mass g) is submitted for histopathological examination and a diagnosis of meningioma was determined.

Postanaesthetic blindness

Postanaesthetic blindness is more common in cats than in dogs and usually occurs as a result of brain hypoxia. The occipital lobes appear particularly susceptible to hypoxic damage explaining why blindness is the most commonly reported clinical sign. Depending on the extent of cortical damage, recovery of vision is possible. An association with the use of spring-held mouth gags potentially leading to decreased cerebral perfusion due to compression of the maxillary artery has been suspected (Stiles et al., 2012; Barton-Lamb et al., 2013).

Contralateral optic neuropathy

The feline optic nerve is relatively short compared to the dog and so its traction is more likely to cause damage to the optic chiasm and subsequent atrophy of the contralateral optic nerve. The most common causes are traumatic globe proptosis and excessive traction on the optic nerve during enucleation (Fig. 38). Presenting neuro-ophthalmic signs include absent menace response, dazzle reflex and pupillary light reflex. Funduscopic signs begin with multifocal peripapillary retinal lesions and progressive retinal and optic nerve atrophy (Donaldson et al., 2014).

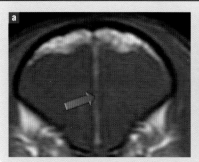 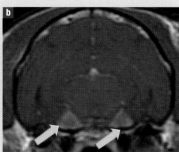

Figure 36. Transverse T1W postcontrast MR images of the brain of a 5-year-old Domestic shorthair which presented with disorientation, absent menace responses and reduced pupillary light reflexes a) at the level of the forebrain, where meninges (falx cerebri) are thickened (red arrow) and b) through the mesencephalon, in which the trigeminal nerves (green arrows) are thickened and markedly contrast enhancing. There was also neoplastic invasion of the kidneys and metastatic lymphoma was diagnosed on the basis of cytology of fine needle aspiration biopsy specimens.

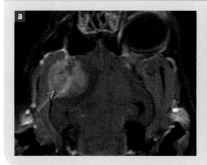 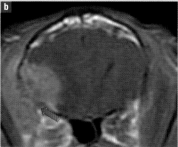

Figure 37. a) Dorsal and b) transverse T1W postcontrast MR images of the brain, at the level of the basal nuclei, of a 15-year-old Domestic shorthair with a dilated pupil and absent menace response of the left eye. There is a large, homogeneously enhancing mass invading the right frontotemporal bone and extending into the calvarium causing a marked mass effect with displacement of the frontal lobes to the left side (arrows). A diagnosis of fibrosarcoma was determined after biopsy.

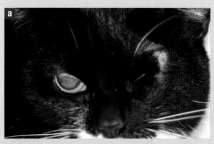 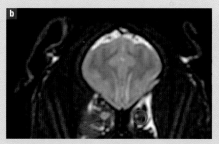 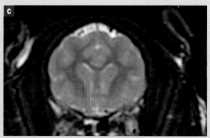

Figure 38. a) The right eye became blind immediately following removal of the contralateral eye (note mydriasis). b) T2W MR image at the level of the frontal lobes. The optic nerve of the enucleated left eye is absent (circled) and there is atrophy of the contralateral, right optic nerve (red arrow). c) T2W MR image at the level of the caudate nuclei. There is atrophy of the right side of the optic chiasm (blue arrow).

References

Biel M, Kramer M, Forterre F et al. (2013). Outcome of ventriculoperitoneal shunt implantation for treatment of congenital internal hydrocephalus in dogs and cats: 36 cases (2001-2009). *Journal of the American Veterinary Medical Association*; 247:948-958.

Barton-Lamb AL, Martin-Flores M, Scrivani PV et al. (2013). Evaluation of maxillary arterial blood flow in anesthetized cats with the mouth closed and open. *The Veterinary Journal*; 196 (3):325-331.

Boydell O (2000). Iatrogenic pupillary dilation resembling Pourfour du Petit syndrome in three cats. *The Journal of Small Animal Practice*; 41:202-203.

Chalkley MD, Armien AG, Gilliam DH et al. (2013). Characterization of Neuronal Ceroid-Lipofuscinosis in 3 Cats. *Veterinary Pathology*; 11:796-804.

Donaldson D, Matas Riera M, Holloway A et al. (2014). Contralateral optic neuropathy and retinopathy associated with visual and afferent pupillomotor dysfunction following enucleation in six cats. *Veterinary Ophthalmology*; 17:373-384.

Giordano C, Giudice C, Bellino C et al. (2013). A case of oculo-cerebral B-cell lymphoma in a cat. *Veterinary Ophthalmology*; 16:77-81.

Goulle F, Meige F, Durieux F et al. (2011). Intracranial meningioma causing partial amaurosis in a cat. *Veterinary Ophthalmology*; 14:93-98.

Guevar J, Gutierrez-Quintana R, Peplinski G et al. (2013). Cavernous sinus syndrome secondary to intracranial lymphoma in a cat. *Journal of Feline Medicine and Surgery*; 16:513-516.

Huss BT, Miller MA, Corwin RM et al. (1994). Fatal cerebral coenurosis in a cat. *Journal of the American Veterinary Medical Association*; 205:69-71.

Markovich JE, Heinze CR , Freeman LM (2013). Thiamine deficiency in dogs and cats. *Journal of the American Veterinary Medical Association*; 243:649-656.

Markovich JE, Freeman LM, Heinze CR (2014). Analysis of thiamine concentrations in commercial canned foods formulated for cats. *Journal of the American Veterinary Medical Association*; 244:175-179.

Negrin A, Cherubini GB, Lamb C et al. (2010). Clinical signs, magnetic resonance imaging findings and outcome in 77 cats with vestibular disease: a retrospective study. *Journal of Feline Medicine and Surgery*; 12:291-299.

Nell B, Suchy A (1998). 'D-shaped' and 'reverse-D-shaped' pupil in a cat with lymphosarcoma. *Veterinary Ophthalmology*; 1:53-56.

Schwab S, Herden C, Seeliger F et al. (2007). Non-suppurative meningoencephalitis of unknown origin in cats and dogs: an immunohistochemical study. *Journal of Comparative Pathology*; 136:96-110.

Sykes JE, Sturges BK, Cannon MS et al. (2010). Clinical signs, imaging features, neuropathology and outcome in cats and dogs with central nervous system cryptococcosis in California. *Journal of Veterinary Internal Medicine*; 24:1427-1438.

Stiles J, Weil AB, Packer RA et al. (2012). Post-anesthetic cortical blindness in cats: twenty cases. *The Veterinary Journal*; 193:367-373.

Wiggans KT, Skorupski KA, Reilly CM et al. (2014). Presumed solitary intraocular or conjunctival lymphoma in dogs and cats: 9 cases (1985-2013). *Journal of the American Veterinary Medical Association*; 244:460-470.

Wyman M, Starkey R, Weisbrode S et al. (2005). Ophthalmomyiasis (interna posterior) of the posterior segment and central nervous system myiasis: *Cuterebra* spp. in a cat. *Veterinary Ophthalmology*; 8:77-80.

Alphabetical index